community life for the mentally ill

community life for the mentally ill

an alternative to institutional care

George W. Fairweather
David H. Sanders
David L. Cressler
Hugo Maynard

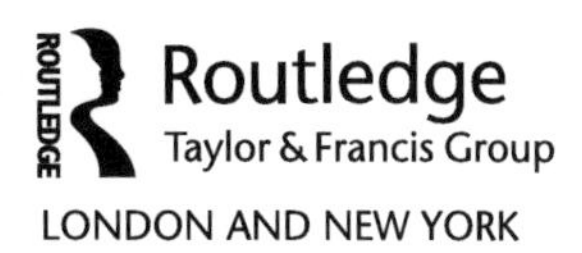
Routledge
Taylor & Francis Group
LONDON AND NEW YORK

First published 1969 by Transaction Publishers

Published 2017 by Routledge
2 Park Square, Milton Park, Abingdon, Oxon OX14 4RN
711 Third Avenue, New York, NY 10017, USA

Routledge is an imprint of the Taylor & Francis Group, an informa business

Library of Congress Catalog Number: 2008005495

Library of Congress Cataloging-in-Publication Data

Community life for the mentally ill : an alternative to institutional care /
George W. Fairweather ... [et al.].
p. cm.
Originally published: Chicago, Aldine Pub. Co. [1969].
Includes bibliographical references and index.
ISBN 978-0-202-36213-7 (alk. paper)
1. Mentally ill—Rehabilitation. 2. Community mental health services.
I. Fairweather, George William, 1921-

RC576.C58 2008
362.196'89--dc22 2008005495

ISBN 13: 978-0-202-36213-7 (pbk)

Preface

This book presents a social innovative experiment aimed at providing new and more participating social positions in American society for mental patients. It presents the events that occurred when a courageous group of former chronic mental patients abruptly left the hospital and established their own autonomous subsociety in a large, metropolitan area. The book continues into the community setting the activities of such patient groups first described in our *Social Psychology in Treating Mental Illness: An Experimental Approach.* From an experimental point of view, it follows the research procedures presented in a recent book, *Methods for Experimental Social Innovation,* by one of the authors.

In order to complete this experiment, it was essential to create a small society in the community where discharged patients could live and work. The problems involved in establishing such a society and its history are described in detail. It was equally important to evaluate the effects of the newly created society upon the behavior and perceptions of its members. Such an evaluation is also presented here. Both the descriptive and comparative aspects of this study are presented as they occurred in real life. For that reason the book is concerned with the medical, economic, sociological, and psychological facets of these former patients' daily lives. Finally, the effects of this small society upon the neighborhood and city in which it was located, as well as its effects upon professional persons, are explored.

All research material has been edited to preserve anonymity. Fictitious names are used throughout, and identifying dates have been altered. Every attempt has been made to disguise the names of the patients. Any name given a patient which is the same as that of any individual in this study is purely fortuitous. The names of professional persons have likewise been changed.

Through the order in which the material is presented, the authors have deliberately attempted to provide readers with the "flavor" of the research activity from its beginning to its completion. However, for those who are not interested in reading the entire work sequentially to capture this "flavor," chapter 1 presents a brief description of the study and a summary of its findings. In this chapter the reader may also find a descriptive account of the contents of subsequent chapters. It is hoped that both the humanitarian and experimental goals of the authors have been communicated effectively in the pages subsequent to this introduction.

No experiment of this magnitude could be accomplished without the involvement of a large number of people. We cannot name all of those who have made a significant contribution to this study, nor can we adequately recognize those who have made such contributions. But to all of them we are deeply indebted. Some persons contributed so much to the total project that—despite the injustice imposed by the brevity of the recognition—their names deserve special mention. First, a debt of gratitude is owed to Dr. John J. Prusmack, the Director of the Veterans Administration (VA) Hospital at Palo Alto, California, where this study was initiated, and to Drs. Thomas W. Kennelly, and John H. Vitale, Director and Assistant Director, respectively, of the Psychology Services there. The aid that they gave the project from its outset to completion was exceedingly important to all of us who worked daily in it. We are also indebted to the heads of all the departments at the VA Hospital, Palo Alto, California, and to the many other individuals there who contributed in one way or another to the completion of this project. And for providing us with information about the rehabilitative programs at their institutions we are grateful to Ladd McDonald, Chief of Vocational Services at Fort Logan Mental Health Center, Denver, Colorado, and Dr. Charles Yohe and Mrs. Billie Larch at Arkansas State Hospital, Benton, Arkansas.

Of course, the work of those who operated the psychiatric ward in the hospital from which all persons participating in the research project came are richly deserving of our thanks. They include Dr. Robert S. Mowry, Dr. Roger D. Jennings, Mrs. Elizabeth A. Rankin, Mr. Keith Wilson, and Mrs. Muriel Grey. Along with this professional staff, Mrs. Remalda Fuentes, Mrs. Nettie Milton, Mr. Francis Norsby, Mr. David Dozier, Mr. Clarence Henry, and Mr. E. Tescero also contributed their invaluable aid. The assistance of this group was important since the maintenance and stability of the ward small-group program on a daily basis was essential to the completion of the project.

To Dr. W. Scott MacDonald we extend our gratitude. By spending the first few difficult weeks with the hospital immigrants in this community venture, he had a unique and important role in helping to create the lodge society. Unfortunately, he accepted a position with another organization once these first few weeks had passed, but it is to his early efforts that the members of this research group owe a great deal. The authors are also indebted to Stanford University for its help in carrying out this project. Particular gratitude is expressed to Sterling Silver, Cassius Kirk, Jr., Donald Price, and Lynn Comeski, who aided the establishment of the lodge society in many ways. It is also important to recognize here the aid of Mr. Cedric Kidder who was a janitorial consultant for those in the lodge society. Finally, special recognition is due the National Institute of Mental Health (NIMH), which provided the funds for this study (Grant No. 3 R11 MH 01259 and No. 7 R01 MH 14690). A list of names of those from the Institute who were helpful in this project is too lengthy to present here, but special gratitude is expressed to the Applied Research Branch and the San Francisco Regional Office.

The authors have had the particular good fortune to know and work with several able collaborators of long standing in the current research effort. Among them was Mrs. Helen J. Pearson who functioned as administrative assistant to the project. In this capacity, her major responsibilities concerned administration on a day-to-day basis of the grant-supporting project activities, especially those important functions of establishing and maintaining relations with the sponsoring institutions of higher learning. Another, Mrs. Betty J. Fairweather, assisted the project substantially by typing transcripts of interviews and scoring data. Finally, aid in completing the cluster analyses of much of the research data was given by the late Dr. Robert C. Tryon and his associates, particularly James Cameron.

There are others who made substantial contribution to the study. Dr. Edward Custer played an exceedingly important role in establishing the medical care for lodge members. We are grateful to Sharon Martin, Barbara Hobbs, and Sharon Doolittle for help in preparing the manuscript. We are also indebted to several publishers for their permission to reprint material first published by them. They are: American Journal of Orthopsychiatry, Harper & Row, John Wiley & Sons, International Universities Press, and Columbia University Press.

But we would be remiss if we did not recognize our lasting indebtedness to those who established the community lodge. Whatever were the benefits that this adventurous group of formerly hospitalized mental patients obtained from this experiment, it was small in comparison to the benefits gained by those of us who worked with them. The daily contacts with them in their struggles to attain independence and to establish their own small society were at times frustrating, unpredictable, and often inspiring, but they were always very human.

G. W. F.
D. H. S.
H. M.
D. L. C.

About the Authors

At the beginning of the investigation reported in this book, GEORGE W. FAIRWEATHER was chief of the Social-Clinical Research and Service Unit of the Veterans Administration Hospital in Palo Alto, and an associate consulting professor of psychology at Stanford University. Subsequently, he moved the research project to Portland State University where he was professor of psychology and director of a research institute. He is now professor of psychology at Michigan State University and is planning an institute to train researchers in the methods of experimental social innovation.

The co-authors were all colleagues of Professor Fairweather during the course of the project. DAVID H. SANDERS, HUGO MAYNARD, and DAVID L. CRESSLER held positions as research associates both at Stanford University and at Portland State University. David H. Sanders is presently associate professor of psychology and psychiatry at Michigan State University; Hugo Maynard and David L. Cressler remain at Portland State University.

Contents

PART I. THE SOCIAL INNOVATIVE EXPERIMENT

1 OVERVIEW OF THE EXPERIMENT

Persons who are hospitalized for mental illness nowadays are often destined to become long-term residents of mental hospitals or to return to the community after a relatively short stay. In either case, the results for those least capable of reassuming responsible community roles are often catastrophic. With the advent of more and more interest in the community treatment of mental illness, a nationwide emphasis upon the mental patient's return to the community has developed. Very often, even with excellent planning and the devoted efforts of mental health workers, finding meaningful and participative community roles for these individuals is not accomplished. For the majority of those who leave the hospital without a family to which to return and for many others who remain in the hospital a long time before leaving, the too frequent result is a lonesome and unrewarding life in the social status of ex-mental patient. Many of these persons feel, and perhaps rightfully, that they have been the unwitting victims of social forces aimed at segregating them from the larger society.

Previous experimental work in the mental hospital (Fairweather, 1964) has shown, however, that many such individuals—at least when belonging to small groups—are capable of taking care of one another, can make realistic decisions about their lives and those of their group, and can adjust reasonably, adequately, and semiautonomously to the hospital setting. But such group living situations, where the strengths and weaknesses of various individuals can be balanced by their working as a team, are not typically available in the community setting. The goal of this research, therefore, was to discover if new and meaningful social statuses and roles for mental patients could be created in the society so these persons could participate more actively in the social processes accorded ordinary citizens in their everyday life. It was, in fact, an attempt to provide in mid-twentieth-century America an alternative to the large mental hospital. In order to achieve this goal, it was necessary for the researchers to create a new small society in the community where chronic mental patients could go to live and work in a supportive group situation.

But it is not alone sufficient to create a totally new treatment program that can be carried out in the community. It must be a demonstrated improvement over current practices before it can be realistically considered by society. It is, therefore, essential that such a program be directly compared with treatment programs currently available to mental patients in the community. So, in addition to creating and implanting an entirely new living and working situation in the community for mental patients, every phase of the new treatment program was carefully evaluated. A thorough presentation of both the background for the comparative research and its results are presented in the five parts of this book.

The first part, chapters 1, 2, and 3, gives a conceptual framework and description of the study. Chapter 1 presents a summary of the research findings as well as an orientation toward the book. Chapter 2 establishes the conceptual position which underlies the creation of a new treatment society. And chapter 3 presents a detailed discussion of the procedure involved in planning and implementing the project, including a description of the patient population, assessment techniques, experimental design, and the general plan for carrying out the experiment.

Part 2 is an historical presentation of the development of the newly created lodge society. Those former patients who constituted the membership of this society experienced an era of maximum professional supervision, presented in chapter 4. Chapter 5 explains the need for and the emergence of a member governing body, while chapter 6 describes the resultant reduction in professional supervision. Chapter 7 portrays the events that led to the complete ownership and operation of the business and living situation by its members, coinciding with the disappearance of professional persons from the small society.

Part 3 gives a description of the interaction by members of the small society with persons in the surrounding community. Chapter 8 places in perspective the social and economic environments in which the lodge existed. Relationships with persons in the neighborhood and the larger community are described in chapter 9. Chapter 10 reports the relations between the innovated society and the university which sponsored the program. Chapter 11 describes the medical care that the members received while living in the lodge.

Part 4 presents an evaluation of the newly created treatment program. Chapter 12 compares the community adjustment of members of the lodge society with matched persons who participated in the typical aftercare programs available to mental patients in the community. Since the residents of the lodge and their comparison group were volunteers, chapter 13 presents an evaluation of the effects of volunteering on the community adjustment of former mental patients. It also explores in considerable detail the effects that previous long-term hospital residence ("chronicity") has upon adjustment in the community once mental patients have returned there. Chapter 14 examines the effects that different community social situations have upon criteria selected to evaluate program effectiveness, and chapter 15 presents a description of the group processes extant in both the hospital and lodge programs.

Finally, part 5 presents some implications of this study for innovative research with the mentally ill and other marginal groups. Chapter 16 summarizes staff and patient views about innovative hospital and community treatment programs, chapter 17 places the research results in the perspective of operating principles for community treatment programs, and chapter 18 discusses the results of the experiment as they relate to the general problem of marginal persons in American society. The discussion is broadened to explain what the research results may portend for disadvantaged citizen groups.

After planning the experiment, which included the creation of the assessment devices and the research design, all individuals on a selected open ward were questioned about volunteering to live in the lodge society. Those who volunteered were randomly assigned to either the lodge group or its control group. Those who refused to volunteer constituted the experimental group used later to discover the effects of the act of volunteering itself.

On a prearranged date, the action phase of the study began. Initial testing was completed for all individuals in the sample, and group meetings by the potential lodge members to plan the imminent move into the community were begun. The members decided who their leaders would be, what procedures for purchasing food were needed, and the type of work each member would do. At the end of 30 days, the lodge group moved into its community residence. The move to the lodge initially occurred with considerable confusion. As with most plans, changes needed to be instituted immediately. Difficulties soon arose concerning the taking of tranquilizing medication, and a system whereby a lodge member gave medication to those persons who would not take it was instituted. The planned janitorial and gardening work was not done well by the members. Work habits learned in the hospital seemed to have been more oriented toward avoiding than carrying out work. Accordingly, work-training programs were initiated. Problems arose in obtaining food and preparing it.

Finally, one member who demonstrated an interest in cooking emerged from the group and eventually became the lodge member continuously responsible for preparing and serving meals.

But management of the food problem was only the first step toward achieving full autonomy in the community. It was soon discovered that the members worked best in teams. Each work team had a leader who became responsible for its work. A business manager emerged with the responsibility for keeping the business records of the organization. To aid the members in establishing competence in the various areas of living and work, the services of a number of consultants also were obtained. Thus the medical problems of the lodge were handled by a house physician, an accountant consulted the business manager about the manner in which the books should be kept, and a janitorial consultant aided the lodge group in improving its work methods.

Initially, extensive supervision of the lodge society was required. This was provided by a coordinator, a psychologist with many years of professional experience in the mental health field. According to the research plan, he was replaced by a graduate student with much less experience, while at the same time a governing body, composed of lodge members, was given increased autonomy in the management of both the social and work life of the lodge members. After several months of leadership under the graduate student coincident with increasing autonomy of the governing body, the student was replaced by lay leaders responsible only for the work aspect of the lodge. The member governing body at this point became totally responsible for the development and operation of the lodge. This committee of lodge members established policy for governing the members and for allocating lodge resources. For example, they set salary levels, approved vacations, determined how the organization's money would be spent, and disciplined troublesome members. Under joint lay and member leadership, an extensive business was created, and lodge living conditions became more attractive to the members. Eventually, the lodge building was closed and the remaining members became a completely autonomous group residing on their own in a new location. Despite this physical change, they continued the work and living arrangements of the lodge organization without the aid of lay or professional persons. Occasionally lodge members did request help from these persons, who then functioned as their consultants.

What did this new society achieve? Did it fulfill the expectations of those who established it? Several questions like these asked at the outset of the study were answered once the full sequence of events leading to autonomy of the lodge society was completed. The first question concerned whether or not a small subsociety of ex-mental patients could be implanted in the community. The results of this study show definitely that such small societies can be established if appropriate attention is given to their location and the norms and values of the surrounding neighborhood, and can even thrive in the appropriate setting. A second question concerned the degree to which a small society providing living and working arrangements for its ex-patient members could increase their time in the community and their employment, as well as enhance their personal self-esteem. Again, this question can be answered in the affirmative. Compared with traditional aftercare programs, the lodge society significantly increased employment and time in the community. The self-esteem of the persons in all aftercare programs was enhanced, since merely living in the community by itself was such an overpowering positive influence.

But what happened to those who did not volunteer to live in the lodge, many of whom gave as reasons for not volunteering that they expected better future employment and improved living situations? The results show that the act of volunteering itself had no major influence upon a person's community adjustment. People who did not volunteer fared no better than people who volunteered but could not go to the lodge because they were in the control group. These results again show the overwhelming value of the posthospital social situation itself.

As expected, the new community society dramatically reduced costs. When all of the expenses were paid by outside sources, the cost was approximately half that of keeping an individual in the mental hospital. And it should be noted here that the members of the lodge society who remained in it eventually became a self-supporting group.

But what of the effects of previous long-term hospital residence (chronicity) which were shown to be exceedingly important in earlier studies (Fairweather et al., 1960; Fairweather and Simon, 1963; Fairweather, 1964)? In this study, longer-term patients continued to adapt poorly in traditional aftercare programs but these differences disappeared in the lodge society. Not only, therefore, did the lodge society enhance the community adjustment of all members, but it also had a comparatively greater effect on those members who had been hospitalized for the longest time.

It is also possible to compare the group processes in the hospital and community lodge societies. In the hospital situation, the group processes were found to involve three essential dimensions: task group leadership, performance of the group, and group cohesiveness. However, in the autonomous community society, the leadership dimension combined with performance to form one dimension and group cohesiveness became the second dimension. Thus, group processes in the community may be explained by two dimensions. The difference between group-process dimensionality in the hospital and in the community appears to be due to the fact that in the hospital the professional staff can never give true autonomy to patient groups so that actual patient leadership can develop. In the community lodge situation, by contrast, the members themselves ultimately had to provide the total leadership for the group. Under this latter condition, excellence in group leadership resulted in excellence in group performance. Under the former condition, because of the social situation in which the patients found themselves, it could not. The results also showed that group formation occurs rather rapidly; 180 days from the inception of a group, its processes are so well defined that an entire replacement of the patient population does not alter these basic group dimensions.

From this study, a series of principles for the operation of community treatment programs was derived. It became clear that as the members developed a greater stake in the social system, they become more responsible. The pride that came with personal independence and the ownership of a business, which is one symbol of successful achievement in this society, was obvious to all concerned. Community-treatment programs thus need to provide as much autonomy to their members as possible. Pride cannot develop with autonomy, however, unless meaningful work, as society defines it, is also available to members, so that the responsibilities implied by autonomy are themselves meaningful. This is extremely important when viewed from the perspective of professional mental health workers. The finding that mental health workers expect patients both in and out of the hospital to fail in their adjustment is often used to justify the continuance of the ex-mental patient in his subordinate social position. The results of this study show that such expectancies are not warranted, and that these negative attitudes urgently need to be changed. Clearly, the paramount implication of this study for both the mental patient, other marginal individuals, and those who manage this society is the urgent need to create new and more participative social statuses and roles for those members who only marginally belong to it.

2 SOCIAL STATUS AND MENTAL ILLNESS

Society has many ways of dealing with the care and treatment of persons who are seen as representing a persistent social problem. Such methods have historically revolved around the dual concepts of custody and treatment. Exactly how a particular society evolves its own means for maintaining social control and stability depends at the broadest level on matters of social policy. These policies, in turn, reflect dominant cultural values that establish the priorities for ordering the allocation of a society's resources. With respect to the problem of mental health, a long-time student of the ways in which mental health care has been allocated in American society has summed up these issues as follows:

> Apparently the treatment of mental illness within the known history of man has been dominated by social, political, and ideological factors. Mental health programs are rooted more in moral and legislative elements than in medical and scientific ones (Freeman, 1965, p. 717).

Basically what is involved in programs for the management and treatment of mentally disordered persons is their rights as members of the society. In recent years, much concern has been expressed about the legal commitment of persons to mental institutions, which clearly reflects the fact that attention is upon the legal status of the disordered person in society, rather than his medical status (Ross, 1959). Extensive revisions of commitment codes in the various states, based on the pioneer Draft Act proposed by the Governor's Conference in 1950, has led to a redefinition of the rights of afflicted persons and the obligations of society toward them. These deliberations are concerned with the way in which society intervenes in the lives of those it has come to define as deviants. Historically, the definition of the disordered person has involved two problems for social control agents: first, the sometimes urgent need to deal with the effects of his behavior on the society; second, the extent to which he is judged in terms of the effectiveness he displays in assuming his rights and duties as a societal participant. Oftentimes, the society's need to control the person prevails over its judgments of his capacity, which tends to keep him in an inferior social status from which it is extremely difficult to emerge.

The patienthood of the mental patient begins when he enters an institution defined by society as one which will help him (Pine and Levinson, 1961; Caudill, 1958, p. 11). This role is taught to him in the institution by staff and fellow patients. It is cultural in nature (Landy, 1960), and he passes through various social processes requiring adaptations that define the new role.

In the modern mental hospital designed to attain institutional control over those exhibiting deviant behavior, a social system has been created which exerts control over individuals through processes that have come in recent years to extend into the community itself. The first of these is the *labeling* process whereby the potential patient acquires a public definition of himself as mentally ill. The medical profession sometimes assists this process through rendering expert judgment to the courts of the society responsible for a public definition of mental illness. A sociological theorist has recently suggested this process is the key to understanding stabilized mental disorder. This process basically initiates the transition of the person from the sick status through that of patient—about whom there are optimistic expectations of recovery—and into the terminal social status of chronic mental patient—about whom there is little expectation of recovery. The theorist asserts that a person so defined becomes "locked" into such a status by the societal reaction to his deviant behavior which ascribes the status by exaggerating the amount and degree of such deviation (Scheff, 1963, 1966, 1967).

The second of these processes involves *socialization* of the patient into the mental hospital society. This process has been dissected in detail in recent years, beginning with Goffman's description of the process in total institutions of "stripping" the self (Goffman, 1957, 1962). The negative effects upon the inmate of these total institutions, one of which is the mental hospital, have been amply described in recent years as the process of institutionalization (Vitale, 1962).

The third, a *"requalifying"* process, consists of the preparation for the return of the mental hospital patient to the community, beginning with the formulation of plans for departure, typically at the initiative of the staff. This process is the patient's introduction to reacquisition of the status of citizen, to the extent that his community may allow it, after a period of psychiatric hospitalization. Sometimes the patient is placed in a temporary citizenship status by the use of weekend visits to relatives or a "trial-visit" period in the community. The latter is often a covert hospital discharge, later acknowledged by administrative action of the hospital and signifying that the patient is no longer connected with the inpatient social system.

However, for those who have spent considerable time in the mental hospital, a fourth process become particularly salient and can best be described as *"weaning."* During participation in this process, the patient is connected to varying degrees with the ex-patient system of what has come to be called "aftercare." The development and elaboration of these community-based facilities, in increasing connection with inpatient institutions, has come about mainly because of the deficiencies noted for chronic patients in the outcomes of hospital treatments (Fairweather, 1960, 1964; Fairweather and Simon, 1963). Poor treatment outcomes and some other factors led to the suspicion on the part of many observers that variables other than the patient's psychological condition had greater relevance to his fate as an ex-patient (Waldron, 1965). Length of hospitalization was ultimately discovered to be one of the most critical variables, with longer hospitalization strongly associated with poorer prognosis (Fairweather, 1960, 1964; Lamb, 1967; Vitale, 1962). Writing in Germany in the early part of this century, Bleuler was among the first to outline the characteristics of dementia praecox which later came to be known as the group of schizophrenic psychoses from which most chronic mental patients suffer. In discussing treatment, he expressed his doubts about the suitability of the mental institution for the treatment of such severe emotion disturbances. In commenting on therapy for the schizophrenic patient, he stated:

> The institution as such does not cure the disease. However, it may be valuable from an educational viewpoint and it may alleviate acute, agitated states due to psychic influences. At the same time, it carries with it the danger that the patient may become too estranged from normal life, and also that the relatives get accustomed to the idea of the institution. For this reason, it is often extremely difficult to place even a greatly improved patient outside the institution, after he has been hospitalized for a number of years. In general, it is preferable to treat these patients under their usual conditions and within their habitual surroundings. . . . Release from the hospital follows the same general principles. One should not wait for a "cure." One can consider it an established rule that earlier release produces better results. . . . The only, and often very practical, criterion is the patient's capacity to react in a positive manner to changes in environment and treatment (Bleuler, 1950, pp. 474–75).

But hospitalization is only a part of the total treatment social system.

The other part includes posthospital treatment programs. Although facilities for outpatient treatment have evolved very rapidly recently, few have encompassed detailed planning for the chronic patient (Kraft, Binner, and Dickey, 1967). Most clinics operated by public agencies have been committed to the treatment of short-term psychotics as well as neurotics. As far as psychotic patients are concerned, treatment in such clinics appears to have been mainly for acutely disturbed psychotics in remission with good prognoses. One community study found a clear social class bias against the use of clinics by members of lower-class groups (Myers, Bean, and Pepper, 1965), into which most long-term patients gravitate if they are not already members.

Considering the financial cost, the operating bias toward verbal psychotherapy, and the unwillingness of patient families in lower classes to enter their members into community treatment, it is understandable that chronic psychotic patients returned to the community are not usually found on clinic rolls, although some are beginning to be now with the development and spread of the day-hospital concept. Although present in a few locations in Europe in the 1930's, the establishment of such facilities was not reported in the United States and Canada until after World War II. After poor treatment success with psychotic patients in the mid-1950's, the Veterans Administration gave considerable impetus to the development of such hospitals. Evaluation showing moderate success of such efforts was not begun until the decade of the sixties (Meltzoff and Blumenthal, 1966). These facilities have often been modified by the time of their availability to chronic patients, so that there are also (and often simultaneously at the same location) night and weekend hospitals. Descriptive accounts of such facilities mainly point to the limited size and scope of the efforts which are possible, especially under the ideological limitation that they are to function only as transitional facilities for chronic patients, with the expectation that such patients will ultimately move more completely into the community when discharged. It is also clear that the ex-patient is still in a patient status while participating in such treatment. Two other types of aftercare facilities also are typically structured with this patient status in mind, namely, aftercare clinics and family care homes (Crutcher, 1959; Muth, 1957; Patton, 1961). Varying in the degree to which ex-patients are retained in the patient status are facilities such as halfway houses, sheltered workshops, and social clubs (Beard, Pitt, Fisher, and Goertzel, 1963; Landy and Greenblatt, 1965; Olshansky, 1960; Wechsler, 1960). One observer has estimated that only 10 per cent of those who might be able to use such facilities are actually being treated, and the clients are typically those with the best prognosis and behavioral potential (Vitale, 1962, p. 257).

If this is the case, who are those who are typically in contact with returned chronic patients? It is likely that they are the established community agencies and institutions. This possibility occurs in spite of the fact that such community resources are hardly equipped to handle emotionally disturbed persons. Indeed, one review concluded that such facilities were poorly financed and badly distributed over the United States, especially in terms of urban and rural distribution, and that personnel were insufficient and untrained for such tasks (Robinson, DeMarche, and Wagle, 1960). Their study of public health and public welfare services, courts, schools, recreation services, churches, family casework agencies, and planning agencies such as mental health associations, welfare councils, and community fund agencies concluded generally that these agencies were poorly prepared to promote even preventative mental health programs, much less support programs for chronic patients. Nonmedical supportive treatment by community agents such as teachers, probation officers, public health nurses, sheriffs and judges, public welfare workers, group leaders, and clergymen may go on, however, as recent studies have suggested (Cumming, 1967; McCaffrey, Cumming, and Rudolph, 1963). The argument of these researchers is that when the chronic patient fails to meet his normal role obligations in the community, which is particularly the case with chronic schizophrenic patients, disruption of different kinds ensues in the social, economic, and familial contexts so that application is made to public agencies (not psychiatric treatment facilities) for assistance. These agencies thus function as collection points for many chronic patients who are, to paraphrase the authors, in an inadequate, "burned out" phase of psychotic disturbance rather than an active, agitated phase which might result in rehospitalization.

Of all the "pathway organizations" for chronic patients to reenter the community, the sheltered workshops have experienced perhaps the greatest surge in recent development (*Journal of Social Issues,* 16, 1960, whole issue). In a survey in 1965, approximately 480 workshops were located in the United States which had emotionally disturbed persons as clients, and the move to include more and more chronic patients in these facilities has picked up momentum in recent years (Kase, Gadlin, and Black, 1966). The impetus for this expansion of work-oriented rehabilitative facilities has been founded on two factors, at the least. First, the realization that "opening" the hospital has not only led to declining resident populations accompanying high release rates and shortened hospital stays, but that it has also seen rising relapse rates. For example, one of the more startling observations during the period when internal reorganization of mental hospitals away from custodialism was in full swing was stated in 1961: Readmissions to mental hospitals of all types in 1957 rose 9.2 per cent over 1956 (Gurel and Jacobs, 1961). In other words, return of chronic patients to the community did not "stick."

Second, several studies of the lives of chronic patients in the community have shown the critical importance of employment to the returning patient. Lamb (1967) showed that when hospital discharge rates are increased without provision for community employment, most chronic patients remain unemployed and only participate socially to a minimal degree. A previous study of dischargees from hospitals in England revealed further that the few who remain for substantial periods of time were likely to be employed, especially if they lived apart from spouses, parents, or dependency-inducing situations like hostels (Brown, 1959). However, it was observed that the work ability of such independently living chronic ex-patients was relatively independent of their clinical condition. On occasion, specialized efforts at aftercare support for such patients have been made, based on the judgement as to whether or not the patient was employable. Employable patients were assigned to a mental health clinic, while those judged unemployable were included in a day-treatment center (day hospital) program (Vitale and Steinbach, 1965). In this study, normative expectations of clinic patients regarding work were associated with a significantly higher rate of employment. Freeman and Simmons (1963) have clearly indicated that the returning patient's self-expectations emerged in their studies as a more critical variable in affecting community tenure than familial tolerance of deviant behavior, but they also emphasized the importance of obtaining employment for the returned patient. The lack of receptivity in industry has been pointed out by a recent author (Ferguson, 1965), and this lack may function as a further spur to the development of sheltered workshops. Low self- and family expectations about work seem associated with impaired ability to remain employed (Hall, Smith, and Shimkunas, 1966; Schooler, Goldberg, Boothe, and Cole, 1967), and usual conditions of work in sheltered workshops do not seem to discourage such expectations. Such facilities have limited financing and hence are unable to compete with industry in such areas as product development, the work is often piecemeal and monotonous since it involves jobs industry does not want to take on itself, and the professional staff often views the ex-patient as still a patient in status, especially when the reward structure for payment of workshop participants is taken into consideration.

Yet workshops generally have as an overt goal the preparation of the client for competitive employment. Gradually there is realization that sheltered employment in the community may be the best that the chronic patient can attain, although this is not generally admitted publicly. Using work as a rehabilitative procedure in the United States has not typically been viewed as anything more than a transitional device, unlike European cultural attitudes, which see work as applicable to all classes of chronically disabled persons and as a serious enterprise, with meaningful goals, tasks, and rewards as necessary components. As the situation appears to be at present for the returning chronic patient in America, participation in the sheltered workshop is most likely to enmesh him in a system of dependency upon professional aid and advice which consistently reinforces his patient status (Bellak and Black, 1960). Aftercare facilities in general, including workshops, typically provide chronic patients with a protective situation resembling the mental hospital from which they have come, allowing them to remain in the community, impervious to readmission (Vitale, 1962, pp. 257–58). At the same time, therefore, existing aftercare services alter the patient's relationship to the mental hospital but maintain his status as an impaired person. Thus the patient is identified as a deviant in the community and his status as a deviant is prolonged.

Like the inpatient social system the chronic patient leaves, the ex-patient systems typically operate under several rules assuring retention in the "shadow" social system which defines him as "sick." First, the patient must remain in a relatively unchanging subordinate social status despite behavioral changes such as increased competence; such changes are seen as irrelevant to the need for the patient's psychological readjustment. Follow-up studies in England and America suggest aftercare agencies do not differ in these expectations from those which spouses and parents have for chronic returning patients (Brown, 1959; Freeman and Simmons, 1963). One recently published study even goes so far as to reject domestic role performance of returning female patients as a useful criterion for judging the success or failure of discharged patients because of its lack of relationship to psychological functioning (Lefton, Dinitz, Angrist, and Pasamanick, 1967). The authors apparently overlook the possibility that demands of the domestic social situation may have fostered adequate community reintegration *despite* poor psychological functioning. The reassumption of certain normal social roles with the same degree of competence as a group of typical married women was viewed as unimportant, however, because of the attention focused upon the single criterion of psychological functioning.

Other covert rules which seem to govern participation of the chronic psychiatric patient in aftercare facilities pose equal problems in relation to his status as a community member. It would appear that for such a person, full citizenship status comes *after* departure from the system, not *before* his entrance into it as a discharged hospital patient. Erikson's recommendation that the returning patient be given a special status in society as "student" must be seen in a new light in view of this operating principle (Erikson, 1957). Such a recommendation neatly fits in with the current emphasis upon occupational retraining of chronic patients, particularly with respect to sheltered workshops. But such a reorientation of thinking further perpetuates an inferior social status in the community of a returning patient who has now become a "pupil" instead of a patient or client. Pupils must be taught by teachers who know more than they; such a social relationship has typically been that of a superior and a subordinate.

Thus the social position of the returning mental patient in American society appears to be a very disadvantaged one. Recent studies of public attitudes in the United States toward mentally ill persons indicate clear and general stigmatization (Nunnally, 1961, p. 233). To them are attributed both realistic deficiencies (they are often unpredictable) and socially despised characteristics such as stupidity, filthiness, insincerity, and worthlessness. The families of mental patients themselves respond to this stigma. They often deny the disordered behavior which precipitated hospitalization, block the ex-patient's reassumption of a role in the family, or avoid contact with professional mental health workers with whom family members have little in common (Schwartz and Schwartz, 1964, pp. 285–86). The ex-patient himself is likely to conceal his history of hospitalization in an attempt to reintegrate his position in the community while avoiding the barrier of the stigma.

Professional mental health workers who maintain contact with the formerly hospitalized patient typically do so by identifying the patient as a community deviant who entered his inferior status when he was diagnosed as mentally ill. This is a particularly effective social device for sustaining the stigma because the patient tends to be seen in terms of a psychiatric label which too often stresses the pathological aspects of his behavior while overlooking his capacities and potentialities. By treating the ex-patient as a "special" case needing further psychiatric attention, the patient is supplied with additional justification for various kinds of failure in the community (Freeman, 1965, p. 719). This has led Walter Simon (1965) to emphasize the substantial reasons why patients are reluctant to leave the public mental hospital. The community often keeps him in a dependent social status and thus denies him the opportunity to reassume a responsible role as a community member. Simon argues that second-class citizenship has increasingly come to be true of the chronic mental patient returning to the community. From this same perspective, Scheff (1967) and Mechanic (1962) have observed that the patient was marked as a social deviant during the process of psychiatric screening which preceded his entrance into the hospital, and this mark is not erased, particularly for the chronic patient. In his study, Scheff found many aspects of psychiatric screening reflected the fact that the official reaction to the person's deviant behavior is to presume his illness without basing this presumption solely upon his psychological condition. This is similar to the most essential elements of caste membership, which designate from the birth of the person the legal and customary limits which are to be placed upon his intimate social participation, about which he can do nothing for the rest of his life (Davis, 1945).

It should be clear from this review that the social status ascribed to individuals recurrently hospitalized for mental illness has greatly influenced treatment programs for them in the hospital, and more recently, in the community. Hospital treatment programs ascribe to all patients a subordinate social status. Patients are administered to by the physician and professional staff, and their expectations are organized around this lowly social position. When community programs are planned by these same professional mental health workers, such programs usually involve supervised treatment, living, and sheltered work situations where professional personnel and supervisors have jobs which *require,* according to the social definitions prevailing in such situations, that they care for the "ill." In the egalitarian culture of *American* society, this is very detrimental, as Hiller has suggested in commenting about the effects of occupying a marginal status:

> A lowly status leaves its mark on persons as truly as the more applauded position does. An old aphorism states that responsibility makes the person. Although this is an important half-truth, the converse is equally true; for occupational subordination and lack of a voice in reciprocities tend to produce either resignation and a feeling of inferiority or a high sensitivity to the implied inequity. Insofar as a culture emphasizes equalitarianism, there is an imputed adverse comparison in all subordinate positions . . . (1947, p. 509).

The degree of such deviant participation in society has largely been determined historically by delegation of decision-making to a limited number of agents of social control, mainly the professionals in medicine and public welfare. But introduction of the concept of self-determination of patient fate through peer-group formation may be a way of remedying the inadequate use of an existing resource (the patient himself), rather than focusing attention on the need for additional finances, facilities, and manpower. Such a focus may attack many of the recurring problems of management of the psychotic person—mainly his social withdrawal, and the maintenance of the effects of his treatment in the hospital once he has returned to the community (Vitale, 1962, p. 259). For too long, the concept of "illness-and-cure" has restricted the imagination of those charged with the social responsibility of aiding chronic mental patients because it has linked the pessimism with which the patient has been viewed to his social marginality and the low relative probability that he would be able to leave his marginal status once in the community. The supportiveness of the community situation has been determined to be one of the single most important variables affecting his stay there (Fairweather, 1964). "Curing" chronic mental disorder means maintaining a person in the community in a participating social status. The strategy of building a new social institution which creates a new network of social relationships that represent more participative statuses for him may be the only alternative to continued residence in a mental hospital which the chronic hospital resident is often reluctant to leave.

But such a change in treatment procedures will require an extensive alteration in public mores. The Schwartzes have described the problem in cogent terms as follows:

> Two questions face the community: What place *can* it make for such persons, that is, to what extent and under what circumstances can it behave therapeutically toward those who cannot perform adequately in normal social roles? What place *should* it make for them, that is, to what extent should it sacrifice other values so that the mentally ill are accepted and their rehabilitation in the community facilitated? . . . What [practitioners] are asking is that society develop another status for ex-patients, one that will help them learn how to live in society while at the same time not penalize them for their failures to perform adequately during the learning period. . . . This is a vastly different matter and involves not only the acceptance of an ex-patient's inability to function but also his right to experiment in society with finding more satisfactory ways of living. If and when such a role becomes established, it will symbolize a basic alteration in the way mental illness is conceived in our society and a profound change in the way it is handled by laymen and practitioners (1964, pp. 287–88).

Meaningful new social statuses need to be established which define persons who are emotionally disturbed as individuals who need situational support in order to find their highest possible functioning level of adjustment. Such a redefinition would permit the creation of treatment subsystems with new and more responsible statuses. Table 2.1 presents the social statuses available to mental patients today. The chart displays a dichotomy of behavioral autonomy associated with the social status of the mental patient in our society. A middle range of statuses is unavailable because they typically do not exist in the American contemporary treatment of mental illness, primarily because of the subordinate social status now accorded mental patients. Table 2.1 shows that there is a common tendency to classify people as either "sick" or "well," even though a person's social status *should* primarily be determined by his ability to assume particular rights and duties, according to the democratic ideology of our society. In practical terms, the working-out of this ideology requires that the individual be given the opportunity to be mobile, both upwardly and downwardly in his social status. This requirement is directly related to the range of statuses available to him, since a restricted range of available social statuses lessens mobility. Such is the situation of the chronic mental patient in our society today, for whom the opportunity to be upwardly mobile is denied and a singularly inferior social status, whether in the hospital or the community, is the only one available to him.

Table 2.1 fails to convey, because of its static nature, this dynamic fact about mobility. In adequately representing the lack of an important range of statuses available to the chronic patient, it does not show that the individual may vary in the level of functioning of which he is capable at any one point in time. The person's position on the continuum of individual autonomy through time is presented in Figure 2.1. A hypothetical person is seen in this figure to become acutely psychotic, whereupon he is

Table 2.1. Autonomy of Mental Patients' Social Status

	None ←		—— *Dimension of Autonomy* ——					→ *Complete*
Social Situation	Supervised Institutional Situation The Mental Hospital		Supervised community situations			Unsupervised community group situations	Partially autonomous individual status	Autonomous individual status
	Closed locked ward	Open unlocked ward	Living situations (home care, day care centers, day hospitals)	Work situations (sheltered workshops)	Combination of work-living situations	Discharged ex-patient–led group work-living situations—work in reference groups	Counseling or psychotherapy	No treatment
Status Situation	Very limited adult rights and duties		Some adult rights and duties			Otherwise, full adult rights and duties	Otherwise, full adult rights and duties	Full adult rights and duties
Available Social Statuses	Sick person					(Unavailable)	Well person	

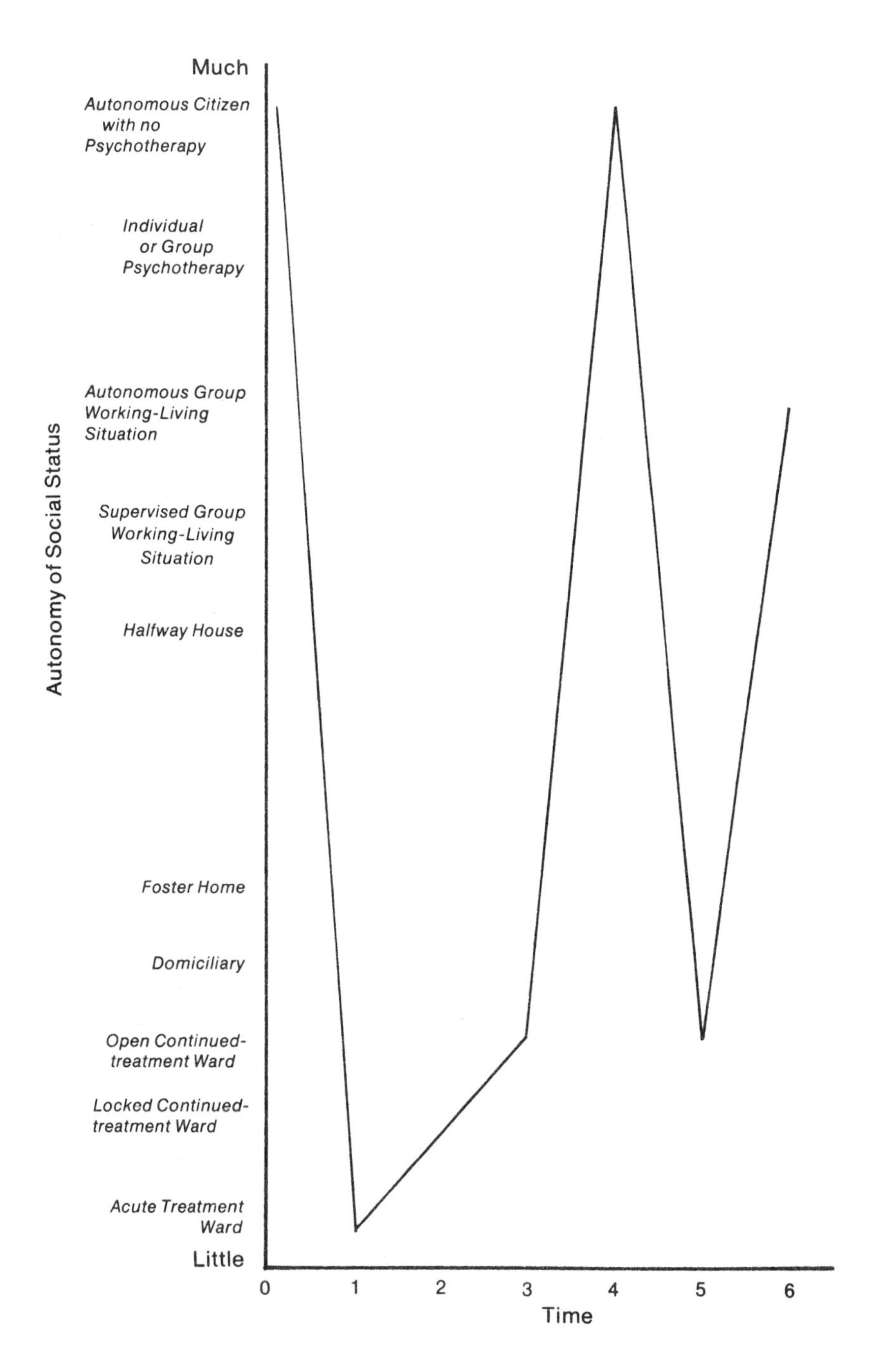

FIG. 2.1.—*Hypothetical course of a mental patient's status over time.*

sent to a locked ward in a mental hospital. Subsequently, he begins showing more adaptive behavior and is transferred to an open ward at the hospital. Later he is discharged from the hospital to the community, but his behavior deteriorates and he is again placed in an open mental hospital ward. Finally, he is able to assume the status of a worker living in a supervised group setting followed by a more autonomous adjustment in a group living and working situation without supervision. This person, at the last observation of his behavior, has shown that his most adaptive adjustment is participating in such a peer-group living and working arrangement in the community.

This latter social status is generally not now available to the ex-mental patient in this society, and will not automatically become available unless deliberate planning and resources are allocated to such an effort. No meaningful mobility for such a person can come about during the natural course of events because the varying degrees of responsibility inherent in different social statuses (other than patient) do not exist for this kind of "sick" person in our society.

When available treatment programs are viewed in terms of autonomy for individual action, the new social statuses that need to be created become clear. They are unsupervised social statuses in the community. To create them, a new social subsystem must be established which would accomplish the following tasks: It must provide alternative nondeviant social roles in the community to the chronic patient; it must maintain sufficient social distance from the community's agents of social control so that regulation of behavior takes place within the framework of the subsociety itself; it must protect him from hostile community forces and from power confrontations which he must inevitably lose, further destroying his confidence and self-esteem; it must reduce the visibility of the chronic deviant's rule-breaking behavior and attempt to regulate it within the normative framework of a cohesive subcommunity; it must assume control over the degree and amount of rule-breaking the subcommunity can tolerate. In general, this newly created social system must be organized in such a way that the largely ascribed social status of the chronic mental patient is displaced by an achieved social status within his own subcommunity which would depend on the individual's residual capabilities rather than on the characteristics of his psychological impairment. In the ensuing pages, judgment may be made on the extent to which such specifications, derived from this theoretical formulation of chronic mental disorder, have been met.

3 PLANNING AND IMPLEMENTING THE PROJECT

In an earlier empirical study, it was experimentally established that problem-solving patient-led groups could maintain their individual members and solve their daily problems in a hospital setting (Fairweather, 1964). This study also indicated that if a new way of living in the community—with greater social participation for chronically hospitalized mental patients—were designed, it would have to have certain special features. Some of these were discovered to be: vertical mobility up and down through whatever differentiated social structure was developed; open access to the social situation in terms of both entrance and exit; meaningful tasks, the accomplishment of which would reward the participants for the effort expended; and a special communication system which could both overcome status barriers between professionals and clients and provide adviser feedback that would continuously influence the solutions to daily living problems which the participants attempted. One way of establishing more participative social statuses for such patients, it was decided,would be to create a new community social subsystem with these characteristics as an alternative to the mental hospital.

These unique features would differentiate it from the usual community social situations provided discharged mental patients. For example, it would be designed so that no professional people were regularly present on the grounds of residence. In this way, some autonomy for the residents would be assured. All professional persons would be consultants rather than the supervisors who typically are responsible for the behavior of the participants. And most important of all, steps would be taken so that all professional supervision would gradually be reduced until a state of complete autonomy from professionals existed. This experiment was planned to accomplish all of these goals. It was designed to create a new social subsystem which redefined the status of the chronic mental patient from that of an ill person to that of a social participant. The new social subsystem would then be implanted in the community as a small, real-life model. But before this could actually happen, it was necessary to plan in as much detail as possible every aspect of the entire experiment from beginning to end.

Obtaining Administrative Agreements

The first step in planning the experiment was to make administrative agreements with the hospital from which the sample of patients would be obtained. Hospital administrative officials were contacted and they agreed to enter into this venture jointly with a nearby university. A psychiatrist in the hospital agreed to continue the small-group ward program described in this chapter (p. 28) and to send patients from this program to the community dormitory as required by the sampling procedures for the study.

Next, it was necessary to make agreements with labor and management concerning the community work roles that these ex-mental patients would have. The support of a nonprofit rehabilitative corporation was sought and obtained. It became the employer of the workers. The university made a management agreement clarifying the workers' relationship with the nonprofit corporation. The nonprofit corporation already had existing agreements with local labor unions and industries which defined its employees as persons involved in their own rehabilitation with respect to employment. They were thus excluded from the usual union-management work contracts. The various insurance coverages, including workmen's compensation, public liability, and a bond for damages to private property, were set forth in the management agreement. A physician, who was an internist and had previous experience as a ward physician in a large mental hospital, agreed to serve as the house physician for such a residence. Later on, other agreements were made with specialized insurance agencies, a car leasing company, and other organizations by either the nonprofit corporation or the university to handle particular operating problems as they arose. Figure 3.1 depicts the final administrative agreements that were reached. A detailed description of the major agreements supporting the operation of the experiment may be found in two subsequent chapters: those pertaining to the university in chapter 10, and those related to the hospital in chapter 11. Some agreements were reached prior to the receipt of the funding grant and some were made later.

The next problem was to obtain money to hire a research staff and to

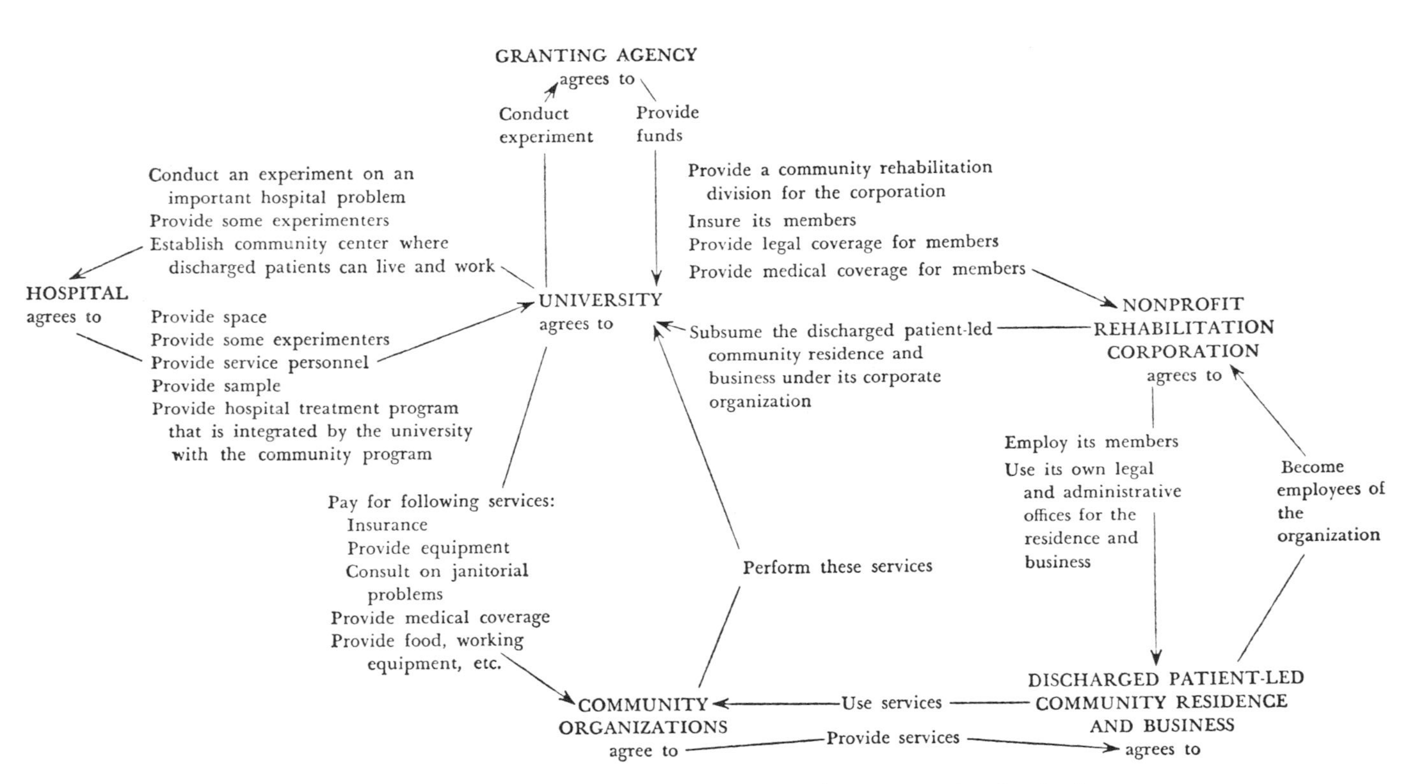

FIG. 3.1.—*Contractual arrangements among the cooperating institutions.*

create the work-living situation in the community. The university applied for a National Institute of Mental Health (NIMH) grant to implement the research plan. The research grant was eventually approved so that the other preparatory phases of the project could be carried into action.[1]

Forming the Research Team

Before the experiment could continue further, it was necessary to assemble a research team. In addition to evaluating the new community program, the team would have two other principal functions: first, establishing and supervising the community work-living situation; second, administering the hospital program from which participants in the community situation would come.

Both the hospital and the community programs needed to be coordinated with the university which applied for the research grant and with the nonprofit rehabilitative corporation which hired the ex-mental patients as employees. Table 3.1 is a chart of the roles in these three organizations. The chief social innovative experimenter was a member bridging both the hospital and the university staffs. He was responsible for the final choice of the research design, hiring the research team, and coordinating the activities of the university, the hospital, and the nonprofit rehabilitative corporation, as well as overall supervision of the research effort. The ward staff which carried out the small-group program in the hospital was comprised of one psychiatrist, one social worker, two nurses, and four nursing assistants. The hospital also furnished one research assistant to aid the chief experimenter in his coordinative function. Consultants to the lodge advised the members about medical and other matters. Table 3.1 also lists a board of directors; its members worked closely with the university and hospital research personnel in assuring the continuation of the project.

The rest of the research team, aside from the chief experimenter, included two research associates who in turn initially supervised the lodge or functioned as ward administrators in the small-group program, a research social worker, a research psychologist, and a research sociologist. All of these had particular institutional affiliations with the university as shown in Table 3.1.

Designing the Experiment

Once the research group was assembled, the research design was put into final form. There were several questions that the experiment was expected to answer which were an outgrowth of the earlier small-group study (Fairweather, 1964). The results from that study suggested that reference

1. U.S. Public Health Service Mental Health Grant Numbers 01259 and 14690.

Table 3.1. Personnel Participating in the Hospital-Community Study and Their Primary Institutional Affiliation

Hospital		*University*		*Nonprofit Rehabilitative Corporation*
Service	*Research*	*Consultants*	*Research*	*Service*
One psychiatrist One social worker Two nurses Four nursing assistants	One chief social innovative experimenter (principal investigator) One experimental assistant	Legal Accounting Insurance Statistical Computer Medical Janitorial	One chief social innovative experimenter (principal investigator) Two social innovative experimenters Three experimental assistants	Board of directors

groups to which ex-patients could belong might be valuable as a rehabilitative vehicle to bridge the gap between the hospital and the community. But what kind of social situation could be provided the group members that would meet two conditions that the experiment just mentioned indicated are essential if small groups of mental patients are to function effectively—namely, a meaningful task for adult males and a supportive living situation? Clearly such a situation would have to provide employment, because work status is the key status for adult males in American society. At the same time, the previously mentioned study also showed the necessity for providing a supportive living situation for these marginal members of society. After exploring the type of work that was needed in the community where the experiment was to be conducted, it was decided that the most appropriate community situation would be a patient-owned and patient-operated business which was combined with a living situation for the workers. Initially, the available facilities suggested a cafeteria business, but since the geographical area in which the study was to be carried out displayed a high and possibly unfilled demand for janitorial and gardening services, eventually it seemed more appropriate to establish a business that would provide these needed services (pp. 49–52). Furthermore, a business organization could create a number of jobs that varied in level of social responsibility, thus providing the opportunity for each member to find a job commensurate with his level of adjustment. A group of ex-mental patients living together was expected to provide the needed social and psychological support in the community suggested by the earlier experimental study.

In addition to studying the effects of such a living-working arrangement upon recidivism, employment, and personal self-enhancement, the experiment was also designed to study the effect of this newly created subsociety upon the hospital from which the patients came and upon the neighborhood and the larger urban environment in which it was implanted. The small-group study just mentioned had also raised specific questions about the group processes themselves, particularly about the relationship among the attributes of a group, such as its leadership, performance, and morale. That study also showed little relationship between attitudes and behavior, both in the hospital and in the community. Specifically, the question arose as to whether or not reference group membership beginning in the hospital and continuing into the community would strengthen the relationships between behavior and attitudes when measured independently in these two situations. It was believed that the low relationships found in the previous study might be increased in magnitude if the community situation were more similar to the hospital situation.

These were the primary goals for which the research presented here was conducted. The questions it was designed to answer were stated finally in the form of the following eight hypotheses:

1. A new living-working social subsystem for treating mental patients can be created and implanted in the community.

2. A community social subsystem which provides a place of residence and work for mental patients will increase time out of the hospital, increase employment, and enhance personal self-esteem when contrasted with a traditional program using those community facilities usually available to mental patients (such as visits to mental hygiene clinics while living at home, or sheltered workshops).

3. The community social subsystem will have its most beneficial effect upon the patients with the longest periods of previous psychiatric hospitalization (the most chronic patients).

4. Patients who do not volunteer to live in the community subsystem will demonstrate no better personal and social adjustment than patients who do volunteer.

5. The new community social subsystem will not require the usual complement of professional personnel.

6. The new community social subsystem will reduce the cost of patient care.

7. The new community social subsystem will yield different interrelationships among the treatment criteria than does the traditional program.

8. The complex social processes of the created groups can be explained by a relatively few dimensions.

To compare the effectiveness of the new posthospital community program with the traditional community programs available to mental patients, it was necessary that all participants should have the same hospital treatment program so that any differences that might later be found between these two community programs (work-living and traditional) could be attributed to them and not to differences in hospital treatment. The hospital small-group program presented in an earlier publication (Fairweather, 1964) was selected as the hospital treatment program. It was described there in the following manner:

> . . . This system required that each patient remain in his assigned task group from the day he arrived until he left the ward. To complete successfully the program, the patient had to progress through four steps. The group was responsible, as a unit, for each of its individual member's progress through these steps. The first step level was personal care, punctuality on assignments, and orientation of new members. When in this step, the member received $10.00 and a one-day pass per week. Each patient ordinarily had some money in his personal funds to be used for expenditures, and the approved funds were taken from these accounts. Step 2 required adequate performance in step 1 as well as qualitatively acceptable work on the job assignment. After successful completion of step 1, patients were advanced to step 2. In step 2 the member received $15.00 per week and an overnight pass every other week. In step 3,

members were responsible for steps 1 and 2 and, in addition, recommended their own money and passes commensurate with individual step level. Members were eligible for $20.00 per week and three overnight passes for the four weekends per month. In step 4 the patient had unlimited withdrawal of money and passes and was responsible for all preceding steps.

The task groups operated in the following manner: Four out of every five days they met in their own room without staff members present. Here they evaluated each other and prepared recommendations for the staff when they met with them on the fifth day. During the autonomous task group meetings, the patients had recourse to request any staff member to appear before the group and to ask him for factual information which was needed to enable them to make a decision. The staff member could not recommend a course of action, but did reveal facts that were needed by the group to arrive at reasonable decisions.

On the fifth day, the staff met with the task group. The group presented specific recommendations about how their problems should be solved. This involved not only recommendations about more adequate group performance but also about how each member's money, privileges, job assignment, and problems should be handled. The staff then adjourned and made decisions regarding the merit of the task group recommendations . . . (Fairweather, 1964, pp. 30–31).

The small-group program took place on one ward within the hospital and was administered by a single staff. All patients in the study participated in this program. Thus the hospital treatment program was the same for everyone in the study. It was the community aspect of the treatment program that was different, so that in comparing a traditional program with a community working and living situation, the differential effects that these two community situations might have in reducing chronic hospitalization and improving self-perception could be ascertained. Finally, earlier studies had shown that neurotic and more chronic psychotic patients might respond differently to treatment than those less chronic (Fairweather, 1960, 1964). For this reason, an experimental design was constructed so that both the effects of posthospital treatment and diagnostic group membership could be evaluated. The final form of the design along with the size of the participating sample is presented in Table 3.2.

It was expected that there would be, of course, individuals who would be randomly admitted to the hospital ward but who would not volunteer to go to the community living-working situation. The question arose therefore about what effect the act of volunteering itself would have upon outcome. Since both the volunteers who did not go to the community living-working situation (control) and those who did not volunteer participated in identical programs, differences due to volunteering would be ascertained by comparing these two groups. The design and sample size used to find the effects of volunteering is presented in Table 3.3.

Table 3.2. Design and Sample Size Used to Evaluate the Effects of the Community Lodge for Three Different Diagnostic Groups.

Diagnostic Group	*Volunteer Lodge Group* Small-group hospital treatment program + Community living–working situation	*Volunteer Nonlodge Group* Small-group hospital treatment program + Traditional community program	*Total*
Nonpsychotics	11	14	25
Psychotics, 0–4 years	27	24	51
Psychotics, over 4 years	37	38	75
Total	75	76	151

Table 3.3. Design and Sample Size Used to Evaluate the Effects of Volunteering for Three Different Diagnostic Groups.

Diagnostic Group	*Volunteer Nonlodge Group* Small-group hospital treatment program + Traditional community program	*Nonvolunteer Nonlodge Group* Small-group hospital treatment program + Traditional community program	*Total*
Nonpsychotics	14	29	43
Psychotics, 0–4 years	24	93	117
Psychotics, over 4 years	38	61	99
Total	76	183	259

Sampling Procedures

The ward in which patients were assigned to each of the experimental programs was an open ward in a large 2123-bed general hospital comprised of two divisions. The division where the experimental ward was located contained 1123 beds, all for neuropsychiatric patients. Patients were assigned to the experimental ward without bias from open wards within the hospital when bed space became available. All patients participated in the small-group program just mentioned. When an individual arrived in step 4 of the small-group program, hospital departure plans had to be made (Fairweather, 1964). At this point in each patient's hospital stay, the lodge program was described to him and he was asked whether he wished to volunteer to participate in it. If he did, he became one of the volunteers in the study and was matched on age, diagnosis, and length of hospitalization with another volunteer. Each one of the matched pairs was then randomly assigned to either the traditional or lodge community programs. This same random assignment procedure was followed for all individuals who subsequently entered the sample. However, since each individual entered the ward at a different time, every person entering the sample after the initial matches was singly assigned to the two community conditions. Thus, initial sampling was done on a matched-pair basis and subsequent sampling by simple random assignment. Such multistage-sampling procedures are discussed elsewhere (Fairweather, 1967). By using this type of multistage-sampling procedure, a sample of 334 individuals was obtained. There were 75 in the volunteer-lodge group, 76 in the volunteer-nonlodge group, and 183 in the nonvolunteer group. The cells with the appropriate numbers for each diagnostic group are presented in Tables 3.2 and 3.3.

Table 3.4 shows a comparison of the demographic characteristics of the samples participating in the two treatment subsystems. By matching individuals on age, diagnosis, and length of hospitalization as closely as possible, the groups were made highly comparable on other characteristics, a result similar to that obtained in earlier studies (Fairweather, 1960, 1964). Table 3.4 shows that the lodge and nonlodge groups are not significantly different with respect to socioeconomic status, educational achievement, employment, drinking behavior, race, marital status, criminal records, military service, hospital admissions, and parental family background. A comparison of the diagnostic groups on the same characteristics is shown in Table 3.5. It reveals that the nonpsychotics are slightly older than the two psychotic groups, that they more frequently have been married, that they have been in the hospital less time than the more chronic psychotics but more than the less chronic, are more often heavy drinkers, and have held more jobs than either of the two psychotic groups. These differential characteristics have also been found in earlier studies (Fairweather, 1960, 1964).

Table 3.6 shows that the volunteers compared with those who did not volunteer for the community lodge have been hospitalized for a significantly longer period of time, have more frequently held lower lower class employment positions, and have held fewer jobs. It seems apparent that the volunteers have made a poorer psychological and social adjustment in their past histories. A second comparison of the diagnostic classifications within the volunteer and nonvolunteer groups is presented in Table 3.7. It again shows that the nonpsychotics are older, have more often been married, were older when hospitalized, had spent fewer weeks in the hospital than the more chronic psychotics but more than the less chronic, were more often voluntary patients, were more often heavy drinkers, achieved higher ranks in military service, and held more jobs than the two psychotic groups.

In general, the matching and sampling procedures used were successful in equating those individuals who participated in the community-lodge

Table 3.4. Comparison of Lodge and Nonlodge Groups on Demographic Characteristics

Variable	*Volunteer Lodge Group*	*Volunteer Nonlodge Group*	*df*	χ^2
Median Age	41	43	1	3.50
Race, %:				
White	81	80	1	0.00
Other	19	20		
Military Service, %:				
Service-connected pension	41	54	1	1.93
No service-connected pension	59	46		
Military service, 0–122 weeks	49	49	1	0.00
Military service, 123 weeks and over	51	51		
Military rank, buck private	28	29	1	0.00
Military rank, PFC or higher	72	71		
Neuropsychiatric Hospitalization:				
Median age at first hospitalization	27	29	1	1.11
Median number prior hospitalizations	2	2	1	0.01
Median weeks prior hospitalizations	233	262.5	1	0.06
Type of Hospital Admission, %:				
Voluntary	44	46	1	0.01
Commitment	56	54		
Parents' Marital Status, %:				
Married and living	12	18	1	0.50
Other	88	82		
Brought up by, %:				
Both parents	42	55	1	1.49
Other	56	45		
Days since Last Contact with Relatives, %:				
0–89 days	64	64	1	0.00
90 days and over	36	36		
Employment:				
Social classification of last job, %:				
Lower middle class and upper lower class	21	29	1	0.95
Lower lower class	79	71		
Median number of jobs held in last 10 years	2	2	1	0.34
Median Highest Grade Completed	11	12	1	0.32
Drinking behavior, %:				
Heavy drinkers	35	26		
Social drinkers	39	48	2	1.52
Nondrinkers	26	26		
Police Arrests, %:				
One or more	59	57	1	0.04
None	41	43		
Marital Status, %:				
Single and never married	64	54	1	1.19
Other	36	46		
Current Monthly Income while Hospitalized, %:				
0–$101	53	47	1	0.44
$102 and over	47	53		

subsystem very closely with those who serve as their control. On the other hand, the volunteers as a group appear to have been more chronically hospitalized than the nonvolunteers and to have demonstrated a generally poorer historical adjustment, a factor that had to be considered in determining the effects of volunteering (p. 240). Both diagnostic group comparisons (Tables 3.5 and 3.7) show that the nonpsychotics have been hospitalized less frequently, are more often heavy drinkers, and have a past history more closely resembling that typically found in the culture.

Assessment Devices

In order to test the experimental hypotheses mentioned earlier (p. 28), it was necessary to create measures for this purpose. The three areas of measurement that were considered to be most important were those having to do with the demographic characteristics of the participants discussed in the previous section, the social processes of the lodge, hospital, and the community, and the measures of outcome.

Internal social processes at the lodge were measured by several different assessment devices. Records of the amount and type of medication prescribed for each person and of actions of the executive committee (p. 49)—a member group that was responsible for the administration of the lodge—were kept. Work-performance rating sheets, check lists for the proper use of tools and equipment, and a record sheet for jobs performed were created. There were also longitudinal measures made of the morale of the lodge members, their expectations, the attractiveness of their living and working situation, and their satisfaction with statuses and roles. These group-process measures were completed in both the hospital and community settings. In addition, a research journal was kept in which important daily events and critical incidents that occurred at the community lodge were recorded.

At three-month intervals, every patient in the study was tested with the same battery of instruments for the duration of his stay on the hospital ward. When a patient entered and left the ward, he completed other tests in a separate room located in the same building as the hospital ward. This type of information was obtained for all 338 individuals in the study. The perceptions of hospital staff personnel about the lodge were measured annually by questionnaires and interviews. The questionnaires were completed by all staff members following a regular staff meeting, while interviews with them were conducted where they worked.

Outcome was measured by follow-up questionnaires, some of which were completed by the ex-patient and some by a respondent who was in current contact with the ex-patient. Since the community work-living situation was mainly established in an attempt to increase time out of the

Table 3.5. Comparison of Diagnostic Groups on Demographic Characteristics for Volunteer Lodge and Volunteer Nonlodge Groups

Variable	*Non-psychotic*	*Psychotics, 0–4 years*	*Psychotics, over 4 years*	*df*	χ^2
Median Age	45.00	38.75	41.11	2	7.84[a]
Race, %:					
White	88	76	81	2	1.50
Other	12	24	19		
Military Service, %:					
Service-connected pension	44	53	47	2	0.55
No service-connected pension	56	47	53		
Military service, 0–122 weeks	36	49	54	2	1.92
Military service, 123 weeks and over	64	51	46		
Military rank, buck private	8	32	32	2	5.96
Military rank, PFC or higher	92	68	68		
Neuropsychiatric hospitalization:					
Median age at first hospitalization	37.75	30.25	25.99	2	8.14[a]
Median number prior hospitalizations	2.38	3.06	2.39	2	0.08
Median weeks prior hospitalizations	148.34	113.69	439.40	2	118.99[b]
Type of Hospital Admission, %:					
Voluntary	64	40	49	2	3.88
Commitment	36	60	51		
Parents' Marital Status, %:					
Married and living	12	20	13	2	1.00
Other	88	80	87		
Brought up by, %:					
Both parents	42	45	52	2	1.22
Other	58	55	48		
Days since Last Contact with Relatives, %:					
0–89 days	70	62	63	2	0.35
90 days and over	30	38	37		
Employment:					
Social classification of last job, %:					
Lower middle class and upper lower class	24	27	23	2	0.19
Lower lower class	76	73	77		
Median number of jobs held in last 10 years	2.88	2.46	1.36	2	15.66[b]
Median Highest Grade Completed	11.63	11.57	11.06	2	1.43
Drinking behavior, %:					
Heavy drinkers	72	33	13		
Social drinkers	28	45	43	4	39.35[b]
Nondrinkers	0	22	44		

Table 3.5. Continued

Variable	*Non-psychotic*	*Psychotics, 0–4 years*	*Psychotics, over 4 years*	*df*	χ^2
Police Arrests, %:					
One or more	68	62	52	2	2.38
None	32	38	48		
Marital Status, %:					
Single and never married	28	49	76	2	21.98[b]
Other	72	51	24		
Current Monthly Income while Hospitalized, %:					
0–$101	60	46	49	2	1.85
$102 and over	40	54	51		

[a] Significant at .05 level.
[b] Significant at .001 level.

Table 3.6. Comparison of Volunteers and Nonvolunteers on Demographic Characteristics

Variable	*Volunteers*	*Nonvolunteers*	*df*	χ^2
Median Age	43	42	1	1.26
Race, %:				
White	80	80	1	0.00
Other	20	20		
Military Service, %:				
Service-connected pension	55	60	1	0.31
No service-connected pension	45	40		
Military service, 0–122 weeks	49	47	1	0.08
Military service, 123 weeks and over	51	53		
Military rank, buck private	29	22	1	1.66
Military rank, PFC or higher	71	78		
Neuropsychiatric Hospitalization:				
Median age at first hospitalization	29	31	1	0.07
Median number prior hospitalizations	2	2	1	0.60
Median weeks prior hospitalizations	239	120	1	7.78[b]
Type of Hospital Admission, %:				
Voluntary	45	39	1	0.70
Commitment	55	61		
Parents' Marital Status, %:				
Married and living	18	21	1	0.45
Other	82	79		
Brought up by, %:				
Both parents	54	54	1	0.00
Other	46	46		
Days since Last Contact with Relatives, %:				
0–89 days	64	74	1	2.45
90 days and over	36	26		

Table 3.6. Continued

Variable	*Volunteers*	*Nonvolunteers*	*df*	χ^2
Employment:				
Social classification of last job, %:				
Lower middle class and upper lower class	29	49	1	8.07[b]
Lower lower class	71	51		
Median number of jobs held in last 10 years	2	3	1	3.87[a]
Median Highest Grade Completed	12.0	11.7	1	1.93
Drinking Behavior, %:				
Heavy drinkers	33	27		
Social drinkers	41	53	2	3.86
Nondrinkers	26	20		
Police Arrests, %:				
One or more	57	57	1	0.00
None	43	43		
Marital Status, %:				
Single and never married	54	43	1	2.70
Other	46	57		
Current Monthly Income while Hospitalized, %:				
0–$101	47	38	1	1.96
$102 and over	53	62		

[a] Significant at .05 level.
[b] Significant at .01 level.

Table 3.7. Comparison of Diagnostic Groups on Demographic Characteristics for Volunteers and Nonvolunteers

Variable	*Non-psychotic*	*Psychotics, 0–4 years*	*Psychotics, over 4 years*	*df*	χ^2
Median Age	47.10	39.60	43.08	2	20.36[c]
Race, %:					
White	91	75	82	2	4.47
Other	9	25	18		
Military Service, %:					
Service-connected pension	70	52	61	2	2.51
No service-connected pension	30	48	39		
Military service, 0–122 weeks	42	42	58	2	5.97
Military service, 123 weeks and over	58	58	42		
Military rank, buck private	5	23	33	2	13.20[b]
Military rank, PFC or higher	95	77	67		

Table 3.7. Continued

Variable	*Non-psychotic*	*Psychotic, 0–4 years*	*Psychotic, over 4 years*	*df*	χ^2
Neuropsychiatric Hospitalization:					
Median age at first hospitalization	35.80	31.27	27.85	2	6.15[a]
Median number prior hospitalizations	3.67	2.25	2.46	2	1.87
Median weeks prior hospitalizations	92.13	80.58	474.05	2	179.22[c]
Type of Hospital Admission, %:					
Voluntary	58	36	39	2	6.13[a]
Commitment	42	64	61		
Parents' Marital Status, %:					
Married and living	19	25	16	2	2.45
Other	81	75	84		
Brought up by, %:					
Both parents	42	56	57	2	2.81
Other	58	44	43		
Days since Last Contact with Relatives, %:					
0–89 days	71	77	65	2	3.51
90 days and over	29	23	35		
Employment:					
Social classification of last job, %:					
Lower middle class and upper lower class	49	46	36	2	3.18
Lower lower class	51	54	64		
Median number of jobs held in last 10 years	3.31	3.06	1.08	2	36.22[c]
Median Highest Grade Completed	11.00	11.77	11.62	2	4.29
Drinking Behavior, %:					
Heavy drinkers	65	22	15		
Social drinkers	28	62	45	4	54.20[c]
Nondrinkers	7	16	40		
Police Arrests, %:					
One or more	67	57	52	2	3.92
None	33	43	48		
Marital Status, %:					
Single and never married	23	40	64	2	22.77[c]
Other	77	60	36		
Current Monthly Income while Hospitalized, %:					
0–$101	44	48	38	2	1.94
$102 and over	56	52	62		

[a] Significant at .05 level.
[b] Significant at .01 level.
[c] Significant at .001 level.

hospital, increase employment, and improve self-enhancement, these three variables constituted the social-change outcome criteria. Many other measures of outcome were also completed by means of questionnaires, including such information as the former patients' evaluation of their living situations, respondents' perceptions of them, and so on. All outcome measures were obtained on every patient at six-month intervals for his follow-up period. In addition to these follow-up measures, structured interviews were obtained from community-lodge members at six-month intervals during their stay in the lodge in order to obtain an accurate account of the members' perceptions. Structured interviews were also obtained every six months from persons who were continuously hospitalized, in order that the accumulated effects of such residence could be explored. In addition, when any person in the study returned to the hospital—regardless of whether he was a volunteer or nonvolunteer, or whether he participated in the traditional or lodge community programs—he was given an extensive interview about his community experiences. Such information was designed to permit a detailed exploration of another type of failure—that which occurred in the community.

Another aspect of the study concerned the relations of the community lodge with the cooperating hospital and with the surrounding community. The effects of the lodge upon the hospital were evaluated by annual questionnaires and interviews completed by professional staff and patients alike. In order to evaluate the effect of the lodge upon the surrounding community, interviews were obtained every six months with individuals who had continuous interaction with lodge members, vendors, other business people, and the house physician. Periodic surveys of customer satisfaction with work done by lodge members were also completed. When the lodge was closed, interviews were obtained from neighbors in the same census tract. These interviews were delayed until the lodge was closed because the neighbors' reaction to a discovery of the ex-mental patient status of those "next door" might have inhibited the growth and development of this new society. Finally, individuals outside the neighborhood who had a continuous but not a close interpersonal relationship with the lodge members completed questionnaires about their evaluation of the lodge society.

Table 3.8 presents a list of the instruments given during the course of the experiment. Each of these instruments will be described in detail in the section of this book devoted to its analysis.

The Final Project Plan

A final research plan for the experiment was developed and followed for the duration of the study. The general plan with dates for specific measures and the planned experimental changes in the research program is presented in Table 3.9.

Table 3.8. Assessment Devices

Outcomes
- Questionnaires for:
  - Respondent evaluation of patient adjustment
  - Patient evaluation of his own adjustment
- Interviews for:
  - Periodic evaluation of lodge by members
  - "Failures" from all experimental groups

Participant Characteristics of Patients
- Questionnaires for:
  - Personal history
  - Expectancies about future
  - Expectancies about the community lodge

Internal Social Processes
- *Of the lodge*
  - *Group—process ratings*
    - Sociometric
    - Role clarity
    - Acceptance of members within group
    - Attraction to group by member
    - Satisfaction with leadership
  - *Research journal*
    - Daily description of group and critical events
  - *Work ratings*
    - Job inspection
    - Training program
  - *Administrative records*
    - Daily report by member in nightly charge of lodge ("OD")
    - Visitors log
    - Departure log
    - Medication reports
    - Number and type of jobs obtained
    - Tool and equipment check sheets
  - *Tape recordings*
    - Staff-member precommunity group meetings
    - Staff-member community evaluation meetings
    - Executive committee meetings of members
  - *Fiscal processes*
    - Accounting books
- *Of the hospital*
  - *Group—process ratings*
    - Leadership
    - Group performance
    - Work
    - Patient improvement (notes exchanged between staff and patients)
  - *Administrative records*
    - Medication reports
    - Entrances & exits from ward

External Social Processes of the Lodge
- Questionnaires for:
  - Relatives' attitudes toward lodge residents
  - Client evaluation of janitorial and gardening service
  - Neighbors' and associates' evaluation of lodge members
- Interviews for:
  - Periodic evaluation of the lodge by those closely associated with it (physician, vendors, etc.)

Table 3.9. General Plan of the Experiment

Program Phase	*Time Scale*	*Research Activity*
Residual of Planning	minus 4 months	Trial of assessment devices under model field conditions
	minus 3 months	Modification and perfection of assessment devices Establish preliminary reliability of assessment devices
	minus 2 months	Establish location of both subsystems Preliminary testing of the samples
	minus 1 month	Draw initial samples for both subsystems Preliminary meetings for participants of both subsystems
Initiate Subsystems	0 months	Initial testing for both subsystems First professional supervisor of community subsystem begins operations
Action	plus 6 months	First general testing of both subsystems First follow-up measures for both subsystems
	plus 7 months	Start training of second professional supervisor for community subsystem
	plus 8 months	Change to second professional supervisor of community subsystem
	plus 12 months	Second general testing of both subsystems Second follow-up measures for both subsystems First measures of community and hospital attitudes toward both subsystems
	plus 15 months	Start training of nonprofessional supervisor for community subsystem
	plus 16 months	Change to nonprofessional supervisor of community subsystems
	plus 18 months	Third general testing of both subsystems Third follow-up measures for both subsystems
	plus 24 months	Fourth general testing of both subsystems Fourth follow-up measures for both subsystems Second measures of community and hospital attitudes to both subsystems
Close Subsystems	plus 28 months	Final measures of community attitudes which were impractical while subsystems were in operation

Table 3.9. Continued

Program Phase	*Time Scale*	*Research Activity*
Evaluation and dissemination		Stop all data collection except for follow-up data Begin scoring, tabulation, and analysis of data gathered to date
	plus 30 months	
		Fifth follow-up measures for both subsystems Begin planning phase of next experiment
	plus 42 months	
		End write-up and publication of experiment

This chart shows that there were pre-established periods for testing every six months. In addition, the research plan also shows that new supervisors were trained and installed in the community subsystem at designated times. This sequential introduction of new supervisors—progressing from professional to lay personnel—permitted a test of the need for professional personnel in such community living-working situations. Thus, supervision was systematically changed from an experienced professional person to a professional person in training, to lay leaders and, finally, as an unplanned event, to complete autonomy for the members. Of course certain practical difficulties in carrying out this plan arose throughout the course of the experiment. For example, a legal suit was brought against the janitorial and gardening service (the ex-patients' business) for damage to a customer's property; this was later dismissed. Perhaps the most difficult problems to resolve were administrative aspects of the program which occurred when the time came to terminate the research aspect of the project and it became necessary to close the lodge. It is a natural difficulty associated with establishing any institution which meets important needs for a large number of people. For example, aside from the ex-patients involved, the owners who held the lease for the lodge building insisted that the project should not end, since it would clearly terminate their income from it. This matter became the subject of legal action which eventually was resolved out of court. Although plans for termination of project responsibility for the lodge had been made at the outset of the study, the greatest difficulty for all those associated with it was closing the lodge itself. For the last several months of the lodge's operation, however, detailed plans were made for the members to become self-sustaining. Those wishing to continue the subsociety formed their own janitorial and gardening service. At the date of this writing, it still continues to provide housing and employment in the community for its members.

After the lodge had been closed and the research program on the ward discontinued, analyses of the voluminous data collected over a four-year span was begun. The varied results from these analyses are presented in the following pages, beginning with a narrative account of the evolution of this unique, ex-patient subsociety.

PART II. EVOLUTION OF AN AUTONOMOUS SOCIETY IN THE COMMUNITY

4 THE ERA OF MAXIMUM PROFESSIONAL SUPERVISION

Preparation for the Move to the Community

The creation of the community-lodge society began when fifteen chronic mental patients were organized as a task group in the mental hospital. This task group participated in a small-group treatment program which has been described elsewhere (Fairweather, 1964). The group's task within the hospital program was to make decisions about solving its members' problems. There was one feature, however, that differentiated this particular group from the other four task groups on the ward—the group spent its work time discussing possible solutions to problems that its members would have to face upon their arrival in the community. This procedure was designed as advanced training for a unique situation that the task group had never faced before—leaving the hospital as a unit. Meeting together for a time prior to moving into the community also afforded the members an opportunity to develop a limited social organization, especially since its members knew definitely they would leave the hospital together for an adventure into the community which could dramatically affect their lives.

Autonomous meetings were thus held daily by the group in order to plan their imminent move to the community. Before each meeting, the ward staff presented the task-group members with written problems whose solution, the staff believed, would be essential for their survival once they had arrived in their community home. The group's solutions to such problems as eating and work arrangements were later presented in writing to the staff member who was to become coordinator of the lodge. He studied them and then met with the members to discuss the reasonableness of their decisions. It was hoped that this method of problem solution (autonomous decision-making and immediate staff feedback) would train the group to make adequate decisions about real-life problems. All autonomous group meetings were tape recorded by the members themselves and the information about these meetings that is now presented was obtained from these tapes.

The initial discussions of the group centered about the degree of autonomy and responsibility they, as ex-patients, would have in the new citizen-oriented community lodge. At the end of their first autonomous group meeting, a social organization was begun when the group elected a general manager and a business manager. Initially, the staff offered two problems for discussion: namely, what would the rules of the society be and how would the group handle daily problems that might arise. Although these questions served to structure the discussions at the beginning, the problems that the group considered to be most important soon emerged in spontaneous questions such as: How would the food be purchased and cooked? What would the eating arrangements be? How would roommates be chosen? Should the members purchase and wear work clothes? Could they use the hospital recreational facilities during their leisure time? How many hours a week would they work? How would they get to and from the lodge? Should they leave the lodge for another job?

Only after many meetings did the group show any concern about the type of work it might do. As the topic of the discussions eventually turned to work, the group decided to try to operate a restaurant. The dining facilities at the motel which they were to occupy had a coffee shop that served the public and the group planned to continue its operation. Consequently, when the focus of the discussions turned to business, it centered about the operation of this diner. Only tangentially was a second business considered—a janitorial service—and this occurred because of the members' concern that the operation of the café might not provide work for all of the members.

As far as the group was concerned, the most important first step in establishing the business was to define the particular roles required in operating a restaurant. Consequently, they proceeded to define and describe the various jobs that such a business would entail. Once this had been accomplished, each member was asked to volunteer for whatever job appealed to him. Those who did not volunteer were assigned roles by the two recently elected officials, the business and general managers. Thus the group proceeded to establish the additional jobs of assistant manager, cook, assistant cook, dishwasher, busboys, waiters, and cashier.

In addition to providing experience in decision-making, the meetings created general group cohesiveness. Five days prior to the move into the community, several problems, including the purchase of linen, planning a week's menu, and the purchase of food, were being discussed. All members of the group agreed to meet in the evening for a third session on that particular day in order to continue seeking solutions to these subsistence problems. However, one member asked the group's permission to be absent from the meeting so that he could go dancing. The group voted fifteen to one (the dancing member's vote) in favor of his attending the planning session. Even though he wished to move into the community with the group, this member stated that he would not attend the special session because he did not want to miss the dance. After he refused to attend the planning session, the group gave the dissident member an ultimatum: If he did not appear at the meeting he would no longer be a member of the group and consequently could not move to the community with them. He attended the meeting. This illustration shows that it required only a few weeks for the group to become a cohesive unit, membership in which required an acceptance of its primary goal—leaving the hospital. In aiding the fledgling group members to reduce their anxiety about the move, the staff thought it would be wise for the members to visit the dormitory so that they could familiarize themselves with their future home. The lodge site and surrounding area which they visited are described at length in chapter 8 (pp. 129–133). The visit had the desired effect. The group made many positive remarks during the visit.

But the planning by the group for the move was not quite so successful. Two important problems were not resolved until the last two meetings. The first was securing items such as clothing and bedding and readying the lodge for occupancy; the second was planning the first week's menu and shopping for the required food. Finally, just a few hours before the move, these essentials were purchased and planning completed.

The First Two Weeks in the Community

The moving day arrived and the plans made by the group and staff were carried out rather uneventfully, despite the high level of anxiety and tension of all concerned. At approximately eight o'clock in the morning, one research staff member took eight members of the group to the lodge. They prepared the house for the remainder of the group who would be arriving later in the afternoon with beds, supplies, and clothing. There was only one minor incident. One of the members of the group, Mr. White, was nowhere to be found when the beds were loaded onto the truck. He appeared as soon as the work was completed. This occurrence marked the beginning of a sequence of similar events for this person (see p. 54).

Once at the lodge, a somewhat confused work organization developed.

Two professional staff members and the owner of the lodge each headed a work team of sorts and the members scrambled around at various people's direction setting up beds and completing other essential tasks. Members congregated in the kitchen whenever a lapse in work occurred. The general confusion was magnified because a plumber, a gas and electric utility man, and a laundry service man were also scrambling around the grounds asking such questions as: Should the gas be left on? Should the motel telephone switchboard be continued in service? Most of these issues had to be resolved by the staff member who was present at the moment and this had the initial impact of making the members dependent upon both staff and outside servicemen for assistance. In spite of the confusion, all members were in residence at the lodge by the end of the first day.

When the research staff member who had been assigned to serve as coordinator for the lodge arrived the next morning, the men began seeking his attention by asking for help with such problems as getting a haircut or money for recreation. Since the questions were literally "thrown at" the staff member upon his arrival, a general meeting to discuss them was quickly called. The coordinator answered only questions of a procedural nature and soon left the group to solve its own problems. But, as was soon to become clear, adequate group decision-making had not yet developed.

During the first few days, the preparation of food was the main preoccupation of the group. Following the meal planning prevalent in the hospital, lunch became the main meal of the day. The main course for lunch was often steak or roast, while the main course for the evening meal was usually hamburgers or hot dogs or beans. None of these meals were too well prepared, since the cook, chosen by the group while in the hospital because he had often bragged of his culinary experience, could neither plan meals nor properly prepare food. Faced with the urgent need to eat more adequately, one of the kitchen workers took over the cooking chores. Since he could not disregard the first cook, he retained him as "cook's helper." Three other men volunteered to become dishwashers. They also cleaned the kitchen and the dining-room areas. Thus, out of urgent necessity, food services emerged as the first organized social activity at the new lodge.

During this early period at the lodge, the general atmosphere was one of confusion and turmoil. There was an awareness that the real-life community was vastly different from the hospital, and a feeling of "freedom" from incarceration prevailed among the men. "Each man should be independent" was a commonly heard phrase. If a man slept late, no one would get him up, since he was now a "full citizen." Although the leader complained that he and two others were doing all the work ("carrying the group"), he did not attempt to alter this perceived inequity. Testing the limits of propriety often occurred. Excessive drinking, refusal to follow medication regimes, and the emergence of new emotional problems were commonplace. Verbal problem-solving behavior learned in the hospital meetings clearly did not translate into appropriate problem-solving action in the community. The members began complaining they had no work to do even though the kitchen and yard needed care, and the floors and windows needed cleaning. There were a number of suggestions from some interested members about what *could* be done—from opening a restaurant to starting a janitorial service.

The staff coordinator finally concluded it was necessary to impose a more demanding social structure upon the group. He decided that work crews would be organized. But it was first necessary for this group to agree upon the type of work they wanted to do. Consequently, the coordinator asked the group to decide whether it wanted to start a janitorial service, a restaurant, or both. The group decided to start a janitorial business for two expressed reasons: it offered the possibility of more jobs for the members, and it would be less physically confining than restaurant work. With this major decision made, the group was then asked to form two janitorial work crews. Two crews were established, but only by the staff coordinator working closely with the group.

The next problem was to establish a governing body for the lodge. An executive committee, later called "ex-com" by the members, was established to make policy and to be responsible for disciplinary problems. The committee was composed of the two work-crew chiefs, the cook, and the two "administrators" elected earlier by the group—the general manager and the business manager.

Since the positive effect of information feedback upon small patient group performance had been demonstrated in an earlier study (Fairweather, 1964), the coordinator decided to hold one general meeting of all persons in the community lodge once a week which would give the group evaluation from a staff member about the adequacy of its problem solutions. This meeting was held in addition to the members' own autonomous daily meetings. The general meeting took place on the last day of the work week and was attended by all members, the coordinator (Dr. Moore) and the research director (Dr. Watson). The weekly group meeting took the form of an informal discussion led by Dr. Watson. It was discontinued several months later when it was clearly no longer needed. Nonetheless, it served initially as a forum where group decision-making could be openly evaluated.

Many decisions were made by the group in these general meetings. Topics relevant to the structure of the lodge and the business were discussed. The rudiments of the folkways and customs of the society began to appear. It established three work statuses and a differential salary scale. Crew chiefs received higher wages than general workers and they, in turn, received higher pay than apprentice workers. The group resolved that a small percentage of the money earned from its business would be placed in a special operating fund which could be used for the purchase of supplies and materials that would be needed by the janitorial service, the major cost of which was borne by research funds. They also decided that prospective jobs were to be inspected upon completion, and that the work-crew chief would have sole responsibility for each job. A checking account was established for the business. Adequate bookkeeping procedures were arranged through consultation with an experienced accountant. This was the first use of a consultant by lodge members—a practice which became more and more frequent as time passed. The group decided that it would purchase work clothing, both coveralls and matching shirts and pants, so that crew members would appear to the public unmistakably as representatives of a bona fide business organization.

Of course, the rationale for decisions made by lodge members was not always self-evident. The decision underlying the lease of a new work truck illustrates this. To lease the truck, two research staff members accompanied three lodge members to a local automobile agency. All arrangements were soon made successfully by the lodge members—with one exception. All three members quickly chose the size and type of the truck, the kind of gear shift, and so on. Then the salesman asked them what color the truck should be. One member said "red," another "green," and the third, "blue." Each member refused to change his opinion and the salesman began to show evidence of frustration as the debate continued. Finally, one member remarked that since they had just organized a new janitorial service, the choice was obvious: "White for purity." The other two members immediately concurred. Shaking his head in disbelief, the salesman wrote the color on the form.

A major problem during these early days of lodge development concerned the disinterest which lodge leaders continued to show in whether a member followed his prescribed medication regime. This situation was uncovered when the staff coordinator discovered that a member for whom high dosages of tranquilizers had been prescribed was not taking his medication at all. Since the procedure for control of this which had been adopted by the members was clearly not successful, it was necessary for the coordinator to develop a method that would effectively prevent further failures in this area. He therefore instituted the technique of assigning one responsible member to give medication to irresponsible persons. In this way, a member-nurse role evolved. Actual count of pills for offenders or suspected offenders was also instituted. When a member who had not taken his medication in the past was again found to be irresponsible, he was assigned to the member-nurse for monitoring of his medication regimen.

After the development of this new social role, the staff coordinator began training janitorial crews on a daily basis, using their living quarters as the training area. To facilitate the training, a second consultant was introduced to the lodge members. This person was a salesman for the janitorial service where supplies and equipment were purchased. He was aware that the workers in the new business were neophytes and had already offered to become a consultant to the group about janitorial work procedures. In this role he demonstrated the proper operation of new equipment and showed the crews how to use waxes and cleaning compounds. His aid was invaluable at this crucial time. Although the need for his consultations diminished over time, he played an active role in the first few months of the work operation when numerous problems arose that were unique to an embryonic janitorial business.

By the end of the second work week, the prospective janitorial crews began to resemble functioning work units, although training by the coordinator was still necessary. The coordinator still required crew members to work on the job until it was done to his satisfaction. He observed their work and inspected each job. Although a serious problem initially, with training, the men no longer attempted to escape from their work. Indeed, they seemed to feel they were ready to try work for pay, since they believed they had become competent in window washing, cleaning sinks and floors, and other janitorial duties. From the coordinator's point of view, however, it appeared that they had simply learned to take each task seriously.

Through this form of persistent and patient training effort, the familiar hospital work norm of appearing to work while doing as little as possible was beginning to disappear. New community work norms were beginning to take its place. Nevertheless, a crew chief still was not able to ask work crew members to do a job without facing numerous excuses from the workers. It was still necessary for the coordinator to provide leadership, particularly where initiative was required and where reporting information to the crews about their work performance was important as an incentive to better performance. A leader with the credentials of an authoritative figure seemed to be necessary at this point in the lodge society's development, because of the unwillingness or inability of the group to take directions from its own members. This caused substantial concern among the research staff, since the hope was embodied in the research plan that as time passed the coordinator could gradually reduce his leadership role by depending more and more on the group's own leaders for initiative and direction.

Settling Down to Business

Jobs were solicited by placing advertisements in a local newspaper, calling apartment houses, inquiring about work from real estate agents, and by personal contacts with friends of the research staff and hospital personnel. The general manager of the lodge and the staff coordinator, in response to several inquiries about jobs, visited the potential customers to estimate what might be an adequate fee for the particular job. These notes from the staff coordinator's research journal [1] reveal another difficulty in establishing the business: The unrealistic monetary standards of these former patients which appeared when Mr. Ring, the general manager, began bidding for jobs.

> The day Black's crew [Black, Ward, Fish], Ring and I went to Wiley's [house], Ring was the most verbose. . . . After being shown what was to be done [by the Wileys], he blurted "I hope you won't think I'm crazy, but I think one hundred bucks." After the strained silence, Mr. Wiley suggested 35–40 and I (foolishly) suggested 30. On the way home, Ring thought we should start at a "ridiculously high" price and dicker to what would be a reasonable price. Several days later he stated the job should have been 100 bucks.

Knowing that it might require a long time before the general manager or any other lodge member could make meaningful estimates of job prices, a cost list for different types of work was developed by the coordinator. The list was given to the business manager who used it in giving approximate prices to customers over the telephone. Eventually, the coordinator had to assume full responsibility for job bidding, since estimating over the phone proved costly to the business. This was true not because of the business manager's lack of ability, but because the description of the job by the prospective customer was often inaccurate and underestimated the work involved.

Finally, the day for the first job arrived. Activities on the first job were a mixture of behavior to be expected from the Keystone Kops and from qualified workers. The verbatim account from the coordinator's notes in the research journal describes this initiatory rite:

> Work started Friday at 9:00 A.M. sharp and everyone put out real good. We worked until noon steadily, although far too carefully and, as a result, slowly. Mr. Rich [worker] needed checks and suggestions on how to solve difficult problems such as how to get clean rags, when and where to move the ladder when cleaning windows, and whether specks were inside or outside the window (which, for some reason, Mr. Black [crew chief] was very slow responding to). Mr. Black went slow at painting and didn't spill so much as a drop on the papers or plastic drop cloth—but he moved at a snail's pace. Mr. Ward [worker] slopped paint on fairly quickly but laid it on unevenly and applied almost equal portions on the walls and the customer's hardwood floors. Mr. Black, in cleaning up, originated a new design in black paint on the customer's rug and unfortunately it was strictly ad lib. . . . Still, by 3:30 P.M. all the windows were in fairly good shape, the painting done, and some of the floors had been cleaned. The customer's reaction was that of strong approval which

1. The research journal consisted of daily notes made by the staff coordinator about group processes and critical events.

was difficult to understand—except that the next time I saw the house, it wasn't nearly so bad as I had anticipated—or remembered.

With the completion of the first job, morale improved. The acquisition of a second job came on the heels of the first because of a recommendation by the first customer. Securing it was another morale booster. To the members this was tangible evidence that they were beginning a profitable venture. However, morale took a sudden downward turn when the second job was terminated by the employer because of numerous mishaps and carelessness. The loss of the second job and the concomitant drop in morale created a crisis. A general meeting was called. Interestingly enough, the topic of the meeting was not the job loss, but rather a shared fantasy about getting large sums of money for many jobs. Anger about the low price bidding of the coordinator was stated openly. These feelings had sporadically been evoked from individual members before the meeting, but this time they emerged openly in the group discussion. Some members expressed the unrealistic idea that their janitorial service was the only one in the area and it could charge what it pleased. Discussing the "low" prices in comparison with their fantasied worth was the group's way of reacting to their first failure.

Despite the low morale, the advertisements and contacts continued to bring in new jobs. Working as employees for pay brought three pressing work problems clearly into focus. They were: crews lacked leadership on the job; the hospital work norm was still in evidence; and the different work crew roles were not yet adopted. Confusion and overlapping work often occurred. For this reason the coordinator began telling each crew precisely what to do. Even after this, work invariably slowed when the coordinator left to go to another job location. Rarely did he find the crew busy working when he returned from such brief absences. Often the crew chief would say that he had "run out of wax" or that "the wax didn't dry," even though in such cases the floor had often not been touched. The crew chiefs were not yet able to fulfill responsibly their role as leaders because they had the same standards as the workers—"take it easy" when the "boss" (coordinator) was not around. The members had not yet adopted the business as their own.

The autonomy and independence that was a research goal was beginning to appear unattainable from the coordinator's point of view without a change in the members' work habits. To accomplish this, the coordinator instigated periodic checks of each work crew at the job site. This close supervision, although frustrating to the coordinator, soon produced a noticeable increment in responsible behavior. Also, the coordinator attempted to reinforce a norm of independence on the job. Such statements as "the job comes first" and "it's your business" were commonplace.

During this period of increasing work activity, an interesting and significant situation arose which was to be repeated on many occasions in the future. The janitorial service was hired to clean a beautiful and expensive home. The men went into the home and performed well below their usual level. They became frightened by all the expensive objects, and in their anxiety they did the very things the customer asked them not to do—banged the sideboards with the buffer, slopped water on the porch and tracked it across the carpeting. Nonetheless, the coordinator inspected the job and the group corrected its poor work. When completed, the home was thoroughly clean and appeared in excellent condition. It soon became apparent, however, that the customer knew the members of the janitorial service were ex-mental patients. He closely scrutinized their work performance. In particular, he had many complaints about their unorthodox work methods.

This incident illustrates a major difficulty for the janitorial service that recurred on many occasions: When the customer knew beforehand that the workers were ex-mental patients he often indicated distrust of them. To compound this distrust, the men often worked in an unorthodox fashion and sometimes their work was careless and sloppy, even though such "errors" were always corrected upon final inspection. If a customer happened on a job while the men were working, he was likely to see at least one of them cleaning himself into a corner, cleaning the lower panes of glass before the upper ones were completed, or doing work that had not been included in the job estimate. These "odd" work behaviors were so irritating to many observing customers that the final product of the work—a clean house, for example—was ignored.

Despite these difficulties, business was flourishing. It was therefore decided to begin a new service—a gardening business. Again the men lacked the skills. Men who stated they were experts in pruning trees could not do so upon actual trial. Consequently, general yard work which did not require sophisticated skills became the new area of work. The first weekly job was obtained at this time. As business calls increased, the need for additional training in those areas where the workers were most deficient—inspection of work, work habits, and crew chief leadership—still continued to plague the organization. Even though some progress had been made, productive training programs and adequate information feedback to apprise the crews of their performance was lacking. To correct this deficiency, check lists of tools required for the job, inspection sheets to evaluate each job completed, and a crew chief's manual aimed at more precise training were created.

A change in the procedure that determined the composition of the work crews also seemed desirable. The coordinator had been shifting members from one crew to another as needed. However, this prevented the development of well-trained work crews. Consequently, an attempt was made to comprise crews of four men each who would continuously work together.

Establishing permanent work crews had a positive effect in a short period of time. Once again it became very clear that a well-defined social structure was essential to good work performance in these early developmental stages.

Early Adjustment Problems

At this early stage of life in the community, a social atmosphere similar to that of freed prisoners prevailed. Lodge members were exuberant over merely being in the community. Several began spending time at a local cocktail bar and supper club. One of the more emotionally regressed members started nightly visits where he imbibed alcohol excessively. He became very sociable. He was "having fun." He discovered women for possibly the first time in his life. As he became more responsive to the outside world, he became more psychotic—throwing rocks at a neighboring service station and at cars traveling on the freeway and starting a fire against the freeway fence. These incidents were reported to the group and investigated by the staff coordinator. Upon exploring the matter, it became apparent that not only was the member's nightly drinking affecting his behavior, but he had not taken his tranquilizing medication for nine days. His psychotic behavior became so pronounced that he was finally returned to the hospital.

The stress of community living had begun to take its toll on the fledgling group. The group member who had disappeared while loading the trucks at the hospital (p. 46) began to disappear at the lodge. He criticized the group's work methods, their use of equipment, and many other procedures adopted by the group. He boasted of his adroitness in the use of janitorial and yard equipment, and, in answer to his boasting, the members promptly appointed him leader of a work crew whose job was to keep the premises clean. After the appointment he failed to show up for work and was just as promptly demoted. It seemed obvious from the outset that this member was unwilling or unable to be a productive group member. In the general meetings held to discuss important issues, he frequently slept or failed to appear. Yet, he maintained a rather affable easygoing manner and frequently said, "I am just lazy." As a consequence of his attitude and inability to adjust to the community situation, this member was also returned to the hospital after only nine days at the lodge. Both members who returned to the hospital stated that they wanted to remain in the lodge despite their maladaptive behavior which ended their stay there. Another member stated soon after he arrived at the lodge that he wanted to return to the hospital. Four days after arriving at the lodge, he became isolated and depressed. He repeatedly asked to be returned to the hospital, and his wish was granted. Thus the original group of 15 members had dwindled to 12 in a little more than a week's time.

As a consequence, concern by members for their peers began to emerge. Members expressed the belief that the loss of three persons in such a short period of time was a "tragedy" that could have been avoided. As a result of these discussions, the members initiated an orienting program for new persons who entered the lodge from the hospital, in an attempt to lessen the shock that apparently occurs in the move from hospital to community. Toward this end, they assigned the orientation role to an interested member.

Because of the noticeable difference between the hospital and the community which culminated in the three failures just mentioned, the lodge members also became aware that not everyone could remain in the lodge. They also noticed that those who failed did so in the first few days. For this reason they adopted a rule specifically requiring that each new member be placed on a two-week trial period upon entrance into the lodge society. After this trial period, if he had demonstrated that he was unable or unwilling to work in some capacity, he was required to return to the hospital regardless of what his desire might be. The decision about his acceptance was made by the executive committee who interpreted the rule to mean that anyone coming to the lodge had to agree to work while there. People refusing to work or showing an incapacity for work would have to leave, according to the committee's interpretation.

Soon after the institution of this rule, three new members joined the lodge. Two of them satisfactorily completed their two-week trial periods. The third newcomer lasted for two days and then was returned to the hospital. Mr. Taylor, the returnee, quickly discovered that work was an essential condition for living at the lodge. The first day, instead of working on the job, he sat down on the ground outside a customer's residence and threw lighted cigarette butts on the porch. He was immediately returned to the lodge where he was later publicly criticized by his crew chief for being a "goof-off." The new member was a rather convincing paranoid schizophrenic with ten years' previous hospitalization. He offered the opinion that the leaders of the lodge society were too well treated compared to the followers and that he should immediately be appointed to a crew chief's position despite the fact that he could not work the power equipment essential for his job. Even so, most members attempted to convince him that he should remain in the lodge and try to work. They failed in this attempt and he returned to the hospital. Later, when offered the chance to leave the hospital again and to return as a crew chief at the lodge, he initially accepted and then rejected the offer because of a condition attached by the lodge members. They required that he undergo a training program to achieve proficiency in the use of power equipment.

During this time, Mr. Mateo, who was one of the original members, left the lodge to live with his parents. Since coming from the hospital, he had worked about three hours every day washing dishes. Because of the increase in the lodge's business, he was told that in addition to his dish-washing job he would have to be assigned part-time to a janitorial crew. He immediately requested a two-day vacation to visit his parents and when he returned with them he left the lodge. He informed the general manager, Mr. Ring, at the time of his departure that he was going to return to barber college—an action that Mr. Ring perceived as an escape from the lodge, since Mr. Mateo had failed to complete the barber's course several times in the past. Willingness to work as a prerequisite for acceptance in the lodge was becoming a well-established norm. Both Mr. Taylor and Mr. Mateo were unwilling to work, while at the same time exhibiting few crippling psychiatric symptoms. On the other hand, severity of emotional problems and psychotic behavior were not considered barriers to membership as long as the person behaviorally displayed a willingness to work.

At the end of the sixth week, the coordinator (Dr. Moore), who had been responsible for the lodge from its inception, announced his resignation. He stated that he would depart in approximately two weeks. His resignation was announced in a general meeting where the group was also told that the staff member who had been responsible for the hospital side of the research project would now become the new lodge coordinator. The reaction of the group was ambivalent. Mr. Murray, the business manager, stated that he would miss the departing coordinator. An argument developed between Mr. Black and Mr. Rich about the relative merits of the old and the new coordinators. This was the beginning of a period of difficulty for the members that would only be resolved two weeks later when the new coordinator appeared. Flurries of business activity punctuated by periods of inactivity occurred during this time. The morale of the group again declined. Although obtaining jobs for pay was temporarily slowed, there was much work that needed to be done around the lodge. Even though various projects were approved by the men themselves, no one took the initiative in beginning work on them.

Then a prolonged period of inactivity occurred. It produced various kinds of agitation among the members of the group. On at least two separate occasions, the general manager, Mr. Ring, resigned his position, only to be reelected immediately to his office. The executive committee, which had been organized as the policy-making body with the hope that it would become the governing body of the organization, only rarely convened to make decisions. Almost all leadership was abandoned. Excessive alcoholic indulgence emerged as a serious problem. During this time, Mr. Ward, an alcoholic, became an acute problem. Although he occasionally drank in his room, he began a prolonged period of seclusive drinking. After numerous private attempts by the coordinator to convince Mr. Ward to stop drinking, the executive committee was convened to urge the members to solve the problem. Their solution was to adopt the rule that "drinking on the grounds" would not be tolerated. However, no action was taken with Mr. Ward, who continued his drinking as blatantly as before. At this, the executive committee decided that their "no drinking" rule could not be enforced and hence should be rescinded. Next they decided that if a member's drinking interfered with his work, he would be given a warning the first time, a second offense would result in loss of pay, and on the third infraction he would be asked to leave the lodge. Despite the new rule, no action was taken about Mr. Ward's drinking behavior. The next day Mr. Ward was found by another member lying in a very shallow pool of water in an intoxicated condition. He was put to bed and then returned to the hospital where it was determined that he was suffering from the d.t.'s. Finally, the coordinator met with the group and imposed a rule against drinking on the grounds. The coordinator further informed the group that he would personally enforce the rule because the executive committee had not done so. Thus it was clear by the end of two months in the community that this embryonic society still required outside leadership to enforce its own social rules.

The First Shift in Supervision

When the new coordinator arrived on the scene, the remnants of leadership remained in the hands of the general manager, Mr. Ring. Upon occasion this member-manager assumed leadership which he then relinquished unpredictably. When challenged by other group members, he would resign his position but just as quickly reclaim it, saying that there was no one else who could occupy the role. Such disorganization required a new restructuring of the social situation. New work procedures were clearly needed. Methods for determining the implements needed on the job and procedures for loading equipment onto trucks were the first innovations developed. Written forms were used as memory aids wherever possible. The greatest change, however, was that the new staff coordinator assumed actual leadership of the lodge. He first broadened the powers of the executive committee so that this group could assume actual leadership of the lodge to replace the arbitrary decisions which continued to be made by the intermittent leader, Mr. Ring. As the first step in this new plan, an organizational chart was devised and posted on the bulletin board. Table 4.1 shows this new "chain of command" and the broadened responsibilities of the executive committee. The new coordinator also posted on the bulletin board, so that all members could be aware of them, the existing rules and regulations for living at the lodge. Even though most of these regulations had been created by the lodge members themselves, the listing of them by the coordinator was intended to formalize these expectations of the members; they may be found in verbatim form in Table 4.2.

Table 4.1. Organizational Chart of the Lodge

Dr. Cochran				
Executive Committee				
Ring (Chairman)	*Murray (Secty.)*	*Smith*	*Jones*	*Black*
Crews and Crew Chiefs				
Business-Admin.	*Kitchen-Food*	*Crew No. 1*	*Crew No. 2*	*Crew No. 3*
Murray	Smith	Black	Jones	Ring
	Hunt	Rich	Fish	Stacey
		Parker	Lee	Steele
		Strong	Gonzales	Walker

Executive Committee's Responsibilities	
1. Medication	Jones
2. Orientation and welcoming of new members	Jones
3. Lodge Reports (daily & weekly): a. O.D. Reports; b. Visitors Log; c. Sign-out Log	Ring
4. Janitorial Reports (daily): a. Job sheets; b. Job check list; c. Job inspection list	Ring (via janitorial crew chiefs)
5. Executive committee actions	Ring
6. Coordination and dispatching of jobs	Murray
7. Kitchen and food	Smith
8. Grounds	Black
9. Living quarters	Ring
10. Inventory (janitorial)	Ring
11. Laundry	Murray
12. O.D. Schedules	Jones

Approximately two weeks after the new coordinator arrived, a general meeting was held during which he announced that all decisions would thereafter be made by the executive committee. The group accepted this reaffirmation without dissent. After the general meeting, the coordinator presented the executive committee with its first problems to solve. Mr. Ring assumed the chairmanship of the executive committee and, accordingly, the committee delegated much of its authority to him since he was already the lodge's general manager. However, the new coordinator informed the committee that regardless of how it delegated its duties, *the committee itself* would be responsible for governing the lodge. While Mr. Ring often attempted to usurp the authority of the executive committee by discussing problems only with the coordinator, on each occasion the new coordinator referred the problem to the executive committee for solution. As the members of the executive committee assumed more responsibility for administering the lodge, Mr. Ring's influence diminished. After a disagreement with an aggressive and much admired new member who was

Table 4.2. Rules for Living at the Lodge

1. No drinking on grounds or in local area in public—only at recognized places for such purposes (bar, private home, etc.).
   a. No drinking anywhere during the regular work day is permitted.
   b. Any member found to have been drinking 3 times will be asked to leave the lodge.
   c. No form of alcohol is to be brought onto the grounds for any purpose.
2. No gambling on the grounds.
3. Everybody must work and be ready for work at the start of the regular work day no matter what activities they participated in during the previous evening.
4. There will be no women brought onto the grounds.
5. People (visitors) must be invited to the lodge before they can come onto the grounds.
6. Those fellows who are indigent will receive $10 per week. If $10 or more per week is earned, no money will be paid to him from the indigent fund. If he earns less than $10 per week, the difference between what he earns and $10 will be paid to him weekly from the indigent funds.
7. Those fellows receiving no pension or compensation as well as those receiving less than $10 per week are classified as indigent.
8. All lodge members must abide by the decisions of the Executive Committee.
9. Any group decision may be vetoed by Dr. Cochran, but this will be done only when, in his judgment, the group decision might jeopardize the functioning of the lodge or janitorial service.
10. Admission to and departures from the lodge are strictly voluntary. Any member may leave at any time. It is the function of the Executive Committee to merely recommend or advise in such matters. Where possible, a request to leave should come before the Executive Committee for recommendation.
11. All new members coming to the lodge are automatically placed on a two-week trial period (LOA from the hospital). At the end of that period, the man will be asked if he desires to remain or return to the hospital. The Executive Committee, at the same time, will decide if the man should remain or return to the hospital. If both the committee and the man agree on his remaining, he will remain and start receiving wages. If the committee feels he should remain but the man wants to return to the hospital, he will return to the hospital. If both the committee and the man agree on his leaving the lodge, he will return to the hospital and receive no wages. It is noted that at any time during the two-week trial period, the new man may return to the hospital for any reason he so desires.
12. All members receiving any type of medication must take their medication as presented by the physician with no deviations.
13. All members will serve as O.D.'s unless otherwise excused by the Executive Committee for a definite reason.
14. Any member desiring to take work passes from the lodge to seek work in the community outside of the Janitorial Service, for the eventual purpose of leaving, must first receive permission from the Executive Committee. He must then abide by the Committee's decision. If work passes are approved, the member will receive no wages for the time off from work at the lodge.
15. All members (roommates) will be responsible for the cleanliness of their own rooms.
16. All new members are to be oriented by the Executive Committee member assigned and must complete the training program to the satisfaction of the coordinator and crew chiefs before he is assigned to a crew.
17. The Executive Committee, as the decision-making body of the lodge, is respon-

Table 4.2. Continued

sible for members' behavior and for taking necessary disciplinary measures.

18. Any member leaving the lodge may return at a future date, providing there is available space and it is approved by the Executive Committee. They will be on a two-week trial period upon their return and receive no wages.
19. Any crew member who is dissatisfied with his crew assignment or his assigned duties, is to make this known to his crew chief. This will then be reported to the coordinator, who will decide whether or not it warrants Executive Committee discussion and/or action.
20. If any money is to be borrowed, it is to be referred to Dr. Cochran providing it involves $5.00 or more. Money can only be borrowed for dire emergencies and is not to be used for drinking purposes or taxicab fares.
21. Members may change room assignments only upon the approval of the coordinator and the members involved in the change.
22. Night work and Saturday work will be accepted based upon the judgment of the coordinator. The members assigned to this work will be on a voluntary basis and they will receive future time off for the extra work done.
23. Money received for night work only will be distributed amongst only those members participating in this work.
24. The assigned O.D. may not leave his post unless he receives the approval of an Executive Committee member and a replacement is found.
25. Any O.D. who is relieved of his duty at his own request for personal reasons must make up this time in the reasonable future.
26. Anyone leaving the lodge during any day of the week other than for his work assignment must sign out and sign in upon his return, no matter where he may be going.
27. All members are to be well-shaven, in uniform and reasonably neat and clean while working in the community.
28. All new members, prior to being placed on the O.D. list, will first become Junior O.D.'s and be assigned to a Senior O.D., with whom he will serve and be instructed in the O.D. duties and responsibilities for at least a two-week period.
29. A regular Executive Committee meeting will be held every other Wednesday evening at approximately 6:00 P.M. Meetings, however, will be held more frequently if the situation warrants it.
30. All Executive Committee decisions are to be reported to the group-at-large as soon as possible after the decision is reached.
31. Members may own and operate automobiles or trucks only with the approval of Dr. Cochran. If a member owns an automobile or truck, he may not use it during the regular work day unless permission is received.
32. All cleaning and washing of personal clothing (other than uniforms) are the responsibility of the individual members, both financially and otherwise.
33. Members are to use their own rooms for sleeping purposes and not the O.D. office or recreation room.
34. Any member using the recreation room bathtub and/or shower is responsible for cleaning it up and removing the towels and wash cloths.
35. The telephone may be used for local personal calls only. Any long distance personal calls are to be made from a pay station.
36. No smoking in food or restricted areas. No smoking is permitted in bed.

rising in the lodge leadership hierarchy, the executive committee expelled Mr. Ring from membership by demoting him from crew chief status—a social position necessary for membership on the committee.

Once the members of the executive committee knew that they could effectively discipline members for rule infractions, they began exploring different ways in which rewards and punishments could be used to shape individual behavior. Punishments took the form of warnings or reductions in wages. Rewards came from promotions, such as that from worker to crew chief, or from increases in pay, or both. For example, the committee suspended a member from his nightly duties as O.D. because of irresponsible behavior and later made him eligible for the O.D.'s work when his behavior improved.[2] In another case, a member was not given a salary for two weeks because of poor performance on the job and the committee further recommended that his job be changed. His performance on the new job improved and, consequently, his salary was increased. These new actions by the executive committee had such an immediate effect that no major infractions occurred for a period of several weeks. Their effective decision-making began to unify the group. This growing responsibility of the executive committee for the lodge's members is well indicated in the new coordinator's research journal notes:

> Shortly after Mr. Walker came to the lodge, I received a call on a Saturday morning from Mr. Sears, indicating that Mr. Walker was in the local county jail, ostensibly for drunkenness. I came down to the lodge and we called the police, who verified that he had been arrested on Friday evening and was, in fact, in jail for drunkenness only and no other charge. His bail was $29. I immediately called an executive committee meeting to decide what to do with Mr. Walker, i.e., allow him to remain in jail, pay his bail, send him back to the hospital, etc. The executive committee decided to grant him a loan of $29 to pay his bail from our operating expense fund which would be paid back via deductions from his salary. Secondly, during the time he was waiting to go before the court after release, he was to be restricted to the lodge and would not be able to sign out at all and would work only at the lodge itself. Thirdly, it was agreed that he was to serve whatever sentence that would be decreed by the judge and if it was a suspended sentence, he was to serve it at the lodge on a similar restricted basis.

As part of the plan to reorganize the lodge, the coordinator communicated all information concerning jobs, individual and group performance, role changes, finances, and the like, to the entire group. Thus executive committee decisions were reviewed by all members at the general weekly

2. Since no staff member was permitted on the grounds after the day's work, a member of the lodge was assigned responsibility for the grounds and the other members. This position was called Officer of the Day (O.D.) after a similar role held in the hospital by physicians.

meeting. In this way, the entire group was made fully aware of changes in procedures and the rule infractions of the members as they occurred. This procedure not only kept the members informed, but some changes in the executive committee's decisions were made as a result. At the same time, a concentrated effort was made to create effective communications between the coordinator and the members. At first, most of the discussions were initiated by the coordinator, but eventually some members began to initiate conversations with him. Discussions were most often held between the coordinator and the lodge leaders—the business manager, cook, and janitorial leaders. Despite his attempts, the rest of the members communicated with the coordinator only when they needed something or when they had committed an infraction of a rule.

Morale improved rapidly during the initial tenure of the new coordinator. The improvement was due to several factors: an increase in the number of available jobs, the social reorganization itself, and increased customer satisfaction with the work of the janitorial services. Members had become more job-oriented. For example, one crew spontaneously volunteered to correct several poor jobs completed by another crew and did so. Joking among members became commonplace. All were concerned about doing a good job and promoting good will, even though some members did not do a good job and the group did not always promote good will. The high morale, developing pride, and job orientation all tended to create a social atmosphere for effective problem-solving. This is demonstrated by two events during this period of lodge development. The first involved the kitchen crew, when an assistant cook, whose performance had been on the decline, suddenly returned to the hospital. His departure left the kitchen crew short of necessary workers. Four members volunteered to take his place working on Saturday so that the kitchen crew chief could have his regular day off. The second incident involved Mr. Black, who persisted in referring to the lodge members as patients. The members asked Mr. Black to discontinue this practice. After a reprimand by a member in the presence of others, he stopped referring to members as patients.

The new coordinator also attempted to establish an eight-hour work day. This was the first attempt to import the work norms of the community into the lodge. When this was first tried, since few paying customer's jobs were available, the group was required to complete work on the lodge grounds. During this period, a fence and two storerooms for tools and equipment were built. Within two weeks, the work day became eight hours long. In addition, a second change in work-performance norms was developing: workers began to feel that quality work should be done even though the job might take longer than anticipated. To accomplish this, attempts were made by the crew chiefs themselves to reduce carelessness, sloppiness, and slowness on the job.

By the time the new coordinator had been on the job a month, rules that regulated drinking and job behavior were being strongly enforced by the executive committee. A verbatim account from the coordinator's journal suggests how these new work norms were developing at that time:

> The two janitorial crew chiefs, up to now, have been extremely critical of their deviant members. I have noted that the workers in the crews have been taking more pride in the group's work and they themselves have become as critical as the crew chiefs. . . . I think the workers who are out on the jobs feel a little more at ease with the clients and certainly Mr. Black and Mr. Jones (crew chiefs) handle themselves well with the clients.

One of the key mechanisms that allowed the executive committee to act with good judgment was the feedback of information from the customers. The members found that poor behavior on the job could result in being fired and excellent job performance was often well rewarded. This immediate communication by the customer of his positive or negative evaluation of the job helped shape the work habits of the members so that they more readily conformed to those of the general community. Acceptable behavior on the job excluded any type of deviant behavior which might result in the loss of a job or that would offend a customer. At the same time there was tolerance for deviant behavior within the lodge environment itself. Thus the group readily accommodated an occasionally hallucinated or deluded person in the lodge setting, but they would not tolerate such behavior on the job.

The idea of quality work, working hard, and pleasing the customer were being strongly advocated by the newly appointed crew chief, Mr. Sears, who had replaced the deposed general manager, Mr. Ring. Mr. Sears' rise to power started after only a few days at the lodge. He rapidly became popular because he impressed the members with his persuasiveness, suggestions, and leadership. Not only was his leadership demonstrated in his role of crew chief and in informal social situations, but also as a member of the executive committee, of which he eventually became chairman. His ability to lead the men effectively and to relate to them was so impressive that it seemed the time had finally arrived when a member could take over some of the duties of the staff coordinator.

The Trials of a Peer Coordinator

A plan was created to train Mr. Sears to assume supervision of the lodge. The staff coordinator would gradually relinquish his role as leader of the lodge group and become instead a consultant to Mr. Sears. The peer coordinator (Mr. Sears), however, would be directly responsible to the staff coordinator for the operation of the lodge. Mr. Sears was approached with this plan. He said he would try it. His training, however, was not initiated for approximately another month because the staff coordinator wanted to be certain that Mr. Sears' initial positive reaction was not a fleeting one. Such a change in leadership offered the opportunity to study the effects of this small society under the leadership of a layman who was himself an ex-mental patient.

The decision was announced to the lodge members at a general meeting that Mr. Sears would commence training as a coordinator. The members were told that his salary would remain the same until he completed training. Then it would probably be increased. Surprisingly, this announcement was received without comment from other members of the group. After the meeting, however, several spontaneous and facetious remarks were made. One member said, "Hi, Doc," to Mr. Sears; another referred to him as "Junior"; a third member called him "my driver" and asserted that he could drive the truck better than the staff coordinator. This duty became the first training task for the peer coordinator. During the subsequent two-week training period, he learned his way around town by driving the truck, took responsibility for its maintenance, and using it, obtained janitorial supplies from the supply warehouse. He was instructed in scheduling jobs, filling out work forms, making job estimates, and checking on medication. As part of his training he was required to perform competently in all these aspects of the coordinator's job, without the staff coordinator being present. Initially, he remained a somewhat dependent individual, preferring to be viewed as the staff coordinator's assistant rather than as the lodge coordinator.

After his training was completed, however, Mr. Sears performed satisfactorily and showed initiative in solving many vexing problems. For example, he created an improved training program for new members in which their job proficiency had to be approved by all three crew chiefs before the neophytes could be assigned to a work crew. Mr. Sears still had some question regarding how much responsibility the staff coordinator would allow him to take and how independent he could be. At first he asked the staff leader questions relating to his work, such as, "How does this job look to you?" and "Is this job okay?" Later, he wanted to know if he could "chew the men out" when it was appropriate. On one occasion, he went on to say that he had been drinking beer and asked the staff leader, "What are you going to do about it?" The staff coordinator told him that even in his new position he was governed by the rules of the lodge, one of which pertained to drinking behavior. Accordingly, his beer drinking was reported to the executive committee for their action.

This testing of the limits by the new peer coordinator was merely a prelude to a major test which occurred about a week later. The situation is described in the following verbatim account from the staff coordinator's research journal.

> At 7:15 A.M., Monday, I received a call at home. Mr. Sears stated that he had been out all night and asked that I drive the truck to take the fellows on the San Agustin jobs and that he would appreciate this very much since he had not slept all evening. Not knowing what the situation was, I did not say yes or no, but merely told him to complete the local route and I would discuss this with him when I saw him. He returned to the office at about 8:30 A.M., at which time he was wearing a shirt and tie, plopped himself down in a seat, and asked if I was going to take the boys to San Agustin. I responded by saying no, I would not —that this was his job, his responsibility no matter how he felt, and that I myself had gone to bed at 3:00 A.M. the previous morning. I reiterated the rule indicating that he and the others could do whatever they pleased at night time but that they must be ready for work the following morning. He did not comment, but merely left the office indicating that he would change his clothes and be ready shortly. He returned approximately 10 minutes later and apparently his attitude had changed quite drastically. It was obvious that this was the big test. . . . His role had now been established.

Afterwards, he performed duties without supervision and manifested a sensitivity to both organizational and individual needs. In addition, he showed a facility in handling customer complaints. He was keenly aware of the processes within the group and became chairman of both the general weekly meetings which all members attended and the executive committee meetings. The number of jobs increased under his leadership and the quality of the crews' work improved noticeably. The lodge became a businesslike organization. Individual specialization began occurring. Mr. Rich, for example, was officially designated as the "stove man" because he became an expert in cleaning stoves. Mr. Black became an expert in cleaning rugs and he was often sent to jobs where rug cleaning was necessary. And, of course, Mr. Sears, the member coordinator, had become the expert in administration.

New procedures were evolving rapidly. A plan for vacations was adopted. Each member was entitled to one week's leave for every six months of work. The executive committee initiated a training program for O.D.'s (p. 62). The new members entering the lodge would start their O.D. duties by serving with an experienced O.D. while they were in training. The senior O.D.'s wrote evaluative reports on these trainees. New members did not begin training until they had lived at the lodge one week so that they could become accustomed to the community situation.

Another development took place in regard to the operating expense fund (10 per cent of the gross income for a given pay period) which was set aside purportedly for the purchase of supplies. It had been used upon a few occasions for temporarily paying damages to customers' property until the insurance payment for the damage was received and for minor repairs at the lodge which were later reimbursed by the lessors. However, during the tenure of the peer coordinator, the executive committee approved a loan to one of the members in order that he could purchase a pair of work shoes. The loan, at no interest, was to be repaid in three installments which were to be deducted from his future earnings. Shortly thereafter, other members requested funds for the purchase of clothing and the use of the members' savings for personal loans became a tradition at the lodge.

As Mr. Sears' contacts increased with customers, suppliers, and others in the neighborhood and general community, he was treated by them as the manager of the janitorial service. He was almost never perceived by the customers and vendors as an ex-patient himself, even though they were fully aware that the work crews were ex-patients. Mr. Sears readily accepted this perceived status and he was pleased at being viewed by people in the community as a full citizen. The perception of the peer coordinator is exemplified in the following excerpt from the staff coordinator's research journal.

> Shortly after my return from leave, the owner of the service station jokingly said to me that he guessed I was out of a job as Mr. Sears was now "running things." . . . When I told him that Mr. Sears was also an ex-patient who had come up through the ranks he was quite surprised. I am sure he felt that an ex-mental patient could not run an operation such as this. He then became very positive indicating that the fellows were doing extremely well and there had been no problem.

After two months of performing at an optimum level, the strain of ever-increasing responsibilities began to show in the peer coordinator's behavior. His fall from grace and eventual collapse started slowly when he did not arrive for work one day because of excessive drinking. Soon after this incident he was married and began living in an apartment in the neighborhood. He came to work as any citizen might who had steady employment. Although this situation could have been a step toward maturity, it created an almost insurmountable financial problem for him. He secured a loan from the lodge operating expense fund to pay for the rental of his apartment. Because of the increased expense of living in an apartment and supporting a wife, Mr. Sears was obliged to secure two additional large loans from the lodge fund, neither of which he was prepared to repay from his weekly salary.

Not too long after his first absence from work, he did not appear at the lodge for three days. Again, drinking was the reason. After this, the behavioral deterioration progressed rapidly. He began complaining about the paper work he had to do. He made sarcastic comments on official papers. His drinking continued to increase. He became intolerant of other members' behavior. He made unrealistic demands upon the men about the quality of their work. On several occasions he walked off the job and the staff coordinator had to be called to replace him. Although his demeanor was typically friendly and courteous when he was not drinking, his behavior could be so destructive at times that finally the coordinator felt Mr. Sears had to change his behavior or leave the lodge. He gave Mr. Sears that choice. Although he chose to remain, soon thereafter the staff coordinator reluctantly relieved him of his job when he learned that Mr. Sears had been driving the work truck while intoxicated. For this serious offense, Mr. Sears was demoted to worker status. After holding and enjoying the highest status in the lodge society, this demotion was especially humiliating. As a last blow to his self-esteem, the executive committee of which he had been chairman told him to "shape up or leave the lodge." He decided to leave.

When the peer coordinator departed, it appeared that the stability of the lodge might be shaken. However, three factors in the situation prevented the disintegration that might otherwise have occurred. First, the staff coordinator was well informed about the detailed developments of the lodge society as an integral part of his consulting role. Therefore, he immediately was able to resume the full responsibilities of the coordinator role. Second, the lodge's social structure had become by this time relatively stable. Finally, the demise of the peer coordinator was not a sudden and unforeseen occurrence for the members. The peer coordinator's maladaptive behavior and consequent decline had been perceived by all lodge members.

Although the changeover to the staff coordinator was not planned, it represented a step backward in the planned progression toward peer group autonomy from all staff supervision. Unfortunately, the reversion from peer coordinator to the previous staff coordinator occurred at an inopportune time as far as the research plan (pp. 40–41) was concerned. The plan required that this staff coordinator be replaced by a second coordinator with less professional experience. Since increased member autonomy was supposed to be introduced by the new coordinator—a graduate student—the last two months of the previous staff coordinator's tenure necessarily had to be spent in maintaining the status quo.

At the time of the transition to the new coordinator, some activities of the lodge members no longer required supervision and others required less supervision than in earlier stages of the lodge society's development. The operation of the kitchen and dining facilities were essentially free from supervision. Mr. Smith, the manager of the kitchen, ordered and prepared all the food. Although the tenure of the current business manager was of recent origin, he no longer required constant supervision. The janitorial and yard crews were far from performing independently, even though they had become more reliable as a consequence of their experience, training, and supervision. Thus, on an occasional job the men still damaged customers' property and most jobs required some supervision from the staff coordinator. This was the state of the organization when the new, less professionally experienced coordinator took over supervision of the lodge. The transition was accomplished over a two-week period during which the new coordinator learned the necessary procedures and finally assumed total responsibility for the lodge operation.

5 A GOVERNING BODY EMERGES

Initial Impressions of the New Coordinator

The new staff coordinator entered the lodge directly from the hospital. That the change in social environments was rather dramatic for him is shown by a description of his initial perception of the lodge. It is contained in his entry in the research journal at the end of his first week at the lodge.

> The difference in the atmosphere between this place and the hospital is very striking for someone who steps into it cold and with no preparation, as I have done. It really has the feeling of a going business, with none of the "marking time" mood of the hospital. In trying to analyze why it produces this impression, I've decided that at least one reason is that the lodge is far more subject to contingencies set by the outside community than is the hospital. The simple fact of sending groups of men out to do productive work in the community for wages has generated a whole series of behaviors which are in contrast to those in the hospital. Because the men at the lodge are engaging in a whole series of activities which are necessary to operate in the community as a business, there is a general atmosphere of purposefulness. The men are engaged in meaningful tasks in the sense they are tasks which will produce a money reward in the society at large. This activity, plus the general absence of "busy work" or "work as therapy" hospital standards, generates the atmosphere I have described.
>
> At present, it is hard to tell how typical this state of the lodge is. I

> know, from John's [Dr. Cochran] reports, that the place has its ups and downs and I may be seeing it during an "up" period and I may be overly impressed. However, it is my impression that the kinds of behaviors which create this impression are simply those which are associated with the place running at all and that, while the effect may be less during a poorly functioning period, most of the features would remain while the place functioned at all.
>
> There is obviously a wide range of difference among the men in performance, activity, etc. Some of them I have not known in the hospital setting and therefore cannot compare on in-and-out-of-hospital behavior. One characteristic seems common to all of the men and is a rather direct result of their changed role in this social situation as compared to the hospital—they are all more self-assured and direct in their approach to John and me than are the people on the ward, except for the psychopath or socially insensate patient who turns up on the ward occasionally. This difference is there to varying degrees in the different men but it is there in just about all of them.

The new research staff member also recorded his impression of the former staff coordinator's role and his new role, as well as some thoughts about the plan for progressive autonomy for the lodge members.

> The main points to be made about the role of John [Dr. Cochran] at the lodge are that it is a very active one and that it is of overwhelming importance. At present, John is supervising all the bookkeeping, doing all the estimates on the jobs, doing all the driving, and inspecting every job. The result is that he is constantly on the move with hardly a spare moment during the day.
>
> John's role is something like that of a good father. He provides the crews with a lot of positive emotion in the way of compliments for a good job, joking and encouragement and he also gets angry when they begin to slack off and gives them a chewing out for it. There is also, of course, the individual attention which Mr. Jones occasionally requires and Mr. Hill's problems. There is actually a good deal of dependency shown by all the members except for Mr. Smith [kitchen crew chief], who is quite a bit more independent in his behavior. In fact, Mr. Smith's job is about the only one in which John is not directly doing some kind of supervision.
>
> The big question with this project is to exactly what degree the group can become autonomous in the business of running the place. It will probably depend as much on the willingness of the members to take the responsibility involved as on their ability to do so. It's clear that Mr. Smith has both the ability and the willingness to be responsible but it is less clear in the cases of the other members—even those like Mr. Jones [business manager]—who have responsible positions. It may be that this environment is sufficiently different from the hospital to effect significant changes to make the group more autonomous. The hospital experience shows pretty clearly, however, that it as much of a problem to get a group to assume responsibility as it is to train them in the necessary

> skills to do a task—in fact, the former problem is more difficult to solve. There will also be the problem of us relinquishing control to the group. Can we let the group bear the consequences of a bad decision? Will it destroy the group because of the community feedback? If we make the group more autonomous, we are going to be making decisions like this and I imagine them to be pretty hairy ones. Part of the problem will be the community sensitivity to the behavior of "ex-mental patients," which would certainly make the group, and us, more vulnerable in the event of a mistake in judgment. This will be something of which we will be very aware and may prevent us from allowing the group to make some mistakes which would not be fatal to it and might even be instructive to the members. In a way it might be a problem of how much autonomy we can stand to give the group without raising our own anxiety to an unpleasant state. If we're lucky, the group's ability to assume tasks will determine the degree of autonomy at a level below the threshold of pain for us. But when has anyone in field research ever been lucky?

The new coordinator's feelings about providing autonomy to the members and his viewpoint regarding the role of the coordinator changed during his first month there, as shown by the following notes in the research journal:

> The performance has been very up and down this past month. It's had peaks and also some very deep valleys. In general I would classify it as very good by hospital standards but probably average or maybe a little below average by out-of-hospital standards.
>
> In thinking back to the notes I made when I first came out to the lodge just after the overlap period with John [Dr. Cochran], it seems to me that I am a little bit less impressed now by the performance out at the lodge although this is partly because, I think, I am more habituated to the lodge performance standards than I was when I first came out. I say this because in thinking as objectively as I can about the performance, it seems to me that in general the work is just as good as when I first came out except for a few notable exceptions and so my feelings that I am not quite as impressed with it I think are partly due to my being more used to the lodge and also partly because I have been pretty damn busy the past month just finding my way about—learning all the small things about the lodge. Learning most of the men and how they characteristically perform and all of the little details that I just wasn't up on when John left and had to find out over a period of time. . . .
>
> I'm still, I think, learning things about the lodge although I feel a lot more relaxed about the place now. I think I know much more about the place and feel much more on top of things. The first part of my month was pretty hectic as far as getting used to things went. I'm not sure that John had a similar experience when he came out here because of course he generated a lot of the procedures as he went along and therefore probably knew about them about as fast as they appeared. It's hard to tell. Also, John is obviously a lot more efficient fellow than I am about

these things and probably a lot more systematic in picking up the knowledge.

I'm sure that I am running the lodge quite a bit differently than John did. This is partly because we are different people, of course, but also because I am consciously trying to move in the direction of more autonomy out here as we agreed to do. I don't mind saying that it gives one a rather uneasy feeling to provide autonomy to the men. It's partly a hospital habit probably but also the consciousness of being much more exposed out here. . . .

I have had some very depressed times at some of the things that have happened but in thinking about it, it seems to me that really—so far anyway—not as depressed as I have been on the ward about things. This is probably partly because I'm new in this and I'm still coasting on the initial mania that I picked up in moving out here. But there have been some times when I've felt pretty low and discouraged about things and in that respect, it's probably important to note how essential it is to get the kind of support from the group that you get out here. In going in, talking to Bob [Dr. Watson], talking to John, being able to phone both of these people—it's an important kind of support. Especially when you first come out here and probably something that should be considered in any kind of enterprise like this—especially for a person like a psychologist who is not trained to do this kind of thing and probably has been avoiding it most of his life and is a psychologist in consequence of that. To be specific about the last point, I mean avoiding things like business dealings, dealing with customers, businessmen and people with whom psychologists just don't commonly deal. I don't mind, at least personally, I don't mind the activity. In fact I enjoy that very much. I think that's been a good source of the manic coasting that's kept me going sometimes. At times you don't get out of the car all day. John says, and I believe him, that we drive about 2,000 miles a month out here. It's very apparent to me how we could do that after being in it a month or so. But that part of it suits me fine. The hours are long but not really uncomfortable once you get into the routine. I hate to get up early and I do come in later than John. I usually come in about 7:30. That's been going on for about two weeks. I think that I began to come in about 7:30 after I began to feel a little more on top of things. For a while I came in about 7:00. Sometimes 10 to 7:00. But now it's pretty much settled down for the past couple of weeks anyway to about 7:30—which for me is early. Although, as I mentioned, the hours are not depressing once you are into the routine.

Challenges to Greater Autonomy

Upon inheriting the leadership of the lodge, the new coordinator began the planned process of giving more and more autonomy to the group. Heretofore, all of the executive committee's decisions were subject to veto by the staff coordinator if, in his opinion, the decision manifested poor judgment on the part of the committee. Even though the veto had been used in only a few instances, the executive committte was constantly aware that the staff coordinator could use it at any time. Therefore, the first formal step toward granting the members more autonomy was the elimination of the staff leader's veto of these decisions. There was one notable exception. The new coordinator retained his veto power for decisions that would in his judgment threaten the very existence of the lodge if they were carried out.

As might have been expected, the new coordinator was immediately faced with two problems that were totally unique in the history of the lodge and prevented a further reduction of coordinator supervision. The first problem arose when the coordinator was inspecting a janitorial job at lunch time to determine the progress of a work crew. His verbatim account of this vivid incident speaks for itself:

> Mr. Black outdid himself today. Early this morning I dropped him off with a crew to do a job in Mt. Pleasant for one Mrs. Waelin, an aged and rather sour crone who wished her floors done, including the stripping and waxing of her kitchen. Since Mr. Black is the original Slow and Steady, I thought it prudent to pack his crew a lunch when I went out to see how they were progressing at noon. I was not disappointed; they had made only modest progress and had only just begun to tackle the kitchen floor. That didn't surprise me. What did was the odor of grape which hung about Mr. Black. I questioned him about this but he denied stoutly that he had had a drop and wouldn't budge from that position. His crew was mum and would give me no information. I couldn't imagine where he had got the stuff to drink. I searched him and the equipment the crew had brought out and found nothing. I finally decided that he may have taken a strong few swigs that morning before coming out to work and that I hadn't noticed it at the time. He had been doing this a little while ago and it seemed the best explanation. Since he seemed steady enough and able to work, I decided to leave him on the job and check again in a short while.
>
> That was a tactical error. The next time I came out Mr. Black was stoned out of his mind and being dragged all over the kitchen floor by his buffer. His crew was lounging outside in a shifty-eyed group. I angrily ordered him out to the truck and surveyed the damage. The kitchen floor was a mess. It had been stripped in spots, here and there, and then carefully waxed and buffed by Black. It looked like the back of a pinto pony. Worst of all, Mrs. Waelin was nowhere to be found and I had to leave her a note promising to make good the next day.

The next day the coordinator learned the source of Mr. Black's liquor.

> The mystery is solved. Mr. Black got stoned yesterday on the Waelin job by drinking the customer's booze. This fact was revealed to me this morning by the customer herself, who called early to inform me of this happy news and to request that I keep those ugly and lascivious fellows

away from her property forevermore. She was adamant on the last point and coldly refused a series of generous offers I made to bring out a crew and set her kitchen floor right. She would have no part of us and asked that I return the check she had left us yesterday (for the original quoted price of the job) so that she could deduct the price of her ruined floor from our wages. Under the circumstances I had not the heart to refuse her and I took out her check at once.

I arrived at her door and knocked. A long wait. Another knock and a shorter wait broken at last by a slight sound to my left. I turn my head to see Mrs. Waelin eyeing me through a crack in a second door and offering me a check through that same crack in what I first take to be a cleft stick but later see is the first two fingers of her right hand. I put on a good face and a cheery smile but she is not amused. She says no, we cannot come back and fix the floor, she had talked to her husband and he says to do what she is doing—namely to write us a new (and smaller) check and then to write us off. So she's doing it, she says. Can't argue with that. She says that she's heard of us and that we are from "the hospital." She says further that I shouldn't be leaving men like that alone in other people's houses—that they drink other people's liquor and God knows what else. I assure her never anything else and about how sorry we are about the liquor and where did she hear about us, but she doesn't say and won't and wants me to leave (latching the door) so I leave. All this I shall report to Ex Com.

The executive committee meeting which was called to consider the drinking incident did not produce more responsible group behavior nor did it offer any real solution to controlling excessive drinking. Mr. Black was simply fined a day's wages. The committee did not show the initiative they had in the past in devising new techniques to control the drinking of a lodge member. A second incident contributed further to the increasing ineffectiveness of the executive committee. It involved a fire in a member's room. The subsequent developments shook the very foundations upon which the authority of the executive committee was built. A verbatim account of the event from the research journal provides the details:

Late this afternoon, just before I was about to leave the lodge, Mr. Jones came to me and said that a fire had been reported in room 11. I went there and found a mysterious scene. It seemed at first as if one of the tiles on the floor had somehow caught on fire and burned or as if something had been burning on the floor. The tile seemed to be melted and charred but the residue seemed more than would have been left by a single burned tile. Mr. Steele and Mr. Parker room together here and I asked them both to come into the room and questioned them. Mr. Steele was particularly suspect since he is a chain smoker and very absentminded about his cigarette butts—he had reputedly put one in his pocket still alight on one instance. The questioning produced no solution until I had a sudden inspiration and asked if there had been a plastic wastepaper basket on the burned spot. When I asked that, the two gentlemen admitted passively that there had been and Steele admitted further that he had been in the room shortly before the fire and had been smoking. He also said that the basket had been full of paper and that he might have dropped his fag into the basket still alight. What had happened, apparently, was that the fire had melted the plastic wastepaper basket and left the remains melted into the tile.

I did two things immediately. I had a number of large cans placed around the central, planted space in the lodge grounds and I called a general meeting. At the meeting I announced that a new rule was in effect that all ash trays must be emptied only in the cans then in place on the grounds, Steele had said that he probably put his cigarette out in an ash tray and then emptied it into the wastepaper basket, since he did remember emptying the ash tray before leaving the room, and that smoking would only be done inside where ash trays were present. I also described the fire incident to the general meeting and announced that Ex Com would meet that evening to take up the incident. The note had already been written. The meeting was a sober one and, apparently, almost everyone realized the danger of the incident and the serious fire hazard that was involved.

Later, I discussed the incident with Bob [Dr. Watson] on the phone and he said that if Ex Com voted to eject Mr. Steele (as was very likely, since he had caused mild fire scares before), we would have to veto the decision. We could see the danger of such a trend toward rejecting all problem members instead of trying to work out a solution for handling them within the lodge. We discussed possible solutions and agreed that, at the least, Mr. Steele would have to be placed in a room with a responsible member of the lodge—some member of Ex Com.

That evening Mr. Jones called me from the lodge after the Ex Com meeting (as I had instructed him to do) to inform me that Mr. Steele had been voted out of the lodge. I told him that the decision was unsatisfactory and that Ex Com should reconvene immediately and make some decision to allow Mr. Steele to stay. When he hung up I called Bob to give him the latest bulletin and we decided that if the decision was again to reject Mr. Steele I should go out to the lodge and attend the Ex Com meeting myself. Sure enough, back came a call from the lodge in a few minutes saying that Mr. Steele had again been voted out. I drove out to the lodge.

When I arrived, the members of Ex Com were gathered in one of the rooms (including Mr. Black, to my surprise—he had been drinking heavily the night before and had not worked that day). They all looked very morose and uneasy and very threatened by my presence. I said a few words about my veto of their decision and pointed out the trouble that all of them had had at one time or another in the past. I described the general lines of the decision that had to be made and asked for a discussion. There was a general balky reaction, with Mr. Smith the most resistive and outspoken, saying that the decisions of Ex Com about rejecting members had never been questioned before and that Mr. Steele was dangerous to the lodge and why wait until he actually burned the place down before acting. Eventually, Mr. Black volunteered to take on the job of supervising Mr. Steele but not until the meeting had become very strained, with Mr. Steele more and more angry and Mr. Lee and Mr. Green showing various small psychotic symptoms. When it was apparent that a decision could be reached I terminated the discussion and excused myself to permit the final decision to be made in private. I waited in the office, thinking it over, while the meeting continued. It seemed to me that Ex Com had been very shaken and threatened by my intervention and I decided, if no one agreed now to take on Mr. Steele as a roommate, that I would drop the veto. The group (that is Ex Com, not the whole lodge) had seemed close to dissolution in the meeting. After a few minutes I saw Mr. Jones leave the room and walk over to the office where I was sitting. He came in and said that Mr. Black had agreed to be Mr. Steele's roommate.

Later I described all of this to Bob on the phone and he commented on a certain shakiness in my voice from the strain of the incident. There is no doubt that the incident strained me. . . .

Today, one day after bravely assuming the responsibility for being Mr. Steele's roommate, Mr. Black was again stoned to an extent which made it necessary to return him to the hospital in disgrace. Sic transit gloria mundi.

There will be no problem, since Mr. Jones has agreed to take over the Steele watch. He is only too glad to do so since it allows him to atone for the guilt he has been feeling for not volunteering the night before. So he has confided to me. He has also confided to me that the morale of the members is at an all time low. Cheerful news. I am not surprised at this in view of recent events but it is distinctly unkind of Mr. Jones to inform me of his survey of opinion while I am depressed by the incorrigible ways of he and his fellows. Of course, Mr. Jones intends to be unkind and we both know it. Sic transit mundo, Gloria.

Growing Division and Unity Within the Governing Body

This outright veto of the executive committee's decision as a blatant incursion upon their privileges contributed to the unwillingness of the committee to assume greater responsibility for the lodge members in the next few months. At the same time, an internal problem that had been in the process of development for a period of several months became a divisive force within the committee itself. Competition had developed between Mr. Jones and Mr. Smith about the business and rehabilitative goals of the lodge.[1] Mr. Jones, who had assumed the member-nurse role at the lodge as the official dispenser of medication (pp. 50, 59), identified very strongly with professional persons and thought that the rehabilitive aspect

1. The term "rehabilitation" was given by members to those aspects of behavior commonly found in the hospital. To the members it often meant "coddling" of others so that they were not held responsible for their behavior.

of the lodge was its only purpose. He was continually arguing this point in the executive committee. Mr. Smith, while most helpful to others, adopted the position that if a member did not perform his job, or brought disrepute upon the lodge in its business operations, he should leave the lodge forthwith and a new man should be brought from the hospital to replace him. When this problem arose in executive committee sessions it divided the committee so forcibly that these sessions had to be mediated by the new staff coordinator. This again placed the coordinator in a position of interfering to a limited degree in the social processes of the executive committee. As a result of this controversy, it had recently failed to make several crucial decisions that would have provided member leadership for the lodge.

Faced with a reluctant executive committee, the coordinator was forced to turn his attention to matters affecting the survival of the lodge. First, he set out to improve the performance level of the work crews by maintaining adequate crew-chief leadership on the job. Since the crew chiefs' performances varied daily, he began planning for the substitution of good for poor leaders to improve work performance. The procedure involved always having a substitute available for one man when another was missing because he was too psychotic to work or was working poorly. This was deemed necessary because such unpredictable behavior happened with great frequency. The method thus involved training a number of men for the same job. The goal was similar to that of having a substitute "bench" in sports—the "bench" should have enough good workers so that a work crew could always be formed regardless of who might not be able to work. At the outset, so few individuals were capable of becoming crew chiefs that it was difficult to have substitute leaders available when the appointed ones failed. However, an influx of new members which occurred at that time provided several potential crew chiefs. It was hoped that an abundance of trained crew chiefs would yield adequate work leadership from the members' own ranks. Less complex job levels, such as stove cleaning, were no problem, since replacements were already available. Thus the principle of always having a substitute for any individual, leader or worker, on each customer job became an established work technique.

About a month after this change was initiated, some minor developments hinted that the hoped-for willingness to assume responsibility might be forthcoming in the members' behavior. In one instance, three workers shifted jobs and simply announced to the coordinator that the shift had taken place to the satisfaction of all parties. A second but more obscure event involved Mr. Smith, the kitchen crew chief. When an unusual delay developed in depositing research funds to the lodge bank account for the purchase of food, Mr. Smith spontaneously provided the money for the groceries. He not only contributed money from his own funds, but he persuaded several of the men at the lodge to contribute. Even though these funds were later reimbursed, this demonstrated the growing independent behavior of lodge members, as well as their loyalty to the goal of lodge survival. Furthermore, increased work autonomy was mainly attributable to the development and utilization of new crew chiefs. This almost eliminated the need for the staff coordinator himself to replace a "missing" crew chief, which had so often occurred before the substitution system was established. Finally, the staff coordinator gave the business manager a freer hand. This produced more errors in the business manager's work, but it fostered an improvement in his willingness to assume such responsibility.

Two other significant developments occurred to minimize further the new staff coordinator's influence in lodge affairs. One change was establishing a driver status for members at the lodge. Two members, both of whom had previous driving experience, developed enough confidence to begin driving the trucks, thus relieving the coordinator of this chore. The new drivers delivered and returned the gardening crews and often participated on the jobs as members of the work crews. These two drivers required a further refinement in the status structure of the lodge. Drivers thus became deputy crew chiefs. This was recognized by the members as a new status, with a rate of pay somewhere between the crew chiefs and workers. The newly established position rewarded the drivers with both prestige and salary. The following verbatim account from the coordinator's research journal illustrates how one of these driver's roles developed:

> Mr. Page . . . has been in training as a driver. He has been very good at it but I think the case of Mr. Page slowly becoming a more autonomous driver illustrates a particular method which is very characteristic of the one we often have to use at the lodge. The method of more or less weaning the men, both as a group and as individuals in particular jobs, to more autonomous behavior. Mr. Page at the beginning obviously needed a lot of support, emotional support, and . . . reassurance in doing his job. He was not certain that he was able to find his way about this area and over a period of time he accumulated a portfolio of maps, road maps, which I drew up for him, of our various steady jobs to which he is now delivering crews by himself. He shows initiative in alerting the crew chiefs for our steady gardening jobs to the fact that they are going out that day. He makes a point of coming in and looking at the board to see who is going to what job so that he knows whom to go and speak to about getting the truck loaded. . . . But it was very necessary with Mr. Page to give him plenty of structure at the beginning and to slowly but steadily relinquish the direct control over him as he showed enough confidence to take it. This is something that I was only able to do by just seeing how he responded. I wasn't able to put any particular plan or schedule into effect except the overall plan of giving him more autonomy. It was simply a matter of asking him each time or rather, allowing him

> each time to have the opportunity to get the crew out on his own and providing him support if he showed any inclination to get it.

The other event that diminished the new coordinator's influence at the lodge was a change in inspection procedures. He began limiting his inspections to spot checks of only certain jobs, rather than examining every job. At the same time, the gardening crew chief began inspecting the majority of his gardening jobs, thus increasing his supervision over the work of other members.

The most striking change occurred when the executive committee began to show more independent behavior, initially related to the removal of the "rehabilitation" leader from the committee (p. 90). The effect was that the work- or business-oriented members in the executive committee became more numerous than those with a rehabilitative orientation. As a consequence, the committee began requiring improvement in the poor work performance of some members. One decision of this now work-oriented committee was its refusal to reinstate the ousted leader of the rehabilitative faction. Mr. Jones, the deposed leader, had recently been fired from his role as business manager because of poor performance on the job, an action which simultaneously removed him from his position as a member of the executive committee (p. 59). In refusing to reinstate Mr. Jones upon his own request, the committee cited his declining performance as business manager, stating that he was not trustworthy. The committee then took the initiative from the coordinator by recommending another lodge member for the business manager's job.

In subsequent weeks, the work faction remained very much in control of the executive committee. It was not that the members did not have some degree of rehabilitative orientation, but rather that no member was as outspoken about rehabilitative matters as Mr. Smith was about work. The executive committee continued to become more autonomous and reality-oriented. For example, it was becoming difficult for members to obtain loans routinely from the operating expense fund. Several members were denied loans that ordinarily would have been approved. The loan refusals were based on previous experience, since some members who owed money had left the lodge without repayment. The best example the committee could cite was the former peer coordinator (p. 64), who had borrowed a total of $280 and paid back only $20.00. The committee also adopted new rules for obtaining loans. The rules specified that (1) loans would be made only for emergency reasons, (2) except under extreme circumstances, loans would not be made to members who owed balances on previous loans, and (3) money owed by members who left the lodge could be paid off within a month after leaving without interest; thereafter, an interest rate of 6 per cent per month would accrue to the balance.

With the advent of the new rules about loans, progress toward total member autonomy had really begun at the lodge. Next, the executive committee decided that they would personally answer requests for information that daily came from various people and firms. Thus the executive committee replaced the staff coordinator in representing the business to the public. The new coordinator quickly agreed with their desire to accept this critical responsibility. The increased interest of the group in supervising its own activities led the research staff to conclude that it was an appropriate time to test their willingness to assume responsibility for the most difficult problem at the lodge—the drinking problem. The sequence of events concerning this test were recorded in the coordinator's research journal:

> I called John [Dr. Cochran] yesterday, in response to an earlier call from him, and he described to me an idea he and Bob [Dr. Watson] had been discussing that day. The return of Mr. Morgan to the hospital raised again the question of what to do about the occasional high-ability boozer who passes through the lodge. We had flunked out before when we tried to get Ex Com [executive committee] to accept hospital control of the wets—John's proposal was that we try the more devious method of limiting the money of drinkers by getting the lodge to act as guardians. The plot would run like this: Faced with a known boozer, the lodge would inform him that he could not return unless he agreed to accept the control of his money by the lodge. If he accepted, all checks received by him would be deposited in a savings or checking account under the joint control of himself and another person (a member of Ex Com or myself) and disbursed to him in some limited amount—say $5 a week—to prevent him from becoming too stoned at any one time. It would be his option to vote himself out of such controls at any time but he would vote himself out of the lodge at the same instant. The details of the strategy (e.g., beating the drinkers to the mail box when the checks arrive) could be worked out if the basic idea was accepted by Ex Com. John's contention—reasonable on the face of it—was that the lodge was already acting as a sort of guardian by dispensing medication to some members anyway. Why not just extend this to handing out money as well? Why not? I liked the idea myself for various reasons. I had not liked the previous suggestion we made to Ex Com because of the involvement of the hospital itself in imposing the controls. I liked this one because I saw it as quite a different proposal which had the following charms: (1) The lodge would be assuming more responsibility for the control of problem members and thus would decrease its dependency on the hospital; (2) The lodge would gain the very considerable services of a high-ability population by creating an institution which would control members without certain self-controls (e.g., Mr. Cole, the best crew chief we have ever had). Even an imperfect control might make such members workable at the lodge; (3) Adding an institution like this would extend the ability of the lodge, as a social system, to mediate between deviant persons and the society. Right now we are flunking out fairly regularly

with binge boozers who get large checks in the mail. These are precisely the cats who would bring our present group closer to optimum group composition. They are also social problems of the first chop.

Filled with these and similar fantasies, I called Bob and told him I was agreeable to the idea and would present it to Ex Com at a special meeting the next day. I thought he [Bob] was more reserved about the whole thing in his manner and he brought up a few problems which might arise at the lodge if the plan did go into effect, such as the pressure on lodge members by the wets when the urge for Demon Rum came on them. I agreed that the whole thing would stand or fall at that time depending on whether Ex Com could hold the line against a party of determined alcoholics with the spirit on them. He also agreed that we should try it, however, and that the gains would be obvious.

This afternoon (a Thursday) I called a special meeting of Ex Com to handle this business . . . and presented the proposal on the money. I said (adopting a strategy discussed with Bob and John last night) that Mr. Morgan was back in the hospital and might be interested in returning to the lodge but had admitted that he could not control his behavior when he got large checks in the mail and had wondered if he could receive help at the lodge in handling this problem. I then outlined the plan to the meeting and pointed out that other former members, such as Mr. Black and Mr. Cole, who had been very valuable men in conducting the business, might be agreeable to returning under the same conditions. I pointed out the advantages and mentioned some of the possible difficulties which might arise from it as mentioned above. I also made it plain that all such persons would have a chance to accept or refuse the guardianship of the lodge and that it would be their own decision to remain at the lodge or to come out under the conditions stated. I tried to be as factual as possible and answered the few questions which were put to me by Mr. Miller, Mr. Kennedy, and Mr. Kline. Then I mentioned that I would be in the office in case the meeting needed more information and left. The impression I had gotten while in the meeting was that Mr. Miller was for the plan and that Mr. Kline was partly indifferent and partly for it as well (he made a number of suggestions on handling the bank accounts). Mr. Lee seemed simply a little puzzled and suspicious and Mr. Kennedy ready to be swayed in any direction by any argument. Mr. Smith was silent throughout and closely examined the carpet between his feet, shading his face from me with his hand.

From where I sat in the office I could see the meeting break up about 10 or 15 minutes after I left. Mr. Kline came over and said that the answer was no. I asked why and he said "Because we don't want this place to get too much like the hospital." Apparently Mr. Smith had led the opposition and had prevailed against a relatively weak positive faction. Mr. Lee later told me that the vote had been 5 to 0 against the plan.

Mr. Jones was on O.D. at the time and, when Mr. Kline brought me the news, was very negative and critical of Ex Com (for which he has no love since they have declared him irresponsible and barred him from the job of business manager). His refrain was that "I thought that this place was

> supposed to help people." Later, when I told Bob of the decision by Ex Com he mentioned that this apparently means that Mr. Smith has won the old battle, between him and Mr. Jones at Ex Com meetings, about whether the lodge was a business or a rehab project. Mr. Jones would take the rehabilitative position and Mr. Smith the other. Mr. Jones' reaction to the decision (which Bob did not know about) seems to substantiate this in a clear way.

The work faction's desire not to be troubled with members who presented drinking problems, unless such members held promise of making a substantial contribution to the business, was demonstrated clearly in the executive committee's final decision.

With the solidification of the work faction and the concomitant rapid growth in autonomy, a major problem at the lodge quickly came to the fore. A conflict arose between the new coordinator's responsibility for the expenditure of research funds and the increasing desire of the executive committee to control such funds. In his research role, the coordinator was required to sign for all purchases, a practice clearly inconsistent with his deliberate attempt to relinquish authority. The focal point of this conflict centered around Mr. Smith, the kitchen crew chief, who resented any interference from the staff coordinator. Mr. Smith began making purchases of supplies without receiving the staff coordinator's written approval required for the utilization of lodge funds. The problem became how to convince Mr. Smith to seek the coordinator's approval for purchases without destroying his independent behavior which the coordinator wanted to encourage. This problem was finally solved by placing $50 in an emergency fund for Mr. Smith's kitchen expenses. However, Mr. Smith agreed that if he should make a purchase which neither the coordinator nor the executive committee had approved, he would pay for it from his personal funds.

The Third Shift in Supervision

It was this attempt to grant greater autonomy to the members while at the same time remaining responsible for their lives and welfare which soon became the most difficult aspect of operating the lodge. By solving problems such as Mr. Smith's through the sharing of responsibility, some restraints were placed on the mushrooming growth of independent action increasingly demanded by the members. This lessening of supervision led, however, rather naturally into the next phase of the research plan, namely, replacing the less experienced staff coordinator with two untrained lay leaders as coordinators of the lodge society. According to the research plan (p. 40), two such persons, with no training or experience in treating mental illness, were hired at random from the state employment service to replace the most recent staff coordinator. After training the new lay coordinators, this graduate student coordinator became their consultant.

The following verbatim account from the coordinator's research journal described his impressions of the new lay leaders and some of the events that occurred during the transitional period:

> The original two men whom we hired for the job were Mr. Hawkins, a retired Marine (Corps) Major, and Mr. Edwards, a former quarry worker who had been partially disabled as a result of a back injury. Both of these men came to work together for the first time on Tuesday, the first of June—Monday being a holiday. It became very apparent over the next week—over the week, that is, of June 1st—that Mr. Hawkins was not at all comfortable in the job that we were asking him to do. He made several arrangements during the first week which made it quite clear that he saw himself as being primarily an office man and organizer and sort of the brains of the outfit, while Mr. Edwards, the second man, took over the outside work—that is, the delivery of crews on jobs and the inspections and so forth. This impression became stronger and stronger as the week progressed in spite of several conferences which the two of them, myself, and Bob [Dr. Watkins] had altogether, and the extended discussions during those times of the lay leaders taking on the entire job which I was then doing by myself. Although Bob and I both stressed this with Mr. Hawkins and Mr. Edwards, Mr. Hawkins obviously continued the kind of behavior which aimed toward him taking over the inside, or office aspects of the job, and leaving the other to Mr. Edwards. This became so obvious that by Monday, the 7th of June, Mr. Hawkins seemed quite depressed about the kind of job he was getting into and I discussed it with him on the morning of the 7th. He told me then that he was evaluating the job and that perhaps it had been more than he had bargained for. I told that to Bob on that same night—the night of the 7th—and the following morning as Bob requested me to do, I sent Mr. Hawkins in to speak to Bob. The upshot of meeting Bob was that . . . Mr. Hawkins was terminated as of June 11. Over the past six days, it had become increasingly apparent that he had been dissatisfied with the janitorial and gardening aspects of the work. It would seem that he perceived these as low-status jobs and did not appreciate the overall rehabilitative intent of the project, although every precaution was taken in describing these aspects of the job to him prior to and subsequent to employment. He stated in final interview, "You did not tell me that I would be mainly running a janitorial and gardening service." This may have more generalizable elements. It occurs to me that people with high-prestige ambitions, who are found predominantly in the more well-educated groups, are poorer risks in administering rehabilitative projects than people from the lower socioeconomic groups. This would be particularly true if Mr. Edwards is able to perform adequately.
>
> So he [Mr. Hawkins] left and Bob hired in his place the following day the third man, who is now the second man at the lodge in leadership, Mr. Hodges. He has taken on a job slightly subordinate to Mr. Edwards and the two of them have worked out quite well together. . . . After one week

together—that was the week of the 14th—Mr. Edwards had to go east to attend the funeral of his father who had just died, and this gave an opportunity for Mr. Hodges to handle the lodge on his own for an entire week. He did so on the week of the 21st and although he was very rushed and somewhat handicapped by his poor memory, he was able to do the job on his own with me helping him in the office and in that way I think that he probably gained a lot of confidence about his ability to handle the job in the event that some emergency would arise and Mr. Edwards would not be there. And he also, I think, learned the job more thoroughly in all its aspects.

About the two men in general, Mr. Edwards is a very active fellow, not very intellectual. He is very phobic of the office work which has to be done —that is, the bookkeeping aspect and the business manager's job in general. This is important, since one of the jobs of the coordinator is to supervise the business manager. Mr. Edwards is very phobic of this and is not at all bashful about saying so, whereas Mr. Hodges is quite used to it from his previous jobs and even has a certain amount of aptitude for it. Now fortunately for this situation, our present business manager, Mr. March, seems very capable and probably could do with minimal supervision. That's a guess. He has not been in the job long enough to really tell, but it seems a happy time for the switch to be made since we do have a very good manager right now in Mr. March.

We have had several discussions with Mr. Edwards—that is, Bob and I have—about the necessity for him learning at least part of the job in the office so that he would be able to handle the supervision in the event that Mr. Hodges had to be absent for some reason. But Mr. Edwards so far has been very adept at avoiding becoming involved in the office. Mr. Edwards also tends to overemphasize the business aspects and let the rehabilitative aspects go at the lodge. This is not entirely bad, but it does have some dangerous aspects to it, namely, the neglect of medication. He is not at all aware of the importance of medication and because of this it may be that we will never be able to turn over entirely the management of the lodge to a lay leader. It may be, it's too early to say but it's at least a possibility, that we will have to exercise some supervision indefinitely, not only because of the lack of concern by lay leaders with the medication of the men and other things like that but also their reluctance to become involved in that type of behavior control. So far both Mr. Hodges and Mr. Edwards, and to a lesser extent Mr. Hawkins, showed this also; both of these men have been only too eager to pass on to us any problems of behavior which occurred. They are not all eager to assume the responsibility for that aspect of the lodge. Right now Mr. Edwards shows a definite tendency to over-extend himself in the business aspects of the lodge. What I mean by that—he does not always pay enough attention to whether or not he is able with the crews he has at present to handle the volume of business which he is so actively going out and getting. This may mean that he is going to be running himself short of crews and not be able to handle jobs as they come up on a particular day. And of course one would expect this to result in a loss of jobs and perhaps a loss of steady jobs and therefore a decrease in monthly income. So far this hasn't happened, but I have had to check him several times by simply mentioning to him that he was accumulating more jobs than he could possibly handle for a week. He is not, I think, fully aware of the limitations of his work crews right now. He is perhaps expecting the men at the lodge to be able to perform at a level which men in general business do. Mr. Edwards is also a rather uncertain and nervous fellow. He has mentioned to us that he has had an ulcer and his personality is consistent with that. He worries a great deal and is forever making some approach to me which is ingratiating [and] which is aimed to sort of con me into sort of a confidence in him. At one point shortly after Mr. Hawkins had been fired, this was on the 11th—a Friday —Mr. Edwards came to me and said that even if we fired him he would probably be down at the lodge the next day anyway just because of his interest in it. This kind of very unsophisticated con game seems to be a characteristic of Mr. Edwards.

Mr. Hodges is very conscientious as I mentioned. He is a rather old man and suffers from a poor memory, but he has worked out all kinds of devices to take care of his shortcomings. On his memory, for instance, he carries a notebook so that he is able to remind himself of things as they come along by noting it in the book and consulting it frequently. He has also run his own business in the past. He said he operated his own general store for about 10 years in Texas and therefore he is quite familiar with bookkeeping techniques and he is not at all overwhelmed by the thought of having to act as supervisor of the business manager.

So far this month things have run quite smoothly in spite of initial difficulties of losing one of our new lay leaders and having to replace him with another and of the absence of Mr. Edwards for an entire week because of his father's death. Things are still functioning quite well. It seems in fact as if the well-known platoon system or substitution system even works well with lay leaders, so that when Mr. Edwards was out I was able to give slightly more help to Mr. Hodges and in that way get him over that.

The general feeling I have as we come to the end of the first month with lay leaders is that it will probably work. It's uncertain what particular difficulties may arise in the future, but it seems clear from this past month that the transition is possible and that it does work to have lay leaders taking over the major part of the work at the lodge. I'm very optimistic right now. My feeling is very optimistic that the lodge can operate in this way and in fact it seems even more a going concern now than it did before.

In many ways the training of the new lay coordinators was similar to the training of new lodge members. It began with a great deal of on-the-job training. The new men together with the most recent staff coordinator inspected all jobs. The coordinator slowly relinquished control so that day by day the lay leaders began assuming more and more responsibility for the operation of the lodge. Within a month's time, the coordinator was spending little time at the lodge. He stopped inspecting jobs. During the training period, the work performance of the members was very good. Coinciding with the training of the lay coordinators, two new members arrived whose presence was destined to affect significantly the future course of the lodge. Mr. March was very intelligent and took initiative in the many duties around the office. He quickly became the new business manager. The second new man, Mr. Porter, appeared to be an outstanding worker and potentially an excellent crew chief. Their arrival on the scene aided in maintaining a high level of performance at the lodge and also helped to allay the anxiety that naturally accompanied a change in lodge supervision.

The lay leaders' role involved only supervision of the work of lodge members. The *governing* of the lodge, including any disciplinary action, was specifically delegated to the executive committee, which by now had become a truly effective administrative group. So began the period of shared lay leader and executive committee authority working with a staff coordinator who had finally become a consultant to the lodge society whose relative autonomy he had worked so hard to achieve.

6 THE ATTEMPT AT SELF-GOVERNMENT

A Jump in Morale and Productivity

The combined arrival on the scene of the two lay coordinators and the two new members (Mr. March and Mr. Porter) initially was accompanied by an improvement in the performance of all crew chiefs. For example, Mr. Miller, the most adequate of the gardening crew chiefs, felt that he was the equal of the new lay coordinators and, as a consequence, became a better leader himself. Thus a rise in morale accompanied the arrival of the lay leaders at the lodge because the men felt more comfortable with the two lay leaders than they had with all previous professional coordinators.

Mr. Edwards, one of the two lay leaders, solicited and obtained many new jobs and increased the customers' cost per job. Charging higher prices was a new experience for lodge members. With pride they perceived increased prices as evidence of improving social status. They felt that charging customers more for their labor and services was an indication that the new lay leaders valued their work more than the professional staff had in the past. The new leadership at the lodge thus created the perception that lodge members were very important people. The following verbatim account from the now consultant's research journal shows the increase in group morale that developed when the lay leaders arrived:

> It is interesting to note that the residents of the lodge view the role played by the nonprofessional coordinator as more desirable than that

> played by the professional coordinator. This is highlighted by the dramatic increase in morale of the members, the increase in business, and the improved work performance of the members when the nonprofessional coordinator replaced the professional coordinator. Apparently the professional, as humanistic as he might be, cannot disengage himself from certain professional, authoritarian, and status aspects which are conveyed, however subtly, to the members. . . . The nonprofessional is seen differently—free of the regalia of the professional, as a friend, a peer, someone who is more understanding and accepting of him, and free from the influence of the hospital.

Even though morale, work performance, and business improved, the lay leaders passed on to the consultant any difficult psychological problems that occurred. Because the two lay coordinators continued to have difficulty in managing such problems of lodge members, the consultant explicitly outlined the managerial responsibilities of the two lay coordinators. This clarification of roles resulted in smoother operation for all aspects of lodge living. Along with this clarity arrived at during the first month of lay coordinators' supervision, there was an essential change in member leadership at the lodge. Members of the executive committee began to perceive themselves as more powerful because of the way in which the new lay leaders interacted with them. For example, the committee began playing a far more significant role in the appointment of crew chiefs. Heretofore, the crew chiefs had been appointed by the staff coordinator. When the lay leaders needed a new crew chief, they submitted the name of a prospective crew chief to the executive committee for approval.

Subsequently, the executive committee began increasing its control over other lodge affairs. It refused reentry to two former lodge members who had previously made a poor adjustment in the lodge society. It began emphasizing good work habits. An increasing number of workers were placed on probation by the committee because of poor work performance. The members proposed for executive-committee approval the purchase of a new television set and a coke machine, which they previously had been renting. They also proposed the purchase of walkie-talkies, so that crew chiefs on the jobs or the lay coordinators driving the trucks could be in constant communication with the office, whether or not they had access to a telephone. Although the committee approved the two purchases, the walkie-talkie proposal was discussed, investigated thoroughly, and subsequently dropped because it was judged by the committee to be too costly.

The lay leaders, for their part, strengthened the work faction of the executive committee because they were far more interested in the business aspects of the lodge than they were in the members' personal problems. With them, the two new lodge members, Mr. Porter and Mr. March, became dominant figures in lodge affairs. Mr. Porter, a strong and aggressive individual, soon became a crew chief in the janitorial service and hence a member of the executive committee. He supported the business faction. However, Mr. March, who was also a strong and aggressive individual had risen to the position of business manager and, as a consequence, also became a member of the executive committee. The rehabilitative position tended to center about him alone. He received no support from the lay leaders and only moderate support on occasion from within the committee. Thus, there was only one new and strong voice within the committee for the rehabilitative position. Nonetheless, Mr. March led a resurgence of the rehabilitative position within the executive committee which is documented in the following verbatim account from the consultant's research journal:

> It's also apparent that there is a more balanced vote in the executive committee now. I'm referring here to the rehabilitation-business struggle that's come up in the past. Apparently now the faction for business seems to be Mr. Smith and Mr. Porter mainly, and the faction for rehabilitation seems to be centered about Mr. March, who occasionally is able to bring in Mr. Miller and Mr. Kennedy.

However, the emphasis upon work had its effect. The lay coordinators vastly improved the lodge's business operation. It's competitive nature is reflected in this verbatim account from the research journal:

> Yet another [example] illustrates the extent to which the lodge had become a business. On one of our jobs some wood chips were bought for $5.99 and sold to the customer for $10.00. It is very apparent that under Mr. Edwards the lodge has become a true American business exercising all the privileges of free enterprise.

Declines in performance which had previously discouraged the two staff coordinators were now being taken pretty much in stride because, in part, all persons involved with the lodge operation were much more aware of the peaks and valleys through which the lodge moved. Furthermore, the lodge now had a history which showed the members that the organization had considerable strength. To them, it was proving capable of withstanding fluctuations in group performance and even cyclical changes in the behavior of its members.

Growing Autonomy of the Governing Body

The executive committee became progressively stronger and more antonomous. An example of this can be found in the way the executive committee treated Mr. Porter, one of the two new lodge leaders. He had been returned to the hospital from the lodge because of his assaultiveness toward several members of the lodge. This was the only instance of such behavior in the whole history of the lodge. Shortly thereafter, Mr. Porter was permitted to leave the hospital once again. The executive committee, at its regularly scheduled meetings, was unable to decide whether or not he should be allowed to return to the lodge. The committee had ambivalent feelings about Mr. Porter because he was an excellent worker and crew chief, on the one hand, but had continuous difficulty in getting along with the men, on the other. He occasionally became almost too angry to speak when workers performed poorly. He also was disliked by many members because of his autocratic and uncompromising behavior. Furthermore, some members were afraid of him because of his recent assaultiveness. Following the tie vote of the first meeting, a second meeting was held on the very next day with the very same result—indecision.

It was the custom at the lodge to bring an issue before a general meeting of all the members when the executive committee could not reach a decision. This was done immediately after the second tie vote of the committee. The feelings of all the lodge members about Mr. Porter became clearly evident by the overwhelming vote against him at the meeting. The membership voted two to one against allowing Mr. Porter to return to the lodge. Undoubtedly his assaultiveness was a major factor in this decision; he had apparently frightened a number of the men at the lodge. This example shows how one member was able to generate so much discomfort among the others by his threatening behavior that these negative feelings in the balance offset the significant work contribution he had made to the lodge's survival.

The revolt against Mr. Porter came primarily from the marginal workers, who were more alarmed by his destructive behavior than they were impressed by his ability—especially since his main preoccupation was to make them work. In a way, Mr. Porter's standards were too high for the lodge. Unlike other successful crew chiefs, Mr. Porter was not able to tolerate inefficiency without losing his temper. However, the rejection of Mr. Porter was not the end of the incident. What occurred subsequently was the work of a clique within the executive committee. Mr. Rich, one of the crew chiefs opposed to the return of Mr. Porter, soon left on vacation. While Mr. Rich was gone, a clique within the committee decided to hold another vote on the question of Mr. Porter's return. As a consequence, Mr. Porter was allowed to return to the lodge by a vote of 4 to 1 with one abstention. This was very clearly a manipulation by a segment of the executive committee who quite consciously and deliberately wanted to circumvent the general vote by all lodge members. The vote was a clear victory for those favoring the work orientation over those favoring the rehabilitative goals of the lodge society.

Subsequent to this manipulation, the executive committee increasingly dominated the activities of the lodge. Far from being unfair, however, the committee became a court of last resort for members when they violated rules of the lodge. An example of this can be found in the verbatim notes recording actions of the executive committee. The following problems were presented to the committee by Mr. Edwards, the lay leader:

> 1. Mr. Ring startled a lady on the job by talking about knife injuries and such and she claims that she doesn't want him on the job again.
> 2. Mr. Ring has been going through people's bureau drawers on the job.
> 3. Mr. Ring has been undermining the entire organization before the public.

The executive committee's notes show that they took the following action: "The executive committee recommends that Mr. March inform Mr. Ring of these charges and invite him to our general meeting on March 6 to defend himself and give reasons why he should not leave the lodge. Vote on this course of action was seven to nothing." As a result of this meeting, a decision was reached—"Decision: we recommend by a vote of 4 to 3 that Mr. Ring be put on two weeks' probation and one weeks' fine. He is guilty of all three charges." At that point, Mr. Edwards introduced new evidence showing that Mr. Ring had told another customer that the Janitorial Service was a "corrupt outfit." Another vote was held and Mr. Ring was requested to leave the lodge by a 4 to 3 vote.

It was often very difficult for committee members to take such action. One member of the executive committee revealed his reaction in these notes taken from the consultant's research journal.

> Mr. March, who was again working overtime in the office to keep things ship-shape, made a really extraordinary speech to me. It was mainly about the issues of personal freedom and the difficulty of having to judge other persons under difficult circumstances. He was speaking specifically about the case of Mr. Ring, saying how much he regretted the fact that Mr. Ring had done what he had done. How much he regretted the eventuality now open about Mr. Ring—that he would have to leave the lodge. And how much he regretted this, especially because he saw the value of the lodge to people like Mr. Ring and knew very well that he had very slim chances outside of the lodge. But still, how complicated this was by the fact that all the other men at the lodge had to be protected also and that it was more important to save the lodge as an institution for the benefit of the greater number of men than it was to risk it being harmed by keeping Mr. Ring. It was a speech, I think, that was full of awareness of the difficulties of making decisions like this on a very high intellectual level. It seemed to confirm the extent to which Mr. March has become a very capable holder of the job of business manager.

The lay leaders themselves (Mr. Edwards and Mr. Hodges) were aware of the control of the executive committee. They observed they had to "woo" the committee in order to obtain the kinds of things they wanted from the lodge. They felt obligated to reach accommodations with the committee and did not feel that they could simply act independently of it. The committee had become very decisive in its leadership, coinciding with high cohesiveness and morale. This stemmed from the committee's growing perception of itself as an elite group within the organization. The high degree of cohesiveness and morale among the executive committee members reveals itself clearly in this quotation from the consultant's research journal notes:

> Another incident—a very important one—showing the cohesiveness and morale at the lodge. On Saturday, the 25th of September, I got a telephone call from Mr. March. He told me that the telephone company had changed our number and also that he had forgotten to make Mr. Smith his check for the weekend. I went out to sign the check and when I arrived I found Mr. Porter, Mr. Spears, and Mr. March [all members of the executive committee] sitting in the office systematically going through our business cards and changing the telephone numbers on them so that they would have the cards ready the next week. They were also taking a whole series of realistic and appropriate actions to make sure that the new telephone number was in the hands of "Information" in case someone should call to get it. They were doing this in the following way: one of the men would go to the gas station nearby to the pay phone and dial the old number as a test call and then check to see whether or not that produced a link to the operator who would then give the correct number. They carried this out until they were quite sure that anyone telephoning the old number would reach the lodge in spite of the change.

The Development of a Regulated Society

As a result of its developing eliteness, autonomy, and power, the executive committee initiated a series of new rules. The first regulations pertained to keeping pets at the lodge, since lodge members keeping pets there had often shown themselves irresponsible in their care. The rules reflected the desire of the committee to allow the members such a privilege, as long as it was responsibly carried out. Responsible behavior became a growing concern of this business community of ex-patients, whose committee next ruled that vulgar language which they believed socially unacceptable to their customers was prohibited in their presence.

Concern for members who put forth extra effort in behalf of the lodge next occupied the committee's attention. The committee voted extra pay for overtime work as shown in its minutes, which reflect both the unique needs of the janitorial service and the extreme form of democracy which the committee was trying to develop:

> Does the executive committee wish to allocate $200 from the operating fund as a working emergency fund whereby we might pay the men $1.50 per hour for special work assignments, which Mr. Edwards [lay coordinator] and Mr. Hodges [lay coordinator] designate as emergency issues and which the executive committee approves of in regular session by popular

vote, and if the executive committee approves of this, may Mr. Miller and Mr. Gardner receive $1.50 each for that extra hour they are working at the new Wilcox job at 7 A.M.?

Made into law and put into effect this 29th day of September 1965 by the executive committee in session.

By a vote of 7 to 0

Mr. March
Chairman

No member could receive extra pay between the hours of 8:00 A.M. and 5:00 P.M., since during this period members who worked were paid according to the established plan of payment at the janitorial and yard service. Overtime pay was also approved for several of the members who worked on Saturdays, so that the janitorial service could retain some well-paying jobs which required work on the weekend. This reflected a major change in work policies—working not for individual customers in private homes but for commercial enterprises, since this was more remunerative employment. The men found they would much rather work for commercial firms than for housewives! This move toward commercial janitorial work also occurred as a result of the influence of the lay coordinators, who had a different view of the business opportunity than had the professional coordinators preceding them.

Finally, again with an eye to increasing the responsible behavior of the lodge members which might affect its relations with the community, the executive committee adopted a series of rules governing ownership and use of motor vehicles by members. These rules established executive committee control by specifying that its approval was required in each member's case and would only be granted if legal and insurance requirements had been met. Thus, responsible behavior required of any citizen was becoming the norm for lodge members, under the executive committee's guidance and direct initiative. The supreme example of this and the committee's crowning accomplishment in this area was a series of thirteen articles setting forth its philosophy about the goals of the lodge and the resultant rules that were to govern the behavior of its members. The articles represent the closing but not yet completed stages in consolidation of the lodge group as a uniquely self-determining small society. They deal with the criteria for selecting those ex-patients deemed suitable for lodge membership as follows:

ARTICLES GOVERNING POLICY OF LODGE MEMBERSHIP

In order to decide definitely what we are running, we submit the following articles governing our policy in selecting lodge members.

1. The lodge is composed of discharged former patients of the hospital who wanted to leave but were unable to for one reason or another. They joined the lodge program in order to leave the hospital and become actively engaged in running a janitorial service . . . in the community.

2. Each man's work is important to the welfare of the business as a whole and each man is expected to do his best on the job he has to do. We feel that no man who does not contribute in some worthwhile way to the business should be allowed to stay.

3. Each member is responsible for himself as well as being socially responsible for the lodge as a whole.

4. We feel that the welfare of the lodge and its members depends upon obtaining the best people possible to share in our work and to build the standards of the business to the highest possible level.

5. Each member is expected to share these principles and have respect for our sincere efforts to build a first-class business, based on efficiency, integrity and service to our customers.

6. We feel that to the extent that the rehabilitative element is allowed to be considered in selecting members, to that extent will mediocrity and defeatism enter in our program and allowances made for work poorly done or left undone.

7. Lodge members dedicating themselves to excellence in the performance of their jobs and the welfare of the business should not have to be concerned with rehabilitation.

8. In order to keep the program from becoming just another hospital ward, we feel it is a business primarily and a rehabilitative program secondly, and the members selected for the good of the business and not for the good of the members themselves.

9. Members are approved or disapproved according to their ability to contribute to the janitorial service and not for personal reasons.

10. It is operated as an autonomy, governed by an executive committee, and supported by two salaried coordinators, whose authority is subject to the executive committee, and a Dr. of Psychology who is available for those members wishing help with their personal life.

11. We feel that we are not in the hospital business and should not be asked to conduct ourselves in the manner of salaried hospital employees and carry the work load of members who have been forced upon us, and who are unable or unwilling to participate in the janitorial business, and who destroy the efforts of those who are willing.

12. We feel that our care in selecting members will largely determine the success or failure of the program.

13. Should a lodge member, after being accepted in the program, become lax in his working habits, or otherwise behave in a way which is judged by the executive committee to be objectionable to the welfare of the business or its members, [he] will be placed on probation for a period of two weeks and if [he] is still found to be objectionable, [he] will be called before a regular meeting of the executive committee and asked to show cause why he should not leave the lodge. If no satisfactory reason is given, he will be dismissed from lodge membership and told to go.

The thirteen articles governing selection for lodge membership were developed by the work faction in the executive committee. Almost all of the subsequent problems presented to the executive committee resulted in a confrontation between the work and rehabilitative factions. The work clique invariably was victorious. This relative emphasis in favor of work rather than rehabilitative goals was exemplified in many decisions, particularly those placing marginal workers on periods of probation because of their limited work contribution to the lodge. The probationary periods carried with them the implied threat of ejection from the lodge if the probationer did not improve his work performance. On two such occasions, the executive committee dismissed lodge members when they showed no work improvement during their probationary period. The committee's rejection of these members resulted both times in vetoes by the staff consultant because he considered such action detrimental to the long-run goals of the lodge. These were the first overt actions by the consultant challenging the power of the work faction in the executive committee. Despite the consultant's action on these two occasions, the work faction remained firmly entrenched. A subsequent incident, in fact, reflected the faction's unequivocal position about work. A list of hospitalized ex-lodge members, who had indicated their desire to return to the lodge, was submitted to the executive committee for its consideration. The committee voted unanimously not to allow a single applicant to return to the lodge because these men could not, in their opinion, contribute to the business of the lodge.

The executive committee's desire for even greater autonomy at this time is illustrated in the following verbatim account from the coordinator's research journal:

> according to Mr. Edwards [one lay leader]—when Mr. Smith overheard Mr. Hodges [the other lay leader] . . . telephoning me at the hospital about some matter, Mr. Smith apparently lost his temper at this because [Mr. Hodges] calls the 'Docs' too often. Summarizing his reaction, Mr. Smith reportedly said, "This place isn't a police station. Why is he calling the 'Docs'?

The Move for Greater Representation of the Governing Body

As time passed, the executive committee became increasingly less representative of the membership of the lodge. Its decisions more and more discriminated against marginally productive workers. These workers never had any personal representatives on the executive committee because it was comprised from the outset only of work crew chiefs. However, up to this point the views of these marginal workers had been represented within the committee by some crew chiefs who showed a concern for their problems—the so-called rehabilitative faction. Thus, members who were not on the executive committee always in the past had had indirect representation on it. When the work faction became the sole power group within the committee, workers—and especially marginal workers—lost their indirect voice in lodge decision-making processes.

As the executive committee increasingly undermined the residual hospital rehabilitative norms that still existed at the lodge and reinforced instead the work norms, nonparticipating members progressively bore the brunt of the committee's "new look." After passively accepting their fate for a long period of time, leadership gradually developed in the ranks of the marginal workers. Mr. Nash, who had resided at the lodge for only two months, became an articulate leader of those men not represented on the executive committee. The harassed workers finally submitted a formal written complaint about their situation to the staff consultant. This document, reproduced in its entirety here because of its pivotal significance, became known to the research staff at the workers' "Declaration of Independence:"

> We have brought the following matter to the attention of Dr. Osmond, in Dr. Cochran's absence. Dr. Osmond suggests that we first present it at this meeting. Should we not be given satisfaction, we then return to Dr. Osmond for him to take action. The subject of this note consists of the following:
>
> Who will be next! During the past months there have been upsetting happenings at our lodge involving a particular conspicuous party and a number of innocent victims who have been set upon viciously each in turn. And the Ex-Com, supposed to be concerning itself with these out-of-order conflicts, has been meekly passing the buck. Yes, passing the buck when it should be doing what's necessary to ensure that we live sociably with each other and maintain good morale. Admit that the Ex-Com is failing this job. Any idea why?
>
> And is it a coincidence that each of the persons set upon is not in the Ex-Com?
>
> Again, *each of these innocent persons is not in the Ex-Com.* So maybe there is method to this madness. We workers cannot place faith in the crew chiefs who have continually passed the buck each time one of us has been humiliated, while you stand off sighing with relief that you haven't been subjected to indignities as we have. *We can stand this treatment no longer.* We're coming out with this to make you be honest about the whole thing. We're standing to be counted rather than continue to take abuse.
>
> *We are making our stand by firmly requesting an in to the Ex-Com meetings around here. We are all concerned and want these meetings opened to us, one and all. It's the democratic way and will give us the means to cope with any further tyrannical threats to our well-being. We the following agree to present this petition that the meetings of the Ex-Com be open to workers as well as crew chiefs. I cast my yes......*
>
> 1. Nash 2. Gross 3. Jones 4. Holt 5. Day 6. Buck 7. Wolfe 8. Parker 9. Kline 10. Walker
>
> Note: We are retaining the original copy including signatures; it can be seen on request.

The committee reviewed the "Declaration" and summarily dismissed it, responding in kind with a document of its own entitled "Executive Committee's Policy on Sit-Ins":

> In reply to Mr. Nash's petition we would like to say that the executive committee is generally in favor of Mr. Porter's policies at the lodge and feel that he has the interest of the business and the welfare of the lodge at heart.
>
> We feel that he is trying to conduct the . . . janitorial service as a business and expects other members of the lodge to do the same. When they behave in a manner which indicates they think they are still in the hospital, and shun all responsibilities, as they did in the hospital, he feels and we feel that they should return there or to some similar place. This is not a hospital and unless the work is done by lodge members, it is left undone.
>
> Any lodge member can be appointed to the executive committee by assuming the responsibilities of his job and doing enough work to be made a crew chief. These are the men who are on the executive committee and these are the men who have earned the right to have a voice in the running of the lodge.
>
> As membership at the lodge is strictly voluntary, those not in favor with its policies are free to leave.

The executive committee's response to the workers' complaint brought the staff consultant into the situation. Since the committee was clearly an unrepresentative body, the staff consultant finally decided upon and drew up new "Rules of Organization" for the lodge and sent them to the executive committee for enforcement. They contained the following provisions:

> *THE EXECUTIVE COMMITTEE: Rules of Organization*
>
> 1. Effective immediately, the executive committee shall be composed of *all* members of the lodge who wish to attend the meetings.
> 2. The executive committee shall meet every Wednesday at such times as all members of the lodge are available to attend the meeting. If Wednesday is an official holiday, the meeting will be held on Thursday. Special meetings must be held at such times as all the members of the lodge are able to attend.
> 3. The meetings of the executive committee shall be held in the O.D. room.
> 4. Each member of the lodge attending a meeting of the executive committee shall have one vote. All votes shall have equal value and there shall be no voting by proxy.
> 5. Any member of the lodge may bring a question, complaint, request or suggestion to a meeting of the executive committee.
> 6. The executive committee shall vote on an issue by secret ballot if requested to do so by any lodge member present at the meeting or by the supervisor.
> 7. The chairman of the executive committee shall be elected by a gen-

eral meeting of the lodge at which *all* members of the lodge are present. On the last general meeting each month, a secret ballot on the chairmanship shall be taken by Mr. Edwards or Mr. Hodges [the lay coordinators]. Members may vote to keep the same chairman or may elect a new one.

8. The chairman of the executive committee shall have the following duties:

1. Announce the time of all meetings of the executive committee to all members of the lodge.
2. Set up and operate the tape recorder at all meetings.
3. Record the decisions, votes and remarks on the executive committee action forms.
4. Keep the log of executive committee actions.
5. Act as chairman during meetings (reading problems, recognizing lodge members who wish to speak, calling and recording votes, etc.).

9. Any member of the lodge may appeal a decision of the executive committee to a general meeting of all lodge members or to the supervisor. If necessary, the supervisor will attend meetings of the executive committee to see that these rules are followed.

It was not without considerable concern about the meaning of this intervention that these rules were imposed on the committee by the consultant. But it was considered vital that the new organization reestablish the lodge as a democratic institution whose operation was to be shared by all members. This action again allowed the workers a representative voice in the lodge's decision-making body.

But this arbitrary action by the staff consultant resulted in some insidious and devious tactics carried out by the work faction of the committee. The crew chiefs were outnumbered during the first several meetings after the new rules became effective. However, in about a month the workers, apparently feeling they had made their point about the *right* to participate, quit attending the meetings. The crew chiefs again became the dominant power group at the lodge. Working within the new democratic rules of organization, the work faction was able to amend two of the nine rules, as follows:

1. Effective immediately, the executive committee shall be composed of the crew chiefs and all members of the lodge who wish to attend the meetings. No executive committee meeting can be held unless there are five or more crew chiefs present.

2. The chairman of the executive committee shall be elected by a general meeting of the lodge, and must be selected from one of the eight crew chiefs.

Mr. Nash, the leader of the workers, was very much aware of the workers' lack of interest in the committee. Because of his concern for the workers' welfare, he submitted a memo to all of them stating that they had once again become a minority on the committee. His memo said:

> Since the meetings have been opened to workers the following points have been made: (1) No worker, present or future, can become chairman for the meetings. (2) It's been proposed to guarantee a wage to crew chiefs but not to workers. *This is some proof of what the executive committee can do so long as workers are not attending to do something for ourselves. There have been usually only 4 present.*

His plea was to no avail. Workers' attendance did not increase during the ensuing months. Because of the workers' disinterest in such participative processes, the work faction of the executive committee maintained its controlling power over decisions during the final period of research-project support. Although it may not be a commentary upon such processes in the surrounding society, it is worth noting that, except for their leader, the workers seemed to be concerned more with the availability of the right to participate in such decision-making processes rather than with the exercise of that right. Once the right to choose whether or not to participate in such processes had been established, actual decision-making was left by the workers to those leaders among the lodge group most interested and concerned with a flourishing janitorial and gardening business. Because of the responsibilities which their roles in the lodge society imposed upon them, these leaders proved to be ready and willing to discharge the trust which the workers by default accorded them.

7 AUTONOMY AT LAST

Efforts Toward Agency Support

A few months prior to termination of research-project support for the lodge operation, the research director tried to interest several federal, state, and county agencies in financing the lodge as a permanent community program for discharged mental patients. This action was consistent with his responsibility for the welfare of lodge members. The response from each of the various agencies was remarkably similar. None disagreed about the need for such a community treatment program but each of these positive expressions was followed invariably by arguments demonstrating why the particular agency involved could not implement such a program. Agencies most frequently gave the following reasons for this inability: they would need additional funds for such a new program (despite the cost reduction shown in the results: p. 210); such a unique program would not fit into the agency's practices; professional staffs would not accept a program which would allow more autonomy for mental patients, since granting such autonomy would require unwelcome changes in professional roles. During this period, the research director also contacted the board of directors of the rehabilitative corporation for whom the members worked (pp. 23–27). This nonprofit corporation was the only organization that expressed an interest in continuing the lodge as a treatment program for mentally ill persons. However, it was completely unable to provide the necessary funds.

The director of the psychology services at the hospital from which the lodge members came believed that the hospital itself might be able to use some hospital funds to support new members in the community. He thought it might also be possible to get special funds for continuing the lodge. This seemed reasonable because patients could be taken from the hospital to live in community residences at less than one-half the cost this very hospital would otherwise expend to continue them as patients (p. 211). Accordingly, the psychology director made this proposal to the director of the hospital, who informed him that authority for the allocation of such funds would be required from the agency that supported the hospital. The agency's central administration was contacted by means of an official communication from the hospital director which presented the results of the investigation in detail. The document concluded by stressing the urgency of the situation, in view of the opportunity not only to provide for the continuation of the lodge at reduced expense to the hospital but also to avoid the financial and human costs of hospital reentry and re-institution of the program at a later date. At nearly the same time, the research director made a personal presentation of the research results to the central administrative staff of the agency. Despite such attempts to convey this information and its urgency, the agency did not provide the action necessary to continue the lodge program. As a result of this inaction, the research staff concluded that the members of the lodge would need to become self-supporting if they were to continue to operate their business and live in the community. Thus it became necessary by default to implement a completely autonomous program, a phase of development in the lodge society completely unanticipated by the research plan.

The Plan for Ultimate Autonomy

When the end of the research phase of the lodge project was five months away, the research staff began planning for this autonomous future. Most appropriately, the lodge would be closed at the conclusion of the lease agreement with the owner of the motel in five months' time, when all members would have to become self-sufficient. Accordingly, this time was used to decrease gradually the amount of research financial support given the lodge, in order to determine how the men would react when they were required to increase support for themselves through their own resources.

Initially, the plan was to reduce by half the amount of money contributed by the research budget for food. A similar reduction in research money to pay for telephone, utilities, gas and oil for the work trucks, laundry, postage, equipment maintenance and repair, work clothing, and other supplies was also planned. The plan required that by the time the lodge was closed, the members would be paying every expense for operating the lodge dormintory and the business. The plan also called for discontinuing research funds given to the men for medication and periodic visits to the local physician. Needy members would have to visit local outpatient or mental hygiene clinics, where the cost would be very minimal or where the costs could be paid by the men from their own resources. The plan expected members would assume the cost of the lodge by contributing from all their sources of income—wages from the business, pensions, compensations, and Social Security disability funds. Of course, the plan assumed that the amount each individual should contribute would have to be determined by the members themselves.

In order to facilitate an easy transition to this more autonomous phase, the research staff set out to determine the various medical resources in the community that might be available to the members, the members' financial and guardianship statuses, and the actual monthly costs for the lodge and the business (pp. 210–212). As a result of this survey, it was decided to extend increasing financial responsibility to the lodge members during the first three months of the five-month period, with the group paying the entire costs of the lodge during the final two-month period. Thus the members would experience two months of autonomous operation before the lodge buildings had to be vacated according to the lease agreement. Based upon lodge costs, the schedule for increasing financial responsibility was established as shown in Table 7.1.

Table 7.1. The Plan for Financial Autonomy

Time	*Per Cent Lodge Members Pay of Total Costs*	*Per Cent Research Project Pays of Total Costs*
1st month	20	80
2nd month	49	51
3rd month	78	22
4th month	100	0
5th month	100	0

Estimated lodge costs included eventual payment by the members for the lay coordinator's salary, all food costs, the cost of the lodge lease, and the cost of leasing work trucks. Finally, the plan specified that eventually members must pay for all medical costs incurred by them. In order to facilitate member payment, it was decided to establish a bank savings account where money contributed by members for payment of their expenses during the five-month period could be deposited.

The completed plan for financial autonomy and member self-sufficiency was presented by the research director to a general meeting of the lay coordinators and the entire lodge membership. The presentation evoked only one or two comments suggesting member anxiety about the future. Most of the members viewed this as just another phase in a project that upon occasion was manipulated by the research staff. They appeared to believe that this move was hypothetical and that the coordinators would continue to "protect" them. The meeting ended with a request that the executive committee convene at the earliest possible time in order to develop a payment plan for the lodge members which would cover 20 per cent of the lodge food expenses allocated by the plan to the group for the first month of this transitional phase. This executive session, like all others, was recorded by the members and the consultant later reviewed the tape recording of the meeting. He then made a report to the executive committee, stating in part:

> My overall impression of the meeting was that a definite beginning . . . was made to solve the problem of how to come up with the $900. . . . The greatest problem was that no one would really deal with the problem as it exists today; and it is a real problem that must be solved.

Not until the staff consultant responded with these impressions of the executive committee meeting did the more responsible members seriously believe that the plan for autonomy was going to be carried out. As a result, the executive committee called a second meeting. The committee devised a payment plan which was a combination of all the proposals that had been discussed between them and the consultant, in an attempt to please all parties. Nevertheless, it was realistic, considering both the relatively small percentage of the costs that they had to pay in the first month and the existing job income of the members. The plan devised by the executive committee basically distributed the financial burden among the members according to their ability to pay. This distribution was to be carried out, however, by supplementing less affluent workers' wages with money from emergency funds in order to achieve an equal amount of money contributed by each lodge member. The concern of the committee for justice to its less "fortunate" members was clearly a factor in shaping the payment plan according to the unique norms and needs of the lodge society.

The research staff expected several lodge members to leave in the face of a plan increasing the financial burden on them for their own support. Nevertheless, none of the 26 members residing at the lodge left during the first month. Whatever shock may have occurred as a result of the announcement regarding plans for the transition appeared to dissipate; there was little talk among the men about the new plan for self-support. Apparently, no one left the lodge at this time because the majority of members still had not really "heard" what had been said and did not take the situation very seriously. They continued in fact to be protected by the lodge environment and project support of it; and the contribution required from their income, based on the executive committee's plan for the first month, was not very penalizing and did not seriously limit their activities. Most grumbling came from those men whose total income was the smallest, although they had the least amount taken from their income according to the payment plan. A separate payment plan was devised by the executive committee for the second month, suggesting the fashion in which the lodge society met pressing problems one by one as they arose. This plan continued equal payments from all members receiving equal wages, with just and agreed-upon allowances for less rewarded workers being compensated by emergency funds.

The Growing Burden of Financial Self-Sufficiency

The exodus of members from the lodge began during the second month of the transition to financial self-suffiency. It started quite slowly and did not gain momentum until the third month. Significantly, the first man to leave did so after the first payroll in the second month, when the amount he had to pay to support himself at the lodge became very real. The share deducted from his pay rose dramatically from 20 per cent to almost 50 per cent.

The second month's plan so drastically reduced wages that some members had to call upon their income from other sources, such as veterans' compensations, pensions, and disability funds, in order to meet the weekly contributions required to live at the lodge. They now realized that their support was no longer guaranteed by research funds. Once this occurred, the anxiety of several men became apparent. Mr. Jones, the first to leave, had been the most anxious of all the members and had also been the greatest grumbler regarding his lack of funds. This was not new for him, since it had been his situation throughout his three-year stay at the lodge. He was financially indigent except for the wages he received while working there. His dissatisfaction with his new financial burden led to leaving the lodge in favor of residence at the home of a former lodge member with whom he had maintained a continuing friendship. After two weeks of living with his friend, he returned to the lodge and requested that he be allowed to reenter, apparently realizing that he could not survive on his own, that it had been a mistake for him to leave the lodge. However, his request to return was rejected by the executive committee because he was now perceived as a financial burden. They knew that his indigent financial position probably would require other members to contribute to his support. His next move was to apply for readmission to the mental hospital from which he had originally come to the lodge.

Such feelings of discontent about the financial burden as Mr. Jones expressed by his leaving continued to smolder during the second month. During a two-week period entering the third month of the plan for self-sufficiency, behavioral regression, psychological deterioration, and clear lack of motivation was shown by some members. The situation was best exemplified by the behavior of Mr. Miller, an excellent crew chief in the past, who now decided to leave. He began to drink heavily, did no janitorial work, and complained bitterly about "working for nothing" and having to "pay to work." He exhibited no desire to become self-sufficient and proceeded eventually back to the mental hospital. The heavy contribution to their own support and the anticipation that it would increase was undoubtedly a crucial determinant in the members' decision to remain or to leave the lodge. One-half the members who were destined to leave during the transition period did so in this two-week period. The payment plan developed by the executive committee for the third month of the transition speaks eloquently and not without some sarcasm, of the burden the members were feeling:

> *EASY PAYMENT PLAN FOR JUNE*
>
> The executive committee in its meeting of June 1, has decided the following in its efforts to meet the obligations of the lodge for the month of June:
>
> Due to the unsettled situation of the affairs of the lodge at this time, with the [nonprofit rehabilitation corporation] still undecided as to its role in the future of the lodge, as well as the fact that several members are making plans to leave if the present set of conditions continue to prevail, we feel that each member who can should pay the equal payment amount of $139.51, and those who cannot, due to insufficient funds, should pay what they can with the exception of $25.00. Each man will receive $25.00 or more for the month unless he is fined or refuses to work.
>
> We feel that the following men, due to their carrying a large share of the work load, as well as receiving a very small or no pension at all, should be given special consideration for their efforts to the lodge, and allowed to keep $40.00 of their monthly take: Mr. Porter, Mr. Spears, Mr. Spahn.
>
> The funds to meet the above expenditures are to be taken from the operating expense fund until July 1, when we will be in a better position to work out a more permanent arrangement.

The arrival of the fourth month brought with it the anticipated total financial commitment from all lodge members. Unlike the previous three months of the transition, the executive committee was not required to devise a payment plan for the fourth month. It was simply unnecessary, since each lodge member was required to contribute the total amount of his monthly cash resources, both from wages at the lodge and other personal income such as pensions. However, along with this total commitment, a method was initiated for returning some of this money to the members in order to cover the cost of their personal expenses. The crew chiefs, because of the nature of their leadership responsibility at the lodge, received $10 per week; the deputy crew chiefs received $7.50 weekly because of their more limited responsibility. These new "wages" were still subject to decrease as a result of any disciplinary action that might be taken by the executive committee or they could be increased if the committee wanted to reward a member for a particularly outstanding performance. Thus, despite the necessity of their total financial commitment, the personal-expense money provided a differential pay scale, with higher amounts going to those in the more responsible positions.

During the first three months of the transitional period, eight of the 26 members who resided in the lodge when the self-sufficiency plan was initiated left the lodge. Seven of the eight left after the change to a 49 per cent payment; no one left the lodge during the phase of 78 per cent payment. With the inception of the 100 per cent phase, two men left the lodge, stating that they "could not afford" to remain any longer. Three others left during the fourth month. Their exits were a direct result of an altercation between two of the three men. The member who initiated the fight became disturbed and was returned to the hospital by the staff consultant. His opponent in the altercation became agitated, left the lodge, and voluntarily admitted himself to a state hospital. The third party left because he became quite fearful and anxious over the incident and over the prospect of not being able to work with his crew chief to whom he had become quite attached, the man who had initiated the fight. He left voluntarily to live with a member of his family. By the end of the fourth month, therefore, thirteen of the original 26 men with whom the transition was begun remained at the lodge.

From a financial viewpoint the total commitment phase of the transition was successful. The remaining lodge members were now paying the total cost of operating the lodge. In effect, they were owners of the entire small society. Now the members honestly could say that they were purchasing their *own* supplies with their *own* money for their *own* business. Thus, within four months the members who remained had become a totally autonomous, motivated, well-organized, and cohesive group of ex-mental patients who could now support themselves adequately in the community.

Relocation and Complete Autonomy

The period of movement toward financial self-sufficiency was also used to divorce the lay coordinators and the professional consultants from the lodge organization. By prearrangement, one of the two lay coordinators left employment at the end of the first month of the transition as a part of this movement. His departure resulted in noticeable effects upon the lodge organization, because he had supervised the member-business manager. Bookkeeping problems developed. It had been hoped that the supervision of the business manager's position would be assumed by the professional consultant who was to remain during the entire transitional period. However, the business manager's duties went unsupervised for a period of several weeks. Ultimately, a scheduled periodic inspection of the books and records by the staff consultant revealed that the accuracy and organization of important clerical and bookkeeping duties were in an initial stage of neglect. On the staff consultant's recommendation, the lay coordinator delegated some of these duties to the most capable janitorial crew chief, Mr. Porter, who became in effect the lay coordinator's assistant.

As time passed, the remaining lay coordinator began showing less and less interest in the daily progress of the business. He delegated many tasks, such as transporting work crews, completing job forms and inspections, keeping the bookkeeper informed of the financial status of various jobs, and other essential work processes, almost wholly to the crew chiefs. For himself, he remained concerned with soliciting business and attempting to establish good public relations. In an unexpected way, the consequence of this deficient motivation, by delegating responsibility to the crew chiefs, aided the group in learning how to manage the lodge's varied living and business problems. It was in effect an unintended training program for members in managing essential responsibilities related to the survival of the lodge society.

The business aspect of the lodge organization continued to deteriorate. The staff consultant was temporarily forced to become the business manager and to train another member for this position. Although he was able to relinquish most of the business manager's duties to the newly trained business manager, close supervision was still necessary. The situation worsened after the newly trained business manager decided to leave the lodge one month later. The executive committee refused to appoint another lodge member to assume the business manager's role, stating that none of the remaining members were qualified for the position. Thus the committee implicitly recommended that the staff consultant continue in the role. From that point until the closing of the lodge, a period of almost two months, the consultant reluctantly played a relatively passive role in this position, keeping only the minimum records required for maintaining accurate books.

By the middle of the fourth month of transition, the lay coordinator's time was almost completely devoted to troubleshooting in order to correct many errors that were being made on customer's jobs. Work procedures (pp. 58–59) so painstakingly developed to avoid such errors were being disregarded because of his growing disinterest in these aspects of his position as coordinator. Despite this damaging effect upon the business, with the imminent closing of the lodge, the remaining members were faced with two alternatives: either close the lodge, terminate the business, and let each member go his own way or relocate as a group in a new residence where the business could continue to operate under the supervision of the lay coordinator. The lay coordinator preferred the latter and the members chose the same course. Despite some reservations about such an endeavor, the lay coordinator's involvement in the lodge with the members had become so important to him that he did not want the organization to become extinct. The move depended on his willingness and that of Mr. Smith, the kitchen crew chief, who would not only have to be cook and leader of the new living system but would also have to replace the staff consultant as business manager. Since Mr. Smith was totally committed to continuing the operation of the lodge, he simply incorporated these added duties into his role. The lay coordinator, for his contribution, assumed the task of finding a residence. Two residences were finally located which were seven city blocks apart. In contrast to location of the lodge in a lower socioeconomic neighborhood, however, the two houses were situated in a middle-class neighborhood across the main freeway (pp. 131–133).

Since the lay coordinator had become the person responsible for the welfare of the members with the closing of the lodge, he had to decide which members would make the move. Because he had already made a commitment to the realtor that only nine men would be living in the two homes, four of the thirteen remaining members had to leave the group and make their own future plans. The coordinator eliminated the four men who he considered to be least productive, who were then given the choice of returning to the hospital or living elsewhere in the community. One man chose to continue living in the community, while the other three decided to return to the hospital. The lay coordinator, apparently believing that his main role in the move had been completed, took little part in the preparations for closing the lodge and for moving to the new residences. Thus, planning for the move became basically the responsibility of the member leader, Mr. Smith, who worked out the plans with the staff consultant.

In preparation, cost estimates indicated that the "new lodge" could be sustained financially using the personal income of the nine remaining members combined with income from the business. In addition, part of the plan for transition to financial self-sufficiency worked out between the staff consultant and the executive committee included setting aside members' funds over the four-month period ending with the closing of the lodge. During this period, several thousand dollars of their own funds were accumulated in a separate bank savings account as a "stake" with which members could begin their completely autonomous venture in the community. The research staff was fully aware of the need, both psychological and financial, for member investment in their own social system when this savings plan was devised. The fund would clearly provide them with a buffer against unforseen emergencies threatening the survival of their small society, particularly during its beginning stages. Consequently, the plan was carried out and the nine men were in a sound financial position at the time of the move.

Next, the group purchased from the university, which was the legal owner of all research project property, the equipment necessary to operate the janitorial and yardwork business, such as floor polishers and rakes. In addition, items such as refrigerators, dishes, and utensils were purchased from local stores. The men had a stockpile of foodstuffs, mainly canned goods, which they brought to the new residences from the lodge. While living at the lodge, they had also accumulated their own furniture, which was sufficient to furnish the new homes. It was agreed that transportation to and from work would be furnished by the lay coordinator, who owned a pickup truck, and by two of the members, who jointly owned a vintage automobile. There was some grumbling among the men when they learned about the seven-block distance between the two houses. The man who complained the most was Mr. Smith, who had the responsibility for feeding all nine men. Nevertheless, he resolved this by deciding to serve all meals for the entire complement of men at the residence where he lived. His assistant, who lived in the second house, planned to keep some food on hand for snacks.

As a final preparation, the actual physical move from the lodge to the new residences was accompanied by a formal legal disassociation of the university and the research-project staff from the lodge members and their leader—the lay coordinator. A document was drawn up and signed by the lay coordinator acknowledging that the research personnel and the university itself had terminated their supervision of the lodge living situation and the business. It stated that these two parties were no longer responsible for the members of the lodge nor for the operation of the janitorial and yard service. At the same time a special agreement was executed between the nine members and the lay coordinator. This agreement, signed by all concerned, revealed in its formality the seriousness with which the move was contemplated, and contained the following provisions:

NEW LEASE ARRANGEMENT

Be it known by all concerned that the following arrangements have been made:

1. Whereas the janitorial and yard service has found it necessary to vacate the premises, and
2. Whereas new quarters had to be found to locate the business and equipment, and
3. Whereas it has become necessary to sign a lease in order to obtain said new quarters, and
4. Whereas we do not want any single person to be held responsible for fulfilling the lease should said janitorial and yard service cease to function,
5. Be it known that should the lease be broken, the outstanding payments will be made from the janitorial and yard service Bank of Colera checking account and/or the Wiltner Savings & Loan Association savings account, and should this not be possible, each member associated with said service at the time that the lease should be broken will be held responsible for an equal share of the balance.

The Responsibilities of Freedom

The description of the events that followed the move to the new residences, because the move was not a part of the original research plan, must be based upon information received through accidental meetings between some of the lodge members and members of the research staff, some infrequent requests for advice, the agreement by a few lodge members to recorded interviews, and by all to completion of follow-up questionnaires. During the first month, information came from one visit and a few telephone calls. This limited information revealed that within three weeks after the move, two members had left the lodge. One decided to continue living with his mother, with whom he had spent a brief vacation. The second man took his leave very abruptly and made no attempt to contact any member of the lodge. During the first week after the move, Mr. Smith telephoned on several occasions to get some needed information about business procedures and bookkeeping records. One visit was made by the former staff consultant to the new house in order to obtain the old bookkeeping records that Mr. Smith was using as a model for the new set of record books.

Mr. Smith reported no major problems. The house appeared much more comfortable and "lived in" than when they had first occupied it. Although they were having some minor financial problems, Mr. Smith reported that they had not as yet taken money from their savings account. Furthermore, he appeared to be sincerely interested and concerned that the men take their medication properly. This was surprising, since throughout his stay at the lodge he had always been opposed to the members taking prescribed medication. He felt it was a symbol that they were "sick" and he was strongly opposed to perceiving working men as people who were ill. It was quite apparent that his personal involvement in the success of the new autonomous community program was so great that he was willing to change some of these cherished ideas. He also revealed that within two weeks after the move to the new residences, two of the crew chiefs demanded higher wages. When their demands were not met, they left. They soon returned, however, because the lay coordinator increased their wages.

The research staff had little further knowledge about what was occurring in the new residences until Mr. Porter visited the research office six weeks after the community move, dressed in a suit and looking very businesslike. He seemed quite anxious to relate something to the members of the research staff who crowded around him upon his arrival. He briefly told of an expanding business and of his influential and responsible role in the "new lodge." He also told the research staff that peace and tranquility were short-lived at the "new lodge." After the move, the lay coordinator began arriving later for work, leaving early, and drinking heavily. At the end of the fifth week he disappeared.

Mr. Smith and Mr. Porter had already begun to take over many of the duties of the lay coordinator before his departure, and afterwards they completely assumed the management of the community enterprise. The changes in the operation of the business and the organization of the two residences into interdependent units were formalized in a document signed by Mr. Smith and Mr. Porter.

The formal relationship between the two member leaders was elaborated in a series of twenty detailed "articles." Primarily, these provisions concerned a distribution of power over the organization. Mr. Porter became the unequivocal work leader, storing the equipment where he lived, receiving the job income, determining the pay of the men for their work, and reporting this information to Mr. Smith, who became the business manager of the "new lodge." Consistent with these responsibilities, Mr. Smith kept the books of the organization, controlled all funds related to both the business and the houses, except for the income from the work, and wrote all checks on the business account for its current bills and payroll. He retained exclusive control over the savings account accumulated as a "stake" before the move, out of which rentals for the two houses were paid. Personal and house maintenance expenses were paid by the work leader for his house out of current income and by the business manager for his house out of board payments by its residents. Cooking and grocery purchases became the responsibility of each leader at the house where he resided. The members agreed that there would be common ownership of all property and equipment pertaining to the business. At the time this relationship was established, two members lived with Mr. Porter, and five were living with Mr. Smith.

At the end of two months in the new residences, by prearrangement before the move, structured interviews with these two key member-leaders, Mr. Smith and Mr. Porter, were recorded. They reported that the residents viewed the new situation as more homelike and congenial. Morale was maintained at about the same level that existed when the "old lodge" was closed. The neighborhood was perceived as much nicer than the one where the "old lodge" was located. They expressed their satisfaction with having their own residences and business, using such phrases as "being in the community," "working with the community," "back living with the public again," "normal." In his interview, Mr. Smith said: "The other [old lodge] had a certain institutional atmosphere, but here in this neighborhood, in this house, it's, I would say almost like normal living in a family." When questioned as to why it was only *"almost"* normal or what it lacked to be normal, he responded, "Well, women, I guess."

The men were more aware, now than in the past, of what the community around them thought of deviant behavior, and certainly demonstrated more interest in how the neighbors perceived them. One of the men expressed it quite succinctly when he said, "You are closer to the community and you don't want to have people say those fellows are a bunch of goof-balls or punks." This was supported by their attempt to apply more stringent rules for their members in the new situation. In this respect, they were more concerned about their personal appearance and the upkeep of their residence. About the latter, one interviewee said, "Everyone knows he has to keep the place neat, and they do keep it better." The level of their increased social awareness was best expressed in the adoption of two entirely new rules; namely, that the curtains had to be drawn while the men were dressing or undressing, and that there was to be no standing, pacing, or loitering in front of the house—this behavior was permitted only in the backyard.

The manner in which ex-mental patients are perceived by a large segment of the public was also brought forcibly to their attention. This event occurred in the group's relations with their neighbors. It is revealed in a verbatim account from Mr. Smith's interview:

> *Interviewer.* Any other reasons for you to say almost normal other than the lack of women?
> *Smith.* No, other than the fact that we are from the hospital and people know that and we are naturally not accepted as we would be if we were just a normal family.
> *Interviewer.* Umhm. Have you had indications of that?
> *Smith.* Well, since Mr. Wolfe made that remark there has been radical change in their attitude around here. [During a conversation with some of the neighbors, Mr. Wolfe had remarked to them that he and the other men were discharged mental patients.]
> *Interviewer.* Has it been negative?
> *Smith.* Yes. Very negative.
> *Interviewer.* In what way?
> *Smith.* Well, we're avoided a good deal more than we used to be. I mean the acceptance [initially] was instant. The kids were over here almost all of the time. In fact, they were too much. They were almost taking the place over. Once they [the parents] found out, that stopped right away. There is a certain reserve—it isn't a hostility—it's a certain reserve that I have noticed.
> *Interviewer.* Coolness?
> *Smith.* Yes. They don't want their children over here and they know we know it, and we're just going to make the best of it—that's all.
> *Interviewer.* Have you had any complaints of any nature?
> *Smith.* Not that I know of. No. Everybody has been very nice to us.
> *Interviewer.* But they are keeping their distance?
> *Smith.* That's right.
> *Interviewer.* As I recall, you said Mr. Wolfe made that remark about three or four weeks after you were out here.
> *Smith.* Yes. Yes. The kids were here every day. They took a great delight in the place. But as I say, it hasn't been all bad because you can't get any-

thing done with a house full of kids. It's been really a good thing in a way but—

Interviewer. It has its disadvantages.

Smith. Yes. They are still friendly. They speak and they all holler at you across the street, but they just don't come in any more.

Interviewer. I see. Were the adults coming in?

Smith. No, the adults weren't coming in. Just the kids.

Interviewer. And the kids, I guess, adhere to what the parents say?

Smith. Oh, yes. In fact, their mothers will punish them if they come over here.

Mr. Smith and Mr. Porter viewed their current roles as much more important than the roles they played at the "old lodge." The rules regarding work had been drastically revised. Although only those men who worked were being paid for their work, there was no longer the rigid rule that in order for a member to reside at the house he had to work. This philosophy in the new situation was redefined so that no member had to work who did not want to work. They were willing to "support" a member and foster his dependency as long as he paid his monthly rent to support the house. In many ways, however, the new situation was perceived much like the old. There were no basic difficulties with the internal economy of the house; their leisure time was spent in much the same manner; the business was earning approximately the income earned in the last month at the old lodge; and the men were doing the same type of work as before. Furthermore, they were having no difficulty in taking their prescribed medication; hence, behavior problems were at a minimum. Both agreed to be interviewed after another six months had passed.

After these two interviews, a major source of information became Mr. Porter's weekly visits to the research office. Ostensibly, the purpose of his visits was to report on the latest happenings of the community group. The research staff encouraged and reinforced his visits because of the information he possessed about the group. However, within a short time, it became obvious that he wished to visit the staff for a second reason, namely, to secure support for his business decisions as work leader of the janitorial service.

Mr. Porter raised on one of his visits the possibility of getting more men from the hospital for the two houses. He emphasized that if he had more workers he could obtain more jobs and make the service grow. Accordingly, the research staff attempted to obtain candidates for the vacancies. Initial contacts with several of the wards at the hospital produced only one patient who agreed to join the group. Later, a former lodge member joined the group, one of the four who returned to the hospital a few days prior to the closing of the lodge. Mr. Porter also mentioned the difficulty he was having in traveling to and from customer's jobs. After the lay coordinator left with his pickup truck, an old car owned by Mr. Porter and Mr. Spears was the only vehicle available. Mr. Porter finally leased a work bus-van at about the same time Mr. Smith purchased a late model pickup truck to be used for shopping and meeting other household needs. Thus, within two months after the move, the group had two vehicles for work purposes.

The continuing success of the "new lodge" was apparently communicated to a number of ex-lodge members. Mr. Smith, the business manager, started receiving telephone calls from them inquiring about the "new lodge." Ex-members then began appearing and requesting admission. A few members began visiting regularly, "inviting" themselves to meals. Finally, to illustrate the positive attraction the new lodge had for former members, one eloped from a mental hospital in order to enter the "new lodge."

Early in the fourth month at the "new lodge," a member of the research staff telephoned Mr. Smith to obtain his opinion about the prospective placement of another ex-lodge member who had requested admission. Mr. Smith announced that Mr. Porter, the work leader, had disappeared. This latest crisis had been compounded because one of the two new members who had recently been admitted to Mr. Porter's house had returned to the hospital. Apparently he had become increasingly depressed and began drinking heavily. The loss of the new man coupled with Mr. Porter's disappearance left only two men residing in the second house. Mr. Smith emphasized that Mr. Porter had been gone three days and the men had not worked during that time. Although they had lost only a few customers, he was aware that they were in jeopardy of losing the rest if Mr. Porter did not return. Mr. Smith was concerned that, if they lost all their jobs, a total disintegration of the house might ensue. Mr. Smith speculated that he might take Mr. Porter's place.

Three days later, Mr. Smith contacted the research staff again. He revealed that he had assumed responsibility for both houses; that he was returning the bus-van (formerly used by Mr. Porter) to the leasing company; that he had been able to retain some of the jobs; and that he had begun driving the men to and from their jobs and was supervising the janitorial work. Mr. Smith, a person with six and one-half years of previous hospitalization for mental illness, diagnosed as a "chronic schizophrenic," was now totally in charge of all aspects of work and life at the "new lodge." Thus, three and one-half years after the beginning of the lodge project, Mr. Smith assumed the same role and status that was originally accorded a professional psychologist. If the rights and duties of the leadership status were fully accorded him in the new circumstances, he would have many of the same frustrations and rewards that past professional and lay leaders had experienced. If the trends established in the past continued, this disabled group of chronic ex-mental patients might gradually and haltingly expand their activities further into the community.

The last research interview with Mr. Smith reveals the extent to which such developments took place. By the time of this interview, he had been sole coordinator of the "new lodge" for four months.

Interviewer. Okay, Mr. Smith, what would you say about the morale out here at this time?
Smith. I think it's good. Mr. Rich is getting a little—used to it—being inside. He said he was unhappy about being inside, but I think he is more or less resigned to it.
Interviewer. Was he lower several weeks before that?
Smith. Yeah, yeah. He was a little unhappy but I haven't heard anything lately about it.
Interviewer. How about the other fellows?
Smith. They seem to be pretty contented. Mr. Spears keeps thinking we're going to throw him out, but it's all an illusion. He seems to like it here.
Interviewer. Umhm. Is he around today?
Smith. Yeah. He's in his room.
Interviewer. Oh. Well, how is the morale compared with when I interviewed you last time in October? How would you say?
Smith. Ah, well they are all making a little more money than they did and they seem to be pretty happy.
Interviewer. So you would say the morale is better than the last time we talked about it?
Smith. Yes.
Interviewer. How does it compare with the morale when you were back at the lodge—that is, the morale now?
Smith. Well, they still like it better here.
Interviewer. For what reason would you say?
Smith. It's more like a home and not so large. Not such a big area.
Interviewer. How does the space compare?
Smith. Well, it's a little lighter. Of course there's fewer fellows and there's plenty of room for what they need and it's a little more compact.
Interviewer. By that you mean—is it too small?
Smith. No, there's plenty of room for the amount of men here.
Interviewer. Okay. How about the cooking and food arrangement—how do these compare?
Smith. Oh, we've got it worked out pretty well.
Interviewer. I know last time you mentioned it was a little difficult to make the adjustment.
Smith. Well, yeah, it was. It's a little different arrangement, but it's worked out pretty well now. It's running pretty smoothly. . . . We have a much bigger cooking area.
Interviewer. Right. How about the housekeeping and gardening as compared with the motel?
Smith. Well, as you can see there isn't—Bill [Mr. Hill] used to do a certain amount of it. Mr. Rich doesn't take much interest in housekeeping at all. Mr. Tucker does a little work in the garden but a minimum. He gets the lawn cut and then he's through. He don't want to do any more. But I've

been able to spend more time on it with him now that I don't have the other place to worry about and I think we can make it.
Interviewer. Shape up?
Smith. Shape up a little better.
Interviewer. How about inside—the housekeeping?
Smith. Well, as I said, Bill [Mr. Hill] used to do some of that but Mr. Rich now is—he vacuums the living room and gradually I think he will—he's getting better. He didn't take any interest in it at all.
Interviewer. He just answered the phone—was that it?
Smith. Yes, he answered the phone and washed the dishes and then he was through. He does a little vacuuming when he feels like it. He's been a little restless lately. He's been taking a walk around the block. His feet have been bothering him. Something like that, but he is taking a little more interest in it.
Interviewer. How about the medication here as compared with the motel?
Smith. Well, I put up their medication every night. Mr. Tucker takes his own. Mr. Spears takes his own. The others I put up every night and it's ready in the morning.
Interviewer. Any trouble with it?
Smith. No.
Interviewer. I know you had a little difficulty with Bill [Mr. Hill].
Smith. Yeah, but that's the only one.
Interviewer. No medication problem with Harry [Mr. Rich]?
Smith. No. The only thing he might forget—it's always out—but he might forget to take it but I've been—I usually remind him. His doctor has cut him down to two pills. . . .
Interviewer. How about behavior problems? How do they compare with—
Smith. Well, it's been very good. They've been very good. I haven't had any trouble at all. A little drinking going on, but it's all well behaved.
Interviewer. No one out of line?
Smith. No. No fights. Mr. Spears had a little trouble getting adjusted but it's worked out very well—
Interviewer. I remember you mentioned this was a difficulty—about a month after you got out here Mr. Wolfe talked to the neighbors and that sort of became a problem. Anything such as that occur?
Smith. No. I've had to gradually get more strict with them. They've become almost unmanageable.
Interviewer. I assume you are speaking of the children?
Smith. Yes.
Interviewer. Is there any problem between the children and the fellows or the adults?
Smith. No, except they've become almost uncontrollable. They did to a certain extent at the other place.
Interviewer. You mean the kids?
Smith. Yeah. I have to put a lock on the back gate and I have to keep them out of the house completely. They were here two dozen times a day for a hand-out and we've cut that down to once a day now.
Interviewer. You mean they are coming now?

Smith. Yes.
Interviewer. They are back.
Smith. Oh, yes. You didn't know that?
Interviewer. No.
Smith. Oh, yes. See their mother forbid them to come over here. Of course they came over anyway.
Interviewer. I see.
Smith. Then their mother decided that she wouldn't stand in their way. So, they took that as a signal that they could practically move in. Her permission was all they needed. So I've had to put up a certain restriction, otherwise they would drive us out of the house completely. But she apparently has no further objection to them coming over here.
Interviewer. Do you know why?
Smith. Well, they have an uncle in the state hospital for one reason. Whether that has anything to do with it I don't know.
Interviewer. Okay. And they found out you weren't so bad after all, huh?
Smith. Yeah. They have a nut in the family so that may have had something to do with it. There may have been other reasons too. I don't know—
Interviewer. You say they got so out of hand that they could have driven you out of the house. What did they do?
Smith. Well, they'd leave the gates open. They'd throw papers all over everything. They are back and forth in the garden on their skates and they would come into the house when I wasn't here. They helped themselves. It just got too much. So—
Interviewer. Did they mingle with the fellows or—
Smith. Oh, yeah.
Interviewer. Or just come in and take what they wanted, so to speak?
Smith. Well, mainly they are here—you know—to get something to eat. They would come in and help themselves. They needed some kind of discipline.
Interviewer. So now they are only allowed in once a day?
Smith. They don't come in at all. I don't allow them in the house at all.
Interviewer. Oh.
Smith. Because they won't leave—well, at one end there's about eight of them and they figure they can all come in—what I do for one I have to do for all of them, so at the present time I'm keeping them out entirely.
Interviewer. Umhm. It sounds as though they were more out of hand than the kids at the lodge.
Smith. Well, the kids at the lodge were fewer—hardly more than three. There's ten in the family. Eight of them were old enough to be active.
Interviewer. I see.
Smith. They have friends that they think are welcome here, too. So it's ten or twelve kids and what I give one they all expect.
Interviewer. So it has blown completely out of proportion.
Smith. Yes. They are unhappy about it but they still get a hand-out every day and twice on Saturday.
Interviewer. Twice on Saturday?
Smith. Yeah. So they can't complain too much.

Interviewer. On the previous two-house situation, I gather from what you've said before you're pretty happy that it's resolved now?
Smith. Oh, yes. That was a great load off my mind . . . because I spent time down there that I felt I should be spending here. It's a relief to have it over with as well as the expense.
Interviewer. Umhm. Does it affect the other fellows in any way or were they not involved in it other than Mr. Spears?
Smith. No, I don't think they were affected in any way.
Interviewer. They didn't care one way or the other?
Smith. No, they didn't care. There was a little more room. That's the only reason I can think of.
Interviewer. Any complaints from the fellows about the room situation as a result of the change over?
Smith. No. He just took Bill's [Mr. Hill] bed—
Interviewer. This is Mr. Spears?
Smith. Yes. They—as I said—had a little difficulty getting adjusted, but it's worked out very well.
Interviewer. He's fairly acclimated now?
Smith. Yes. He feels that he's always going to be thrown out or put away in the hospital. He asked me today when he was—when they were going to put him back in the hospital—
Interviewer. Well, any new rules that have been established as a result of the new situation—that you can think of?
Smith. No, except they are not allowed to loiter in front of the house. Of course that's more or less been that way.
Interviewer. Right. You mentioned that last time.
Smith. Yes. And I don't believe—they do a little drinking but there's no special rule. In fact we've had no special problem to call for a rule.
Interviewer. And as far as you can recall there's no other special rules other than the one about loitering?
Smith. No.
Interviewer. Any new teams or arrangements?
Smith. Oh, I don't allow them to wear—to come in the living room undressed. They have to wear their shoes. They can't come to their meals undressed, but it's always been that way.
Interviewer. Well, that I wasn't aware of last time so—but you mean it's been that way since the beginning?
Smith. Yeah. I mean the other place they couldn't come into the dining room with no shoes on or no shirt—I mean they have to be well dressed or when they go out they have to be fairly well dressed.
Interviewer. Umhm. You mean out into the community?
Smith. Yes.
Interviewer. And they have no difficulty in handling this?
Smith. No. Whatever I ask them to do they seem to be willing to do without any trouble.
Interviewer. . . . Are there any new routines in living?
Smith. No. We have a more standard—get up about 5—eat and go to work. Come home. They usually don't do too much in the afternoon.

Interviewer. Umhm. Well, one of the new routines then, in a sense, I think you mentioned to me: they work until about 11:30 or 12:00 and there's no work in the afternoon.
Smith. Very seldom. Once in a while we get some but very seldom.
Interviewer. Is it that you don't have it or that they don't want to do it?
Smith. They don't want it. We have lots of work. We have really all we can handle and more. We have people wanting us all the time that I have to turn down.
Interviewer. How come you work in the afternoon from time to time? Does the work demand it or what?
Smith. Well, we get a job started that isn't finished but most of our regular jobs are ones that—now we have a job coming up next week that's going to require all day and they'll work in the afternoon. They'll do it once in a while.
Interviewer. They are agreeable to this?
Smith. Yes. Just so it doesn't happen too often. I got started—I thought I'd put in a full day, but they objected to it.
Interviewer. What was the objection, do you know?
Smith. Well, I don't know. They just said they lose interest if they have to work too much.
Interviewer. Umhm. Now you know back at the lodge when Tom [Mr. Edwards, the lay coordinator] was there—I was thinking about this—you know Mr. Porter's group used to go out at 4:00 or 5:00 o'clock in the morning and finish up by 12:00. Do you think this has anything to do with that?
Smith. Oh, yes. Mr. Wolfe especially. He wanted to continue that but that's too hard on me completely. You see I get up at 5:00 now and of course we don't get out of here by that time but he would prefer—he likes that kind of life. The earlier, the better.
Interviewer. So that sort of set the standard for here, you would say?
Smith. Yes, it did.
Interviewer. It's carried over.
Smith. I guess they got in the habit of being done early and they like it that way.
Interviewer. The living arrangements here would you say are more formal or more informal than they were at the lodge?
Smith. Well, a little more coordinated. I don't know about formal but it's a little more like a home—a normal home and I suppose it's a little more informal.
Interviewer. By coordinated?
Smith. For instance, they are all in the same house. Down there they were more or less in a separate unit to sleep but it's fairly close here at all times.
Interviewer. So you've got your finger, in a sense, in everything at once.
Smith. Yes—
Interviewer. How do you see your new expanded role since you've taken on the business?
Smith. Well, I have to be careful I don't take on more than I can handle. I try to have a certain amount of free time and there's always a great de-

mand on my time. I'm trying to do as much as we can without doing too much. At one time there we felt almost harassed or driven because we'd—people were calling up and wanting us to finish a job we'd started and it just got over my head, so I'm trying to be careful now.

Interviewer. How long ago was that?

Smith. Well, shortly after Bob [Mr. Porter] left. I had ideas about building up a big income. He was drawing down pretty good money. But that didn't last long because I was going to have to do most of it myself. I was a little disappointed in Mr. Spears. He didn't want to accept—I don't know if he's really capable of it—but he didn't want to accept any responsibility.

Interviewer. After Bob left?

Smith. Yes. Then there was Wolfe and Davis, but it's pretty much up to me and they'll do—I kind of set the pace and they'll work almost as much as I want them to, but then they'll get discouraged if it's too much.

Interviewer. I see. So you've got to tow the line, so to speak.

Smith. Yeah, and like they say they've got the impression that they are paying me to run this place and they don't want too much responsibility. They say that's what we're paying you for, to take care of these things.

Interviewer. Is that what they say? You mean that money they put in each month?

Smith. Yeah. We're paying you for—to take care of the place for us.

Interviewer. I didn't know that. That's the first time I've heard it. When did that develop? Do you have any idea?

Smith. No, I don't have any idea.

Interviewer. Of course, do they know that you're not getting paid for running the place?

Smith. Yeah. It's just their way—of course they are paying board. I suppose in a way they feel that it's my job. It's more or less like Tom [Mr. Edwards]. I sort of half stepped into Tom's shoes in a deluded sort of way and they'd say that was his job.

Interviewer. Unhuh. Do you, in fact, get more or—

Smith. No, I pay myself the same as them.

Interviewer. Right. Do they know this?

Smith. As far as I know, they know. Most of the time they don't seem to care much.

Interviewer. No matter what you say.

Smith. But when they hand that money over to me, in a sense they feel they are paying me to run the place.

Interviewer. I see. I get it. Well, that's a new wrinkle. That's kinda cute in a way. [both laugh.] It's sort of their excuse maybe for not taking any responsibility.

Smith. Yeah, well if they're happy and contented and do a job on work that we have to do, that's quite a lot.

Interviewer. And you feel satisfied with this? Despite the fact that they say this?

Smith. Yes. It doesn't matter to me. In a way they are running—the money they get is paying for the program.

Interviewer. And you don't feel upset over having this new expanded role? The way it is now?
Smith. No. No. I don't get much choice actually, but it's worked out pretty well.
Interviewer. Of course you have the choice of not doing it versus doing less, but you're satisfied with what you are doing now?
Smith. Yeah. Well, I couldn't very well refuse. Bob [Mr. Porter] left and there it was. I mean, the place would either fall apart or somebody had to do it. Well, anyway—
Interviewer. Have there been changes in the role of the other men?
Smith. No, not a great deal I don't believe, except Mr. Rich.
Interviewer. How did that develop?
Smith. Well, Bill [Mr. Hill] didn't want to be alone, so I moved Mr. Tucker up here and Bill kept going—leaving for extended periods—and there was no one to answer the phone. So we kept leaving him in—
Interviewer. Mr. Rich?
Smith. Yes. To answer the phone and take care of the place while we're away and it's just continued that way.
Interviewer. I see. How about Mr. Tucker? Has anything changed with him—his role—does he work?
Smith. He does a little bit. He helps Mr. Rich now. He dries the dishes and puts them away, cleans the table off. I tell him to cut the lawn. He says he likes to cut the lawn. He likes to work in the garden, but he doesn't do too much.
Interviewer. Does he go out on the jobs at all?
Smith. No.
Interviewer. So his role has changed.
Smith. Yes. Well, I don't know whether—I guess—I don't know whether Bob [Mr. Porter] took him out or not. I guess he did.
Interviewer. Yeah, I believe he did. At least that's what he told me.
Smith. But he hasn't gone out—since he's been over here. We used to take him out to a [night club] but, as I say, Bill [Mr. Hill] complained about being alone, so we left him in and it's just continued that way.
Interviewer. Same with him as with Harry?
Smith. Yes.
Interviewer. How about Mr. Davis. Is his role—
Smith. Mr. Davis is very good. He's shaped up. I was surprised. He and Mr. Wolfe are very good. He'll—he knows what to do and goes right ahead and does it. He doesn't give you any argument. You tell him something to do he goes ahead and does it. I'm very—he and Mr. Wolfe are very—excellent.
Interviewer. Excellent workers, hmmm?
Smith. Yes. The only thing is they don't want to work all day. They just want to do a certain amount.
Interviewer. They both feel that way?
Smith. Yes.
Interviewer. Well, we covered Hill, Tucker, Wolfe, Davis, Rich—oh, Spears. How's Spears' role changed?

Smith. He had a little trouble accepting me in Bob's [Mr. Porter's] job. He objected to it, but he's more or less submitted now.
Interviewer. He's resigned to it?
Smith. He's resigned to the idea and he'll ask me what I want done, but there was an argument there every time at first. I suppose that was natural. He was working with Bob [Mr. Porter] all that time and he and Bob were pretty close friends.
Interviewer. Umhm. How is he now? Any arguments now?
Smith. Not since he moved up here—
Interviewer. Now the situation as you explained with the neighbors and the children—has that been the extent of it with the children and the neighbors or has there been any other difficulties with them or any other relationships with them?
Smith. Well, everybody on the block has been very friendly. They all speak and they seem to be anxious to be friends.
Interviewer. You mean if they see you out they—
Smith. They speak.
Interviewer. They come by or—
Smith. Well, when they come by—we had one lady, one girl down the street stopped—she came in and told us who she was. I think—I never was sure—I think she's a university—from the university, I'm not sure. But they seem to be anxious to be neighborly. The people next door are a little hostile. They object—they have a very young daughter that was in here with another little girl and she fell off the chair one day and cried and she went home crying and that kind of soured it. She was in here drinking soda pop. She was too small, so I don't allow her to come in any more. They are a little hostile but everyone else seems to be friendly.
Interviewer. Sounds like a more friendly situation now than before.
Smith. Yes, I think so. I think they more or less have accepted us and it's a very friendly community—friendly neighborhood.
Interviewer. And there are no difficulties at this point?
Smith. No. We've been very fortunate. Haven't had any difficulties at all.
Interviewer. Have your shopping and buying practices changed since you moved, would you say?
Smith. They are about the same. I go up about twice a week. Sometimes oftener if I need anything and it's about the same. It's a little more convenient here. Shopping is closer. It's about the same as it was down there.
Interviewer. Umhm. Okay. Is the type of work you are doing now in the janitorial service the same as you were doing before?
Smith. Pretty much. We don't do much rug shampooing. It's—we don't do as comprehensive a job as we did before. Of course, it was all more or less new to me.
Interviewer. Umhm.
Smith. I had to learn it from the guys, but I steer away from rug shampoos and stuff like that.
Interviewer. By comprehensive do you mean it's not as complex—is that what you mean?
Smith. Yes.

Interviewer. Okay. Has anyone mentioned leaving?
Smith. No. No, they all seem to be satisfied.
Interviewer. Mr. Davis came back satisfactorily from his week's leave?
Smith. Yes. He says he came back because he ran out of money—
Interviewer. What do the fellows do with their free time, usually?
Smith. Drink beer and sleep.
Interviewer. That's it?
Smith. They don't go to movies much. They stick around pretty close to the place and they might walk up to the shopping center, but most of the time they go to bed early. They get up early—drink a little beer—that's about it. Watch television. Once in a while they watch television—
Interviewer. Have the men been paying their room and board regularly?
Smith. Oh yes. No problem—
Interviewer. Have you had any trouble with the money?
Smith. No, I thought I would. Mr. Spears got—he handed it over and then tried to borrow it back, but I put a stop to that. He got into me for $20.00 and I told him no more of that. So sometimes he gets his back up, but he hasn't so far since he's been here.
Interviewer. Umhm. He got into you for $20.00 since he's been here?
Smith. Yes. His check came and he said he didn't have any money and he'd like to borrow some. I loan all the money and then when—of course James, he gets that extra money, he'll pay me back. I've been trying to get Mr. Rich to hold it down.
Interviewer. Do you loan money out of your own personal pocket?
Smith. No. Out of the funds.
Interviewer. I see. Do you take it off their salary or—
Smith. No. Mr. Wolfe [James] pays me—he'll get $25—
Interviewer. Yeah.
Smith. —and he'll just give it back to me. Mr. Rich's brother-in-law paid me.
Interviewer. That $100?
Smith. The $100 and told me not to loan him any more money but—
Interviewer. It's hard—
Smith. Well, he's broke—I mean, I'm away all day and the money's here. He could help himself. So I loan him $1.00 a day and try to hold it down to that and if—he'll pay it back if the pressure isn't too much. He's got quite a bit of time now. Of course they've all got a little time and then that's the first thing they want to do is drink beer when they get time but—they've got to do something.
Interviewer. Umhm. So you feel it's a fairly good compromise in a sense?
Smith. Yeah. They're happy and they seem to be contented when they get a little beer, so—Mr. Spears is the only one. I asked him when he was going to pay me back and he said, 'I'll pay you back when my check comes.' I said I've already got your check. He has money in the bank. I think it's just a gimmick so I don't loan him any more.
Interviewer. What pay or salary arrangements?
Smith. They are still making $10.00 a week. You see they were making that and they insisted that they couldn't get along with any less. They just

couldn't possibly get along with any less, so I kept it up so far with $10.00 a week except Mr. Tucker. I give him $5.00 and he says I don't do nothing and I get $5.00. But he's happy.

Interviewer. He's happy. I was going to ask you if there was any differential pay. He's the only one?

Smith. He's the only one.

Interviewer. When Bill [Mr. Hill] was here, you got $10.00, Mr. Rich got $10.00, and the rest of the boys $10.00 and yourself too?

Smith. Yes.

Interviewer. There's no differential pay in terms of how well they do, or how poorly they do, or what they do?

Smith. No. No. There's really no incentive to take on more work with an arrangement like that. Up to now I haven't thought of anything better and, as I say, they would probably be willing to do more if I asked them to as long as it wasn't too much. I may decide to take a steady job for Thursday which will give us something every day.

Interviewer. And a little more income.

Smith. Yes. It could be built up.

Interviewer. Has your total income, by that I mean for the business and from the fellows' monthly checks, has this been meeting monthly expenses satisfactorily?

Smith. Oh, yes. I've had to draw on that reserve fund there, but we had some expenses from Porter that we wouldn't have had otherwise. . . . We're not accumulating anything for ourselves paying rent to him . . . we ought to buy . . . but at the present time I don't see any other way.

Interviewer. You're thinking along the line of purchasing something?

Smith. Using the money to buy a house . . . but that's involving yourself for so long—things have been so uncertain for a long time—it's hard to see that far ahead.

Interviewer. Well, it's interesting to hear that—it's the first time that you ever mentioned the idea of purchasing—

Smith. Yeah. It would be nice to have a place that you owned, but it's doubtful right now.

Interviewer. Well, I'm kinda gratified that you've even thought about it. I think it's something nice to think about.

Well, that about winds it up for the very last time. . . .

Indeed, this was the "very last time" that the research staff had formal contact with the small society they had helped to create nearly five years earlier. Lack of agency support for the continuation of the lodge in its old location was in many ways a "blessing in disguise." Both the research staff and the members themselves were forced to confront a possibility which was not even a part of the original research design, namely, testing the viability of the lodge society when financial and consultative support and responsibility for the welfare of the members was completely withdrawn. The original design was not intended to raise the real-life issue of survival in the community, but institutional sluggishness did. The events during the eight months of unanticipated but added formal contact with the lodge group subsequent to the move from its original location yielded far more information about the validity of the research idea than would have been gained by dismantling the society at the conclusion of the original research plan.

As the last interview with Mr. Smith indicated, his combined role as business manager and work leader thrust upon him the identical responsibilities which the research staff had anticipated abandoning with the conclusion of the study by transferring support of the society to an interested agency. The society itself changed significantly. Throughout most of its earlier life, the staff coordinator or consultant was required on occasion to defend the rehabilitative norm by which tolerance of marginal productivity was protected against the business success which so impressed the most influential members of the executive committee. Mr. Smith himself was earlier and consistently one of the most outspoken exponents of the work norm, but in the face of his ensuing responsibilities at the "new lodge" he found his views turned around almost completely. He came to realize his dependence on the other members' financial contribution for the literal survival of the society, despite the lack of some of them in making a significant work contribution. He came to see that, faced with such an issue of survival, he was forced to become more concerned with how members would "fit in" to the small society, more concerned with their individual and personal needs, than he had had to be as a member of the earlier work-oriented society where survival was assured and welfare of persons was someone else's responsibility. He completed the interview by literally negating years of psychiatric hospitalization, talking as an ordinary responsible citizen would of his prospects of buying a house for his charges, and "settling down." There could have been no more fitting reward for the research staff's efforts to create a new social status in the community for these "lost" members of the larger society, to which the discussion turns in the next section.

PART III. INTERCHANGE WITH THE SURROUNDING COMMUNITY

8 THE SOCIOECONOMIC ENVIRONMENT OF THE LODGE

A complete account of any social subsystem should include a description of the social and economic surroundings in which it is placed because the environment is a part of the subsystem's definition (Fairweather, 1967, p. 77). The lodge was an innovative social subsystem aimed at solving the problem of chronic hospitalization for mental illness. The social and economic environment in which it was implanted was very important because some outcome criteria, such as employment, necessarily involved the active interaction of the participants with the surrounding community. Since social events outside the lodge affected the well-being of its members, the lodge had to be compatible with the larger community. Thus, the success of the lodge depended on the social and economic character of the environment in which it was implanted.

The description will have two aspects. One will be the social character of the area as it is revealed in various demographic measures; the other will be the economic climate in which the lodge existed. Both discussions will deal with five demographic divisions of the geographic area in which the lodge was placed. These divisions, adapted from Carr (1948), extend from the largest practical demographic unit of interest to the smallest. They are the following:

1. The metropolitan region;
2. The lodge trading area;
3. The urban community;

4. The local community;
5. The neighborhood.

Each unit on the list lies entirely within the one which precedes it and thus is smaller both geographically and in population. Table 8.1 gives a description of the units on selected information from 1960 census data (Bureau of the Census, 1962a, 1962b). Each of these five divisions permits an analysis of some particular aspect of the social environment in which the lodge existed. Thus the metropolitan region serves as a backdrop to the more immediate environment of the lodge but is not so large an area that it loses its relevance to the present study. The trading area was the business arena for the janitorial service, and it derives its importance mainly from that fact. The urban community interacted with the lodge through the usual civic processes and agents like the police, fire department, and the rest. It had that special relation to the experimental social subsystem which exists among institutions in a modern incorporated city. An analysis of the local community serves to illuminate the position of the neighborhood in which the lodge was placed, and a description of the neighborhood itself has relevance to the problem of implanting an experimental social subsystem in a community.

Table 8.1. A Description of the Five Demographic Units

Census Category	*Metro Region*	*Trading Area*	*Urban Community*	*Local Community*	*Neighborhood*
Population	3,425,664	208,521	79,244	22,754	95
Housing Units	1,178,321	67,493	26,451	6,366	34
Total labor force	1,304,158	81,037	31,075	8,261	43
Labor force in Education and Professional Serv.	147,696	11,313	6,598	1,273	7
% Labor force in Education and Professional Serv.	11	14	21	15	16
Median Family Income	5,700	8,000	8,200	*	*

*Not available.

The Metropolitan Region

The experiment took place in the San Francisco Bay Area of northern California. Figure 8.1 shows that the lodge itself lay almost exactly on the boundary of the two Standard Metropolitan Statistical Areas (SMSA) into which the U.S. Bureau of the Census divides this part of the state. These two SMSA's together form the metropolitan region. It is one of the two great urban concentrations in California which encompasses a population of about four million people and well over a million housing units. It is a major center of commerce, industry, and education, containing two

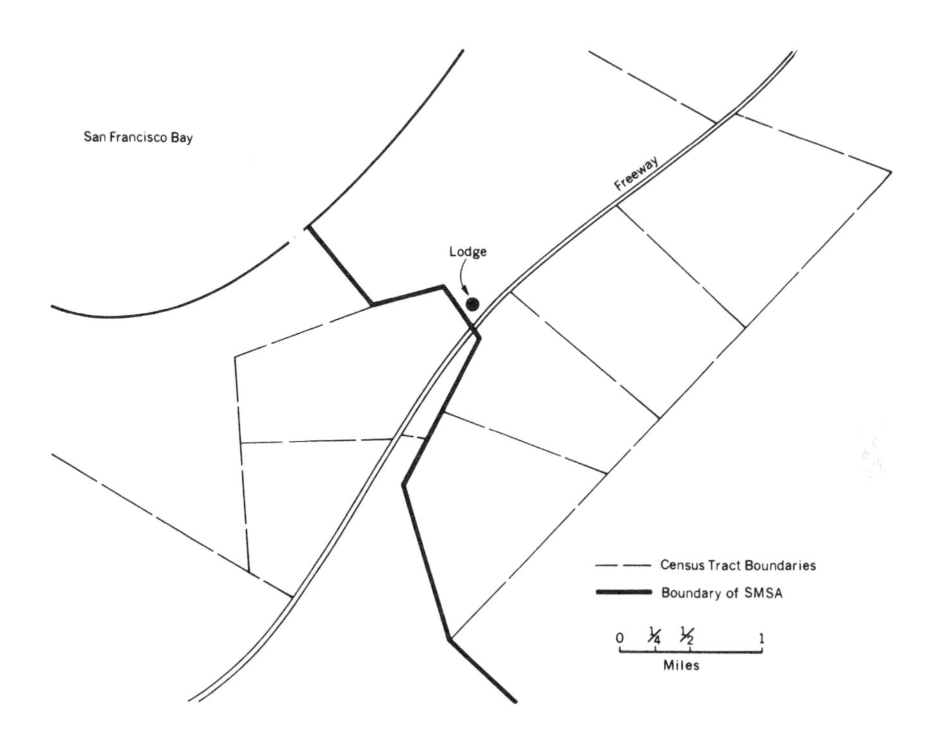

FIG. 8.1.—*Geographic space in which the lodge was established.*

of the state's three major universities. Eleven per cent of its labor force is devoted to educational and other professional services.

By almost any standard, the region is a prosperous one in comparison with the United States as a whole. Over the past ten years, for example, the average annual income per household within the region has been at least $1,000 higher than the comparable national figure, and lying inside the region's boundaries are two of the ten most prosperous "suburban" counties in America. Culturally, the San Francisco Bay Area is unique in California. The major influences in this respect are the city of San Francisco and the two large universities. But there is a new factor emerging in the past decade from the rapid rise of new aerospace industries in the area and the influx of a labor force to serve them. This new factor, the population increase, tends to make the Bay Area more similar to the southern part of the state, but it still retains a distinct cultural and political climate.

In general, a "progressive" atmosphere prevails in the region. Political affiliations are heavily Democratic and the voting behavior in state and national elections usually reflects a "liberal" orientation. Allied to this general cluster of attitudes is an apparently greater tolerance of new groups and movements with goals of political or other social reform. San Francisco and its environs have been, historically, the site of much of this type of activity in the state, and therefore the region might be able to accommodate an innovated social subsystem like the lodge more easily than other parts of the state or country.

The Lodge Trading Area

The largest geographical space with which the lodge interacted directly was the trading area of the janitorial service. This area, within a range of five to eight miles from the lodge site, was the place where the great majority of the janitorial business was done. It was also the place where all of the transactions supporting the lodge as a living unit for its members were accomplished. Only an occasional excursion for these purposes was made outside this area. Several factors, such as the longer travel time to distant points and the plentiful local opportunities and facilities, combined to keep the bulk of the lodge's business inside the five suburban cities and other smaller communities which lay roughly within an eight-mile radius.

The lodge trading area is much smaller than the metropolitan region. With 210,000 persons and 70,000 housing units, the former contains less than one-tenth the social mass of the latter. Following this change in size is a difference in the influence exerted on the lodge by the two areas. Just as the character of the metropolitan region was important in setting the general political and cultural atmosphere in which the experimental social subsystem was placed, so the character of the trading area largely determined the success of the lodge as an economic unit. It is mainly because of the importance of this factor that the lodge trading area is considered here. The operation of the janitorial service was an important half of the "work-living" social subsystem.

The trading area was even more prosperous than the metropolitan region. The 1960 census data, presented in Table 8.1, shows that 14 per cent of the labor force was occupied in educational or other professional services and the median annual family income was about $8,000. The latter figure is $2,300 higher than the comparable one for the region. This high level of prosperity was very conducive to the establishment and expansion of the janitorial service, as will be evident later in this chapter.

The Urban Community

The lodge lay just within the bounds of the incorporated city and very close to the limits of the neighboring one. It was with these two communities that the lodge had its closest relations: with the first because the lodge lay within the city limits and was subject to all the usual agencies of civic government, and with the second because of its proximity and the large number of work and recreation activities carried out there.

These two cities together made up the urban community. Table 8.1 shows that they constitute about a third of the population and housing of the trading area. The trend of greater prosperity as one narrows attention to smaller areas within the metropolitan region continues with this division. The urban community has the highest median family income of any grouping discussed thus far and, similarly, the highest percentage of the labor force employed in educational and professional services.

The Local Community

The local community was a group of five census tracts—the tract in which the lodge was placed and four others directly bordering it. Table 8.1 reveals that this area, lying mainly within about a mile of the lodge site, contained about 23,000 persons and over 6,000 housing units. It is the character of this demographic unit which mainly determined the social and economic status of the neighborhood in which the lodge was located. The real "setting" of the lodge neighborhood from the perceptions of outside observers in the society was the local community. A limited access highway or "freeway" ran through this group of five tracts, dividing them into two roughly equal areas (as shown in Fig. 8.1). This was the most important geographic feature of the unit in its effect on the social position of the neighborhoods. Tracts on the same side of the highway were very similar in most characteristics and were usually very different from ones on the other side of the highway. Generally speaking, in this area the highway separated neighborhoods of high social status from those of low social status.

The Neighborhood

This demographic unit includes the single census tract containing the lodge site. Table 8.1 shows the small population and group of dwellings that it contained. Most of those persons and dwellings were clustered in a small area of the total tract which was around the site of the lodge itself. The characteristics of the tract were mainly those of the immediate lodge neighborhood when it is defined as the smallest and simplest social grouping (outside the family) which exists without benefit of a specific, formal organization. It was the membership in this social unit which gave the lodge its primary social status identification.

Social-Economic Analysis of the Demographic Units

Further analysis of the demographic units just mentioned will follow the work done by Robert C. Tryon (Krech, Crutchfield, and Ballachey, 1962, pp. 319–26). He obtained measures on 33 demographic variables for 225 neighborhoods (census tracts) in the San Francisco Bay Area of California and then performed a cluster analysis on these variables to derive the main dimensions which adequately describe those tracts. All of the 33 variables were abstracted from published data of the U.S. Bureau of the Census.

Tryon's study produced three descriptive dimensions which accounted for most of the similarities and differences among the tracts. Those dimensions and the variables which define them appear in Table 8.2. The original work was done with data from the Census of 1940; when data for 1950 became available, the same census tracts were scored on the three dimensions and the results compared with the first study. The average correlations of scores on these three dimensions for the same tracts in 1940 and in 1950 ranged from .95 to .97.

These high correlations reveal the very high stability of these characteristics of the neighborhoods over time. The measures were taken ten years apart and bracketed a period of great social turmoil since the Second World War and its aftermath intervened between the two censuses. Yet the tracts remained essentially the same in sociological character. Table 8.2 shows that both personal and social situational variables make up the dimensions. The stability of these attributes of the census tracts persisted despite a high rate of migration among tract residents, both in and out of the neighborhoods. This migration exemplifies the high mobility of the American population in general. For example, it is not surprising that within the two SMSA's being discussed in this chapter, over 60 per cent of the 1955 population had changed their places of residence before the 1960 census. This resulted in an average annual population turnover of over 12 per cent. The sociological stability of the neighborhood, in spite

Table 8.2. Demographic Characteristics of the Three Census Dimensions

Dimension	*Demographic Characteristics*
Socioeconomic independence	Higher education
	More professionals and managers
	More female domestic service workers in residence
	More children under 18 years of age
Family life	More single-family dwellings
	More owner-occupied dwellings
	More families with children
	Fewer wives employed outside household
Assimilation	More native-born whites
	More skilled men workers
	More persons of North European ancestry
	More white-collar women workers
	More adult women in residence

of this high rate of change in specific residents, indicates that persons leaving these tracts were usually replaced by immigrants with similar characteristics. Apparently this neighborhood environment, for largely unknown reasons, helped to determine selectively which persons entered or left as residents.

A comparative analysis of the five demographic units (presented in Table 8.1) was performed using Tryon's three descriptive dimensions. The dimension score was established as the mean score of the defining variables for each of the three cluster dimensions. Table 8.3 presents the three dimension scores for each of the five demographic units together with the resultant mean score combining these three dimensions into an index of socioeconomic level. Table 8.3 shows that the neighborhood in which the lodge was located had the lowest scores on all three dimensions—socioeconomic independence, family life, and assimilation.

The overall index representing the socioeconomic level of the five units (the mean score in Table 8.3) is presented in graphic form in Figure 8.2. It shows that as one moves from larger to smaller areas around the lodge, the socioeconomic level of the units becomes progressively higher until one reaches the immediate lodge neighborhood itself. The index than plunges to a very low level. This is a graphic, quantitative demonstration of what is readily apparent to the informal observer, namely, that the particular neighborhood in which the lodge was placed is an island of low socioeconomic status in an area which is particularly advantaged and prosperous. This was a very favorable position for the lodge. It allowed the living system to be established in a neighborhood community which was relatively tolerant of marginal populations and organizations (the lowest socioeconomic group) and yet still placed the janitorial service within easy reach of a prosperous trading area.

The importance of the local neighborhood to the eventual success of the lodge should not be underestimated. From Tryon's results it is clear that these Bay Area census tracts maintained their social identity over at least one 10-year span, apparently in the presence of a selective effect with respect to what specific populations and social organizations would be suited for survival within the area. Judging from this stability of each

Table 8.3. Comparison of Demographic Area on Tryon's Demography Clusters

Dimension	*Metro Region*	*Trading Area*	*Urban Community*	*Local Community*	*Neighborhood*
Socioeconomic independence	.33	.38	.47	.44	.20
Family life	.60	.66	.65	.77	.53
Assimilation	.51	.54	.54	.50	.29
Mean score	.48	.53	.55	.57	.34

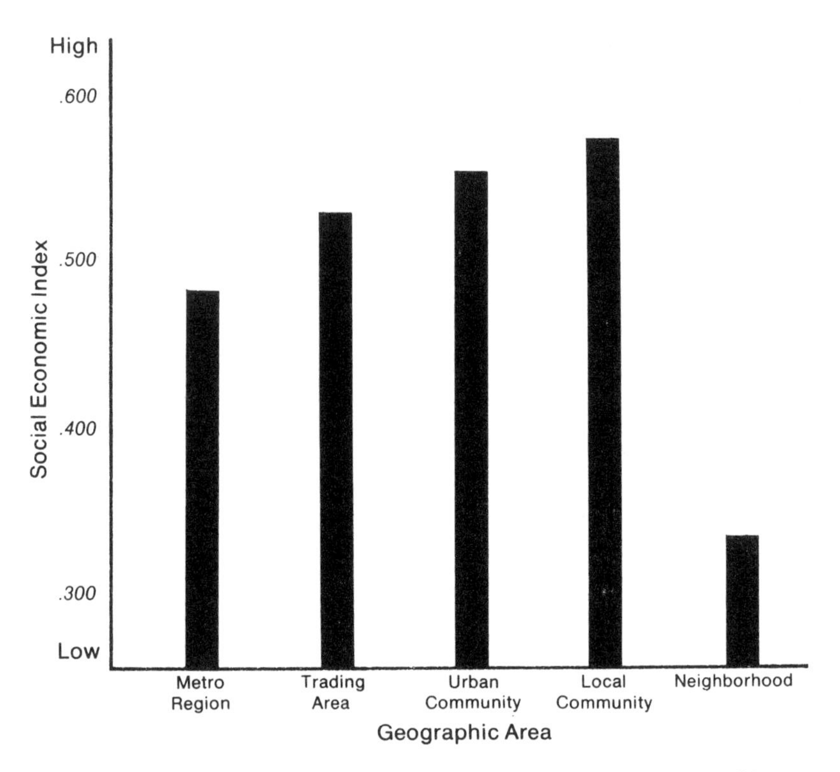

FIG. 8.2.—*Tryon's social economic index in the five geographic areas surrounding the lodge.*

tract's social identity, such populations and organizations had to be compatible with those already existing in the tract, at least to the extent that they had similar social characteristics. Some tracts might lose one identity and gain a very different one through some massive change in population or social reorganization, but the high correlations found by Tryon between dimension scores in these tracts between 1940 and 1950 imply that considerable social stability existed, spanning even such massive social changes as those accompanying a large-scale war.

Such social stability played a major part in the selection of the lodge site by the research staff. It was essential to find a neighborhood which would permit the entry of a group of persons considered marginal to the general society. This meant finding a place tolerant of minorities and of a low social status business operation. These two specifications are intimately related to the variables which define Tryon's demographic dimensions of assimilation and socioeconomic independence. Inspection of Table 8.3 shows how well the neighborhood fitted the requirements of an ideal lodge site from this point of view. It is precisely on those two dimensions that the neighborhood shows the lowest value contrasted with the other, larger demographic areas. For example, on socioeconomic independence, the neighborhood score represents a value only 45 per cent of the same score for the local community; similarly, assimilation stands at 52 per cent, and family life at 68 per cent.

But how did it happen that such an ideal tract for establishing the lodge as a living situation was also so well suited to the operation of a janitorial service, which requires a relatively prosperous neighborhood for the service work? One might expect that prosperous neighborhoods, at the highest socioeconomic level, would be some distance from those—like the lodge neighborhood—which are at the lowest levels. In fact, the lodge neighborhood tract even shared boundaries with some of the most prosperous and high-level tracts in the trading area. To understand how this could occur, we must look at the interaction between the social class and the geography of the area.

In earlier times in American society, the railroad track has been a geographic dividing line separating communities into areas of high and low socioeconomic status. This social fact has even passed into our language. The railroad line may still serve that purpose in many communities, but in the area surrounding the lodge site it no longer does. There is, however, another more modern structure which does systematically divide areas of high and low socioeconomic level in many American communities. It is the limited access highway or freeway. The effect of being on one side of the freeway or the other usually is reflected in the level of income and also in the proportion of residents who belong to minority groups. A few 1960 census figures will show the extent to which this effect of being "on the other side of the freeway" prevailed in the lodge area. As shown in Figure 8.1, the lodge site was almost directly on the freeway itself and was separated from it only by a "frontage road" running parallel to the limited access highway. Along the stretch of freeway about three miles from the lodge site in each direction, there were 13 census tracts, most of which lay entirely on one side or the other of the highway. Two of the 13 tracts were mainly on one side but also extended partly onto the other; for comparative purposes, they will be considered as lying on the side in which they have the most area. The five tracts lying on the lodge side of the freeway showed median family incomes which ranged from $4,753 to $7,563. The comparable statistics for the eight tracts on the other side ranged from $6,950 to $19,129; four of these eight figures were over $10,300. The lodge itself lay in a single tract with one of the lowest figures for median family income, yet it was directly across the highway—a matter of a few hundred feet—from a tract with a similar family income median of almost $12,000.

The figures on the proportion of minority group residents are equally striking. On the lodge side of the freeway the populations of the tracts contained an average of 38 per cent minority group members. On the other, more prosperous side of the highway, the figure was well below 3 per cent. In the tract directly across the freeway from the lodge, less than 2 per cent of the population were minority group members, while in the lodge tract the figure was 42 per cent; thus, there were proportionately 21 times more minority group members in the lodge neighborhood tract than in the tract just across the freeway. In such an environment, a working-living subsystem of ex-mental patients had good prospects of being accepted by the neighborhood as an implanted social institution.

The Lodge Site

The actual site of the lodge (shown in Figs. 8.3, 8.4, and 8.5) was a group of buildings which formerly had been used as a motel. A large main building contained the business office and what had been a coffee shop with commercial kitchen facilities and a dining area. Two additional multiple-unit structures containing 13 dwelling units and a few auxiliary structures, such as garage and storage shed, were built around a large central

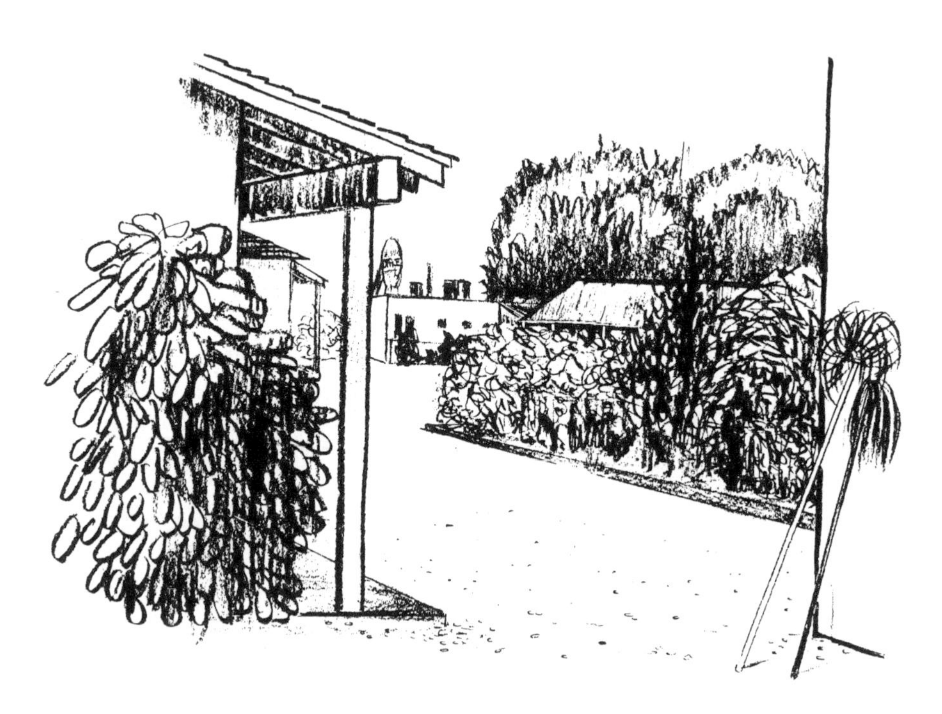

FIG. 8.3.—*Lodge area.*

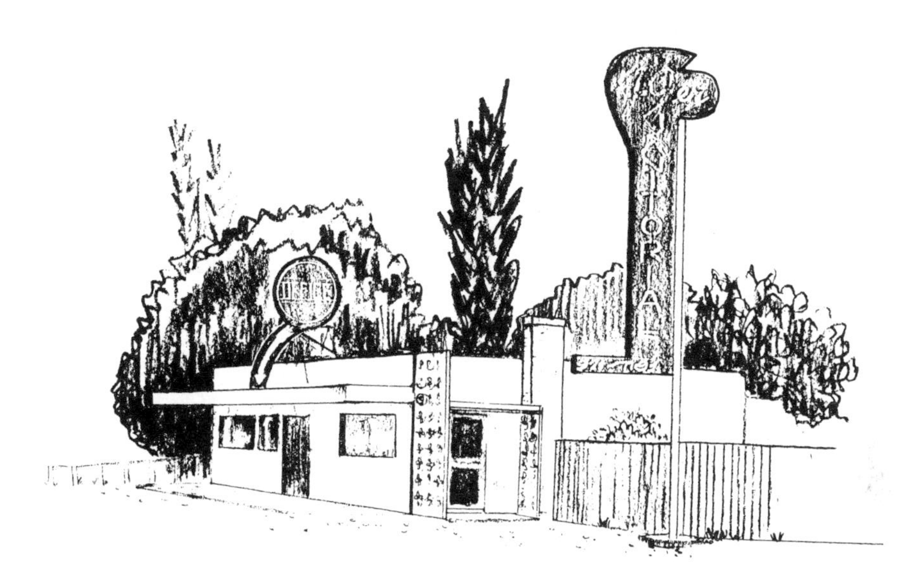

FIG. 8.4.—*Lodge area.*

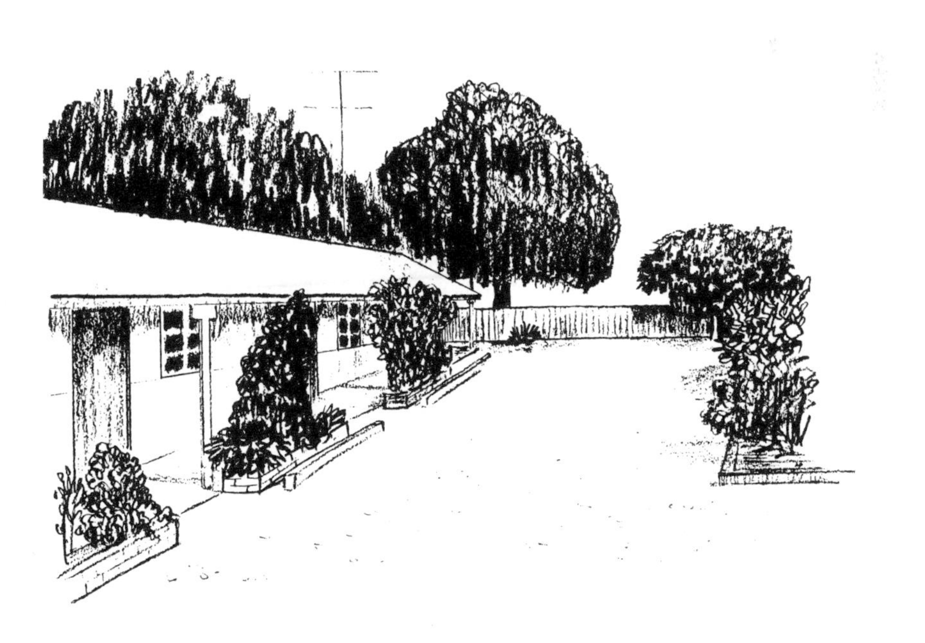

FIG. 8.5.—*Lodge area.*

parking court. The site was pleasantly landscaped, with a planted garden area in the central court and along the front of the dwelling units.

The former motel occupied a corner lot on the "frontage road" immediately adjacent to the freeway just discussed. The neighboring buildings on one side of the lodge were comprised of a group of multiple-unit rental dwellings occupied mainly by a low-income, transient population. Behind the lodge were a few single-unit dwellings occupied by low-income families or by bachelors and college students. These units were often unrented for long periods of time. About half of the housing so situated was owned by a landowner who resided with his wife in one of his own houses in the neighborhood. He was one of the oldest residents of the area, a fact attested to by the naming of a local street in his honor.

Next door to the lodge, on the side opposite the transient rental buildings and on the frontage road, was a large, modern service station, affiliated with a major oil company. The location in reference to the freeway was a reasonably good one, but the station often suffered from poor management and changed hands three times during the period of the research study before it became what appeared to be a successful enterprise.

Beyond the filling station and also fronting on the same road was a large garden nursery which was the most successful and stable industry in the neighborhood. It was operated by a group of six Japanese families who also lived in the immediate neighborhood and made up a large part of the minority-group population in the tract. Many of the older members of these families spoke broken English or none at all, while all but one of the younger members were educated in America and completely assimilated in this society's culture. The only exception was a young housewife who had recently arrived in the country as the bride of one of the nursery employees. The group of families were not all relatives but simply made up a small colony of persons with a common occupation and ethnic heritage.

Next to the garden nursery was one of the city's main branch post offices. Most of its employees lived outside the lodge tract, but one or two of the route carriers and mail sorters sometimes lived in the transient housing near the lodge and one long-time post office employee had been living there for many years.

The Economic Environment of the Lodge

The lodge was established in the last month of 1963 and operated until mid-1966. This was a period of continuous expansion in the American economy, so that the janitorial service operated by the lodge was afforded a good opportunity to survive and even to expand during the time of the study. For example, in the years between 1963 and 1966 the Gross National Product (GNP) of the United States increased at an average rate of 5½ per cent per year in constant prices. More significant for the present discussion was the rise in real disposable income per capita, which the *Economic Report of the President* (1967, p. 41) describes as "the best single measure of consumer welfare." According to that source:

> In 1964 and 1965, real disposable income per capita increased by 5 per cent a year—the equivalent of more than 2 extra weekly paychecks annually. Despite the disturbing rise in consumer prices in 1966, real disposable income per capita continued to grow strongly—by 3½ per cent.

It would be very misleading to use such a statistic to evaluate the ability of the general population in the United States to afford extra services beyond the ones necessary for basic welfare, because a graph of the distribution of income in America shows it to be extremely skewed; hence, mean income figures are greatly affected by the small number of persons with very high incomes. Thus, for example, although there may have been a very generalized disposable income increment of 5 per cent from 1964 to 1965, persons with smaller incomes (who are the most numerous) shared very little in this increment compared to those few who had substantially larger incomes. Fortunately, the lodge was placed within range of a prosperous trading area where persons with relatively high incomes resided. These residents were likely to have a greater use for extra services such as those provided by the janitorial service.

In recent years, California has enjoyed a rate of economic growth which is considerably higher than the national average and, since 1950, its per-capita income has run from three to five hundred dollars higher than the same figure for the country as a whole. In the period from 1962 to 1964, employment rose in the state by 8 per cent and taxable payrolls by 17 per cent. An even greater increase occurred in the area of business services, which includes firms offering janitorial services. In fact, it is apparent that such services expanded at a rate higher than the economy as a whole, both in the state and in the nation. From 1962 to 1964, the number of workers employed in such services in the United States rose by 14.4 per cent; in the same time, taxable payrolls rose by 21 per cent and the number of firms by 12.8 per cent (Bureau of the Census, 1964). The state figures are even higher. For the same period, the increase in the number of such employees in California was 27.4 per cent, and in payrolls 40 per cent, while the number of firms increased by 14.5 per cent.

To look more closely at the economic position held by the janitorial service that operated out of the lodge, figures for areas smaller than the state and for the specific kind of services offered by the lodge business are informative. These figures are available for the metropolitan region and for the lodge trading area for the years 1964 and 1965, a period when the lodge business was growing from a neophyte business into an established enterprise. During that time, the expansion of janitorial service industries —Industry Code Number 7349 in the Standard Industrial Classification

System (Bureau of the Budget, 1957)—was somewhat less inside the metropolitan region than the increase in more general service industries. Within the region, the number of employees in janitorial services increased by 4.7 per cent from 1964 to 1965, while the taxable payrolls increased 6.3 per cent and the number of firms by 7.9 per cent. These figures are equal or greater than the growth rate of the economy as a whole, but they are far below the rate of increase in the area of general services.

But we have only to narrow our attention from the metropolitan region to the lodge trading area to obtain a very different picture; and one which is far more advantageous to a business enterprise like the one operated by the lodge members. In the period from 1964 to 1965, janitorial service industries within the trading area increased in number by 11.3 per cent, employed 15.3 per cent more persons, and paid 16.8 per cent more in taxable payrolls. These figures represent a substantially greater expansion of janitorial services in the lodge trading area than occurred in the surrounding metropolitan region. Most critically, this acceleration in the use of such services occurred precisely in the geographical area in which the lodge did most of its business.

Figure 8.6 shows the development of the lodge business over the entire time of the experiment by six-month intervals. It demonstrates graphically how the business contacts, which at first covered a very wide area, gradually became more and more restricted to an area closer to the lodge site as the business developed over time. The next two charts provide a quantitative description of this developing trade area. In Figure 8.7, one sees that the percentage of job contacts made by the janitorial service declined over time in the local community and in the neighborhood at the same time that they were rising in the two larger demographic units, the lodge trading area and the urban community. By the end of the study the lodge was doing over 90 per cent of its business inside the lodge trading area and 75 per cent of it inside the urban community. These results are a reflection, in data collected during the present experiment, of the rising demand for services noted in the last paragraph. Figure 8.8 illustrates the relative prosperity of the regions by showing the number of jobs per 1000 residents in the same four demographic units. The urban community enjoys the highest rate of usage of the janitorial service, but the increase shown in the lodge trading area (on a much greater population base) is constant and almost as impressive.

The increasing use of janitorial services in the lodge trading area is consistent with the greater prosperity and socioeconomic level of this area compared with the metropolitan region as described earlier in this chapter. Presumably, such services could be purchased more readily by persons with a greater surplus income and they would be more needed by persons with more elaborate living arrangements. Both these conditions existed to a greater degree in the lodge trading area than in the larger surrounding

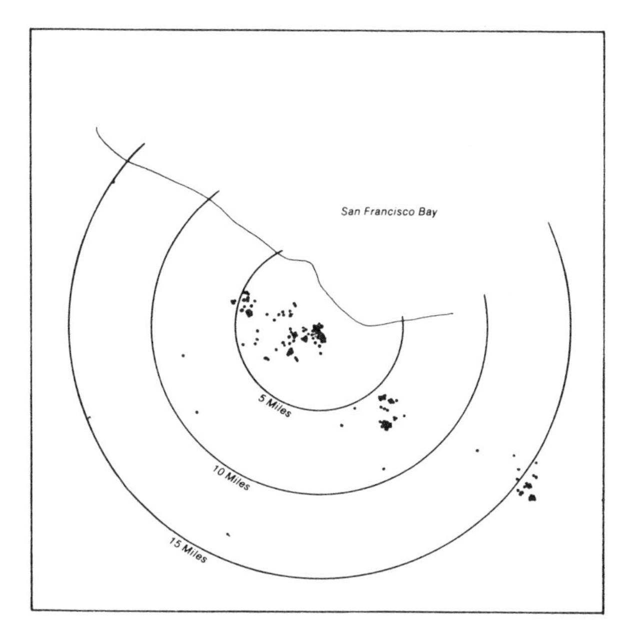

First Six Months

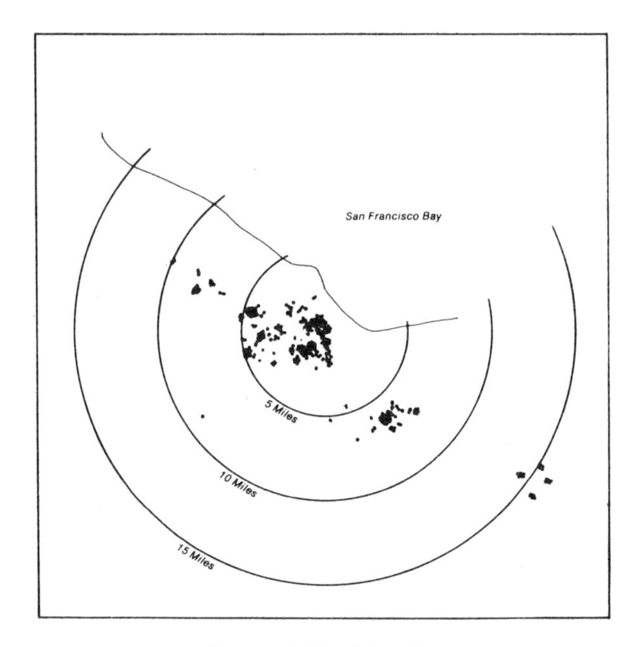

Second Six Months

FIG. 8.6—*Job concentration (each dot represents one job; circles show distance from lodge in five-mile intervals).*

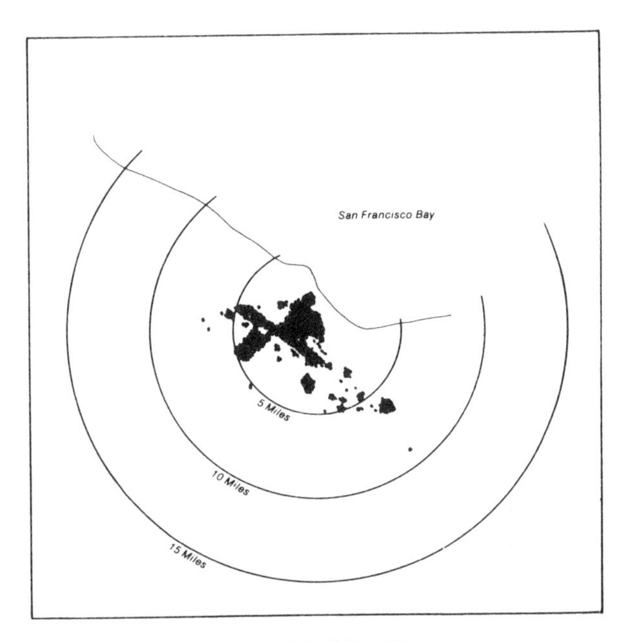

Third Six Months

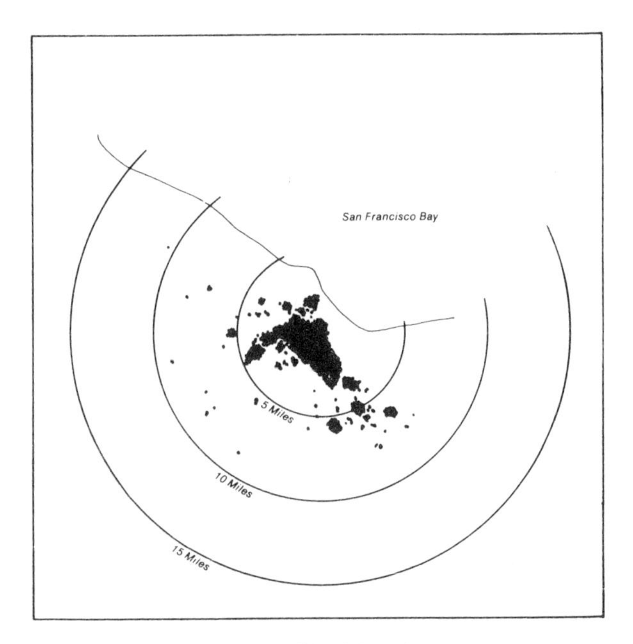

Fourth Six Months

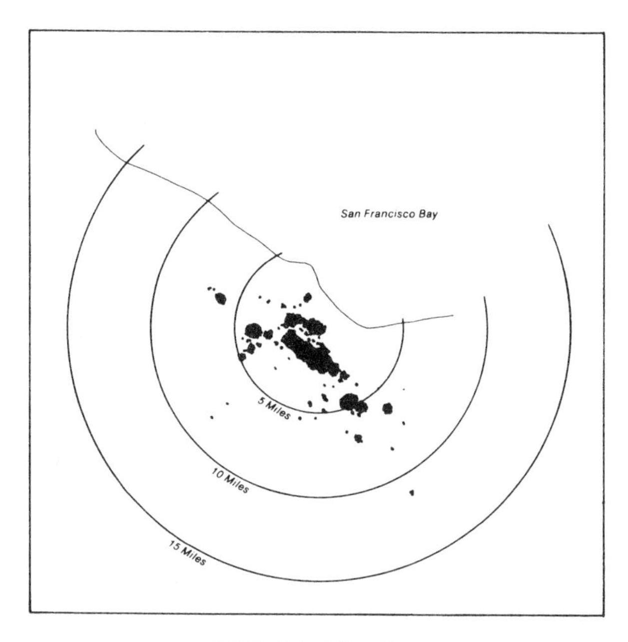

Fifth Six Months

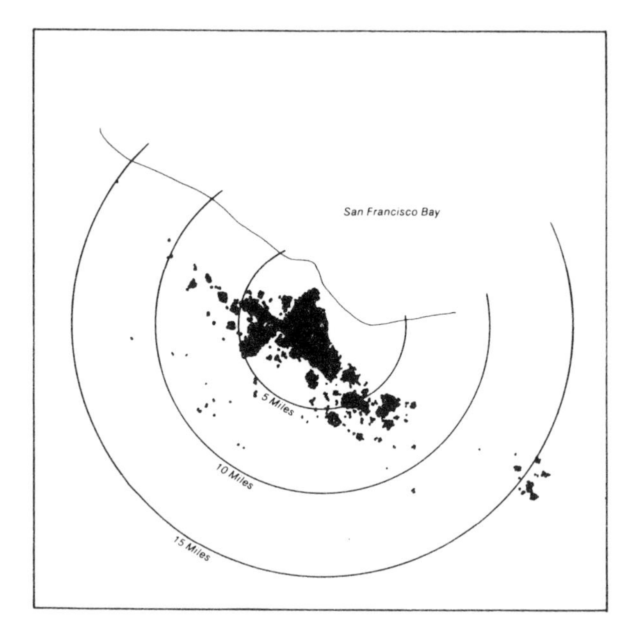

All Thirty Months

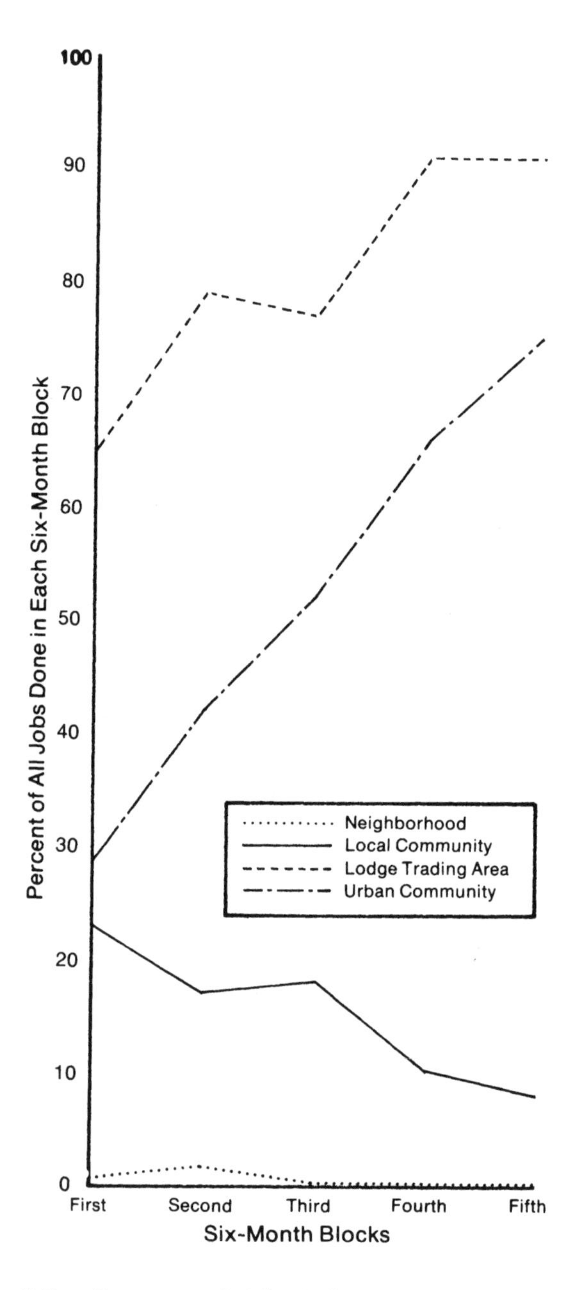

FIG. 8.7.—*Per cent of jobs held in successive six-month blocks in four demographic areas.*

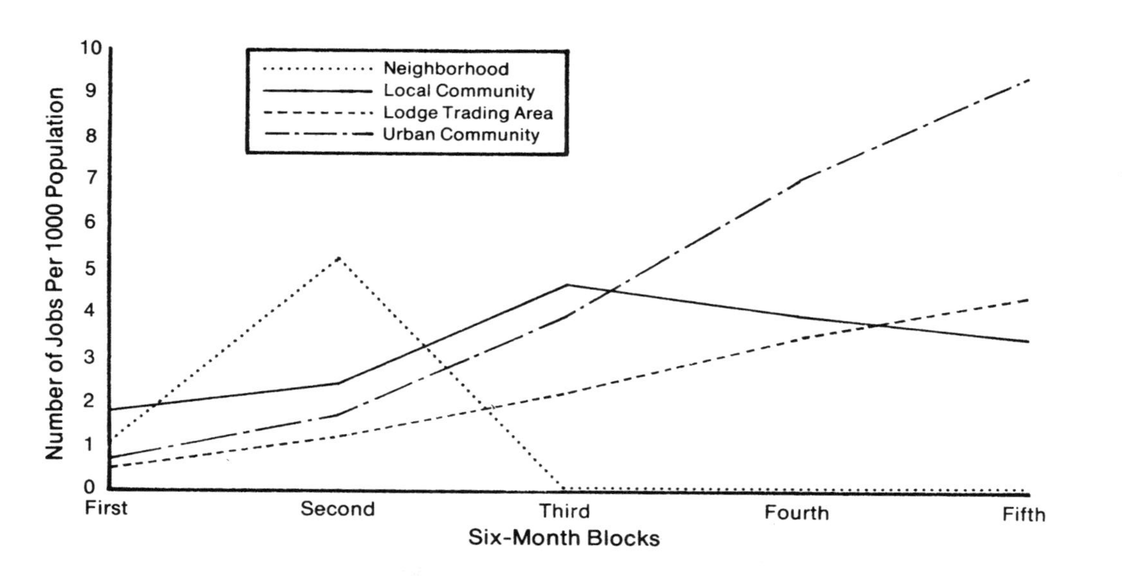

FIG. 8.8.—*Rate of jobs per 1000 population in successive six-month blocks in four demographic areas.*

metropolitan region. The lodge was thus placed to good advantage with respect both to its functions as a living unit and as a working unit. Its location made it socially compatible with the immediate neighborhood, suggesting that it would probably not be expelled, because the neighborhood was of low socioeconomic status and had a high proportion of minority group residents. At the same time, the lodge was close to a group of prosperous neighborhoods which could provide a strongly expanding market for the services which it offered as a working unit. This fortunate but fortuitous combination of circumstances was probably essential to the survival and growth of the new small society.

9 SOCIAL EXCHANGE WITH THE COMMUNITY

Any social institution having a life in a larger community has a wide variety of both formal and informal contacts and exchanges with that community. The lodge had the full range of such contacts during the experiment. As an experimental rehabilitative project, it interacted with the grantee university, with the federal hospital, and with private medical institutions. As a business, it related to various official agencies of local government and to the public who were its customers. As a living unit for its members, it came in contact with the friends and relatives of the men who came to the lodge as participants in the experiment. Finally, the lodge related directly to the neighborhood in which it existed. As a unit, and through the individual behavior of its members, it interacted with the local residents and businesses in the immediate vicinity—an area mainly defined in the previous chapter as the "neighborhood," together with a fringe area of the "local community" which lay closest to the lodge site.

Chapter 10 will present a description of the relations between the lodge and the university, while chapter 11 will concern relations between the lodge and various medical agencies. The present chapter will summarize the remaining social interactions which created the fabric of the lodge's social position in the community. It will begin with the broadest set of such relations, the public who were customers of the janitorial service, and conclude with the most immediate ones, relations in the neighborhood and with the relatives of members.

Relations With Customers of the Janitorial Service

The broadest interaction between the lodge and the surrounding community took place through contacts with the customers of the janitorial service. Chapter 8 showed the extent of the business trading area and the distribution of customer contacts over the period of the study. The trading area was the largest geographical unit in which the lodge had regular direct community interactions.

Customers of the janitorial service were also the most diverse group to come in contact with the lodge members. Like other small firms offering this type of service, the lodge mainly drew its customers from private homes, leaving the bulk of the commercial accounts to very large janitorial service companies. This was generally true, even though the tendency during the last year of the study was to shift more toward commercial jobs because of the better financial return and the better working conditions. Even then, the number of customer contacts in private homes remained higher than commercial ones because of the high number of "once only" jobs done in private houses; commercial jobs were more often contracts for regular service. Table 9.1 shows the number of different customers in two successive years who were private or commercial accounts. The private homes make up 83 per cent and 92 per cent, respectively, of the different business contacts made by the lodge. Chapter 8 showed that these customers came from a wide variety of socioeconomic neighborhoods in the lodge trading area, and that most of them were situated in the high-income tracts bordering on the lodge neighborhood.

In the experience of the lodge members and the research staff, the customers of the janitorial service seemed to fall naturally into three categories on the basis of their attitudes to the janitorial crews and their behavior while the men were on the job. One group of customers appeared to have no knowledge of the status of the lodge members as ex-mental patients and approached the work crews as members of a reputable, local janitorial service. A second group of customers did know of the hospital backgrounds of the men or else found out about it during the course of the job, either in conversation with the crew or because of their observations of the men at work. A third group of customers were persons em-

Table 9.1. Number and Per Cent of Janitorial Service Customers Who Were Private Home or Commercial Clients

	1964		1965	
Type of Job	(*N*)	(%)	(*N*)	(%)
Private home	73	83	170	92
Commercial	15	17	14	8
Total	88	100	184	100

ployed in the field of mental health who knew of the lodge because of their contacts with the experimenters or other hospital personnel.

Generally, the policy at the lodge was not to make a point of mentioning the ex-patient status of the men in the usual course of business but to answer honestly any questions put by the actual or prospective customer. One goal of the experiment was to free the men from the role of "ex-mental patient." The object of the strategy was to avoid both the penalties and advantages of advertising the former status of the lodge members.

The lodge members usually preferred to work for customers who did not know of their former hospitalization at the time of hiring. Such customers often were not present when the work was being done and would readily *trust* the crew to complete the work under the supervision of the crew chief. In many cases, the crew was asked to lock up after finishing if the customer did not expect to return before the end of the job. Under these conditions, the crews usually performed well and any corrections found necessary upon inspection of the job could be made before the customer returned. These were usually the conditions under which commercial work was done and this was one of the reasons that such jobs were preferred at the lodge. Customers of this kind generally made only reasonable demands and, except for an occasional person who was impossible to please, only complained if the crews truly had done poor work.

The least satisfactory customers were those who were mental health workers. It seemed apparent, both to the work crew and to the staff and lay coordinators, that customers who were mental health workers had very little faith in the ability of the lodge members and did not trust them to do a competent job. Often, such customers would insist on observing the work of crews very closely and might even direct the members in their tasks and change the assignments made to the workers by the crew chief. In one case, a customer, who was a nurse in the mental hospital from which the lodge members had come, made a special trip home at noon to check on the work she was having done by the janitorial service (p. 318).

Working under these conditions usually generated a whole series of ill effects on the performance of the work crews. The intervention of the customer often undermined the leadership of the crew chief and weakened the group's ability to operate as a team. It also aroused hostility from those members who, as time went on in the experiment, were more and more jealous of their autonomy and resentful of anything resembling hospital control. Experiences of this kind only served to confirm the opinion of many lodge members that mental health workers were unreasonable and authoritarian people. There were notable exceptions to this rule. One of the favorite customers at the lodge was a psychiatric nurse who had an uncommon ability to relate to the men in a friendly and natural way, and the crews always made special efforts to do a good job for her. In general, however, jobs for mental health workers were very unpopular.

This was so much the case that when the last job of this kind was done, the lodge members had a small celebration.

The tendency of mental health workers to interact with the lodge members in a way showing distrust of their competency is consistent with the findings reported in chapter 16 that hospital staff had very low expectations for the posthospital adjustment of such patients. These expectations were probably based on their hospital experience supporting perceptions that patients are dependent persons who cannot act without staff supervision and tend to return to the hospital in a fairly short time if discharged. This finding suggests there is apparently little appreciation of the part played by the hospital staff and the hospital social system in shaping and maintaining the dependent behavior of the patients who live there. With such perceptions of patients and ex-patients, the mental health worker tends to fall immediately into his supervisory role with the lodge members, whether they are able to act autonomously or not. For their part, and despite all their resentment of the consequent loss of autonomy, the lodge members were usually unable to resist complying with a mental health worker who approached them in an authoritative way. They were as well trained by the hospital social system in this regard as was the typical hospital staff member.

There is further evidence suggesting the special features of the relation between lodge members and mental health workers in the experience with customers who knew of the ex-hospital status of the men but were not employed in a medical setting. This type of customer often behaved in a way similar to hospital personnel and often with results equally disastrous to the crews; but no general dislike of this type of customer resulted at the lodge. The crew members were entirely open about their identity when conversing with customers and often mentioned that they were ex-patients. Generally, this had no effect on their relations with the person if the work was going well, but if the work was poor, the customer was more likely to react with greater patience than with annoyance. The same was true of persons who hired the janitorial service with full knowledge of the background of the men.

There were, of course, incidents in which a customer suspected that the men were ex-patients and the stereotype of the "mental patient" led to a significant change in attitudes and behavior. One such incident is especially revealing because it occurred when the peer coordinator was in charge and, because of his responsible position, he was not perceived as an ex-patient by the customer. The incident is related in the research journal by the first staff coordinator at the lodge:

> *Statewell Incident of 5/25:* All of the men were taken to the initial day's work at 9 A.M. that morning and both Mr. Sears [peer coordinator, p. 64], and I then left after he showed them what was to be done. I reached the lodge first, as he had some errands to run. After he arrived, Mr. Murray

[business manager] indicated that Mr. Swanson, [a construction] foreman on the Statewell job, had called at approximately 10 A.M. stating that he was quite dissatisfied with the fellows on the job—that "they were running around" and did not know what to do. In addition, he said that professional window washers used squeegies and brushes and not spray cans and rags. He also indicated to Mr. Murray that he was concerned about thievery. All this sounded quite preposterous in light of the fact that they had only been on the job for one hour as well as the fact that these fellows had worked on large jobs before and it was apparent that they were not running around but probably were still in the process of organizing the work, as it was within the first hour on the job. The question also arose, what was Mr. Swanson doing observing them within the first hour. Prior to going out there, we postulated he had found out that they were patients or ex-patients.

Mr. Sears went to see Mr. Swanson at lunch time and questioned him on the whole situation. Swanson said he had seen several fellows staring out the window. This is from his vantage point outside the contractor's shack, which is many yards away. Mr. Sears said it was obvious that he had no legitimate criticism and pointed out to him that Swanson himself had indicated that no water was to be used inside as it might spoil the quarry tile, and, therefore, we were not using squeegies and brushes. This he acknowledged as remembering. He then fairly bluntly, but in a discreet manner, asked if these fellows were patients, which we had suspected, and Mr. Sears responded with, "They are ex-patients—they have been discharged from the hospital and have no connection with the hospital whatsoever at this point." Swanson then indicated that he thought they probably knew what they were doing, and that was that. It was later learned that an electric drill of his had been stolen and Mr. Russell, our [lodge] foreman on the job, reported that Swanson asked him privately if he had any light-fingered men in his crew. It is interesting to note, as we have done in the past, that this man essentially hired our men because of the good estimate, then found out that they were ex-mental patients and, therefore, became highly critical of the work they had hardly even begun and, in addition, he had them classified as thieves. Since that incident, he has become increasingly more positive in that he has been extremely well pleased with the type of work and the time it is taking. We have been able to meet all the demands of the schedule he has laid down for us for completion of work. It is also interesting to note that Swanson treated and responded to Mr. Sears as though he were not a patient and Mr. Sears very readily accepted this role. This was pointed out to Mr. Sears by me after the incident and it was obvious that he was pleased at being viewed by someone in the community as a non-patient.

Continuation of Statewell job: As reported in the last progress notes, things seemed to be working out satisfactorily. However, succeeding weeks brought forth the actualization of my hypothesis concerning clients who find out the fellows are ex-mental patients. It seems as though Mr. Swanson, although a nice fellow, became increasingly more critical in terms of quality of work and time allotted for the job. There were several instances where Mr. Sears had to remind him of agreements made with him con-

> cerning when certain jobs were to be completed. However, in fact, some of the work was careless and his complaints were legitimate, but for the most part not so. We had made additional efforts to please him by working in the evening to meet a deadline, but the most significant problem was when we initiated the cleanup of the outside upstairs windows. It was obvious that we were going to have difficulty with this and he spotted this right off the bat and wanted to know if we could do it. He said if we could not, he would get another outfit in to complete the job. We attempted various techniques, all of which would have worked but would have taken a long period of time. Consequently, we decided to give up that aspect of the job and deduct $150 from the total cost of $990. Subsequently, during a visit out there to pick up some of our equipment we spotted the "new and more experienced janitorial service" that was hired to clean the upstairs windows. Swanson had indicated that it was costing him $275 to have this job done because the bottom windows needed cleaning as a result of water running down them while cleaning the upstairs windows. It did my heart good when we observed the two men from the recently hired janitorial service utilizing pretty much the same method that we were going to use but thought too slow. To boot, after watching them for about 15–20 minutes, it was obvious they were not dirtying the bottom windows because they were only cleaning part of the upstairs windows a small piece at a time. My original thoughts on this were that maybe this was too big a job for us to handle and that we should stay away from this type of office building work in the future. However, after seeing the other outfit working, I was convinced that we could continue to estimate jobs like this, providing we had an adequate number of fellows who could climb the high ladder.

Customers who approached the janitorial service as if it were any other business rather than an ex-mental patient organization were the group who had the most stable set of relations with the lodge members. This might have been so because the relation and attitudes were formed solely on the basis of the business contact and were not subject to the vicissitudes of private knowledge and friendships through which the lodge business came to the attention of other groups of customers. We have mentioned the subjective impressions and naturalistic observations that demonstrated the three types of customers were very different. Data from customer surveys show that the three groups came in contact with the lodge through very different channels.

Table 9.2 presents the evidence. It shows that customers with no knowledge of the ex-hospital status of the lodge members found the lodge mainly through its newspaper advertising, with the next most important avenue the recommendation of a friend who had used the service. Their contact through "other sources" includes listings in the telephone directory, the sign on the lodge building, the business card of the janitorial service, and observing the crew at work for a neighbor.

The customers with knowledge of the ex-hospital status of the members generally heard of the lodge from a friend or from "other" sources. In

Table 9.2. Per Cent of Each Type of Customer by Source of Contact with the Janitorial Service

Type of Customer	News Advertisement		Friend		Business Associate		Other	
	1964	1965	1964	1965	1964	1965	1964	1965
No knowledge of ex-patient status of lodge members	45	49	24	35	17	4	14	12
Knowledge of ex-patient status of lodge members but not a mental health worker	17	21	33	40	17	18	33	21
Knowledge of ex-patient status of lodge members and is mental health worker	0	17	20	8	10	25	70	50

this case, other sources include relatives, other businesses, and their own prior experiences in former dwellings, or through friendship with one of the lodge members. Less than a quarter of the contacts in this group were through news advertising.

The mental health workers mainly listed "other" sources as relatives, hearing of the lodge at a hospital staff meeting, hearing of the lodge at work in the hospital, and the like. Many of the contacts in this group listed as "business associate" referred to other mental health professionals and workers. Table 9.2 shows that at the time of the 1964 survey, early in the life of the lodge, customers in the mental health field never found the lodge through the news advertising but almost entirely through "other" sources and through friends. This is a quantitative expression of a fact well known informally to the experimenters during the study: when the lodge was first established there was an effort on the part of mental health workers who knew of the project to give support to the men at the lodge in their attempt to start a business. There is no doubt that the effort to help was sincere and very generous. Unfortunately, this generosity of spirit was often accompanied by authoritarian role behaviors and attitudes which have been described earlier that promoted discomfort and hostility among the former patients who were not full-fledged workers.

Relations With Local Government Agencies

As a business and as a group living situation, the lodge was the object of interest by several agencies of local government which had the task of regulating the practices of such enterprises. Most of the contacts made by government agents were routine and mainly concerned the enforcement of health and fire regulations. The public health agency became concerned with the inspection of the kitchen facilities, especially because of the original but abandoned plan to operate a short-order restaurant at the lodge (p. 49). The fire inspector made regular visits to advise on adequate fire precautions and to enforce the city code prescribing minimum standards for such premises. Without exception, there were cordial relationships between the lodge members and the agents of these two departments. The attitudes of the inspectors toward the lodge and its members were uniformly positive and they expressed approval of the lodge as an enterprise.

The government agency most impressed with the community lodge, however, was the local police department. As part of the experiment, the chief of police was asked for an assessment of the experimental site each year. In his first reply, the chief of police reported that the lodge site had been "a constant police and neighborhood problem in the past," before the start of the experiment. He said further that the location had been the source, just before the opening of the lodge, of an "increasing number of Alcohol Beverage Control liquor violations, fights, littering, complaints of suspected prostitution and narcotic violations. It truly could have been called a trouble spot and necessitated constant police surveillance." All of this stopped when the lodge members occupied the premises. The chief expressed appreciation for "the manner in which this location is now being operated" and for the cooperation with his department in ending a chronic trouble spot in the area.

Relations With the Route Salesmen and the Neighborhood Service Station

In the course of maintaining the living and working arrangements at the lodge, the members established relations with a number of sales and delivery men who supplied the kitchen and the janitorial service with staple items. The kitchen staff had regular contacts with delivery men for dairy products and for prepared meats, while the janitorial crews dealt regularly with the neighboring gasoline service station and with the salesman for a janitorial supply company.

The salesmen for all these services were seen annually by the research staff in a structured interview which assessed their attitudes toward the lodge and its members. The interview sought to measure the attitudes of the salesmen about the lodge as a rehabilitative unit and as a business venture; about the assets, liabilities, and future of the lodge; about any changes which they might have noticed over time; and about the adjustment of the members themselves and their own relations to these men. Table 9.3 summarizes the per cent of positive, neutral, and negative atti-

Table 9.3. Per Cent of Positive, Neutral, and Negative Attitudes Expressed by Salesmen about the Lodge

Salesmen	*Positive Responses* (%)	*Neutral Responses* (%)	*Negative Responses* (%)
All salesmen responses	77	17	6
Service station	67	23	10
Janitorial	91	9	0
Dairy	95	5	0
Prepared meats	63	26	11

tudes expressed by the representatives of these various firms, together with the overall attitudes of the salesmen as a group.[1]

The most prominent feature of the table is the relatively high proportion of positive attitudes expressed toward the lodge, which verified the general subjective feeling of the members and research staff during the experiment that excellent relations were maintained with the salesmen who made regular visits. The somewhat high proportion of negative responses from the service station attendants was due mainly to the responses of one of the three attendants who recalled some trouble which had occurred early in the project with one of the lodge members who had stopped taking his medication and had become overtly psychotic while living on the grounds (p. 55). Apparently he had caused some trouble with customers at the service station while in this state—about which the research staff never learned.

Generally, however, the service station attendents (and the owner) were glad to have the lodge project located next door. They all testified to the improvement in the appearance of the neighborhood as a result of the repair and painting done by the members, and expressed great relief at the positive change in neighborhood atmosphere already attributed to the lodge occupants by the chief of police. They emphasized this change since it affected their physical security in what had been (and in some ways still was) a rather dangerous neighborhood. Both the improvement and the danger were expressed aptly by one of the attendents during the interview:

> I'd rather have these guys that we have now, because when we had the other—the motel going on, the bar and everything—it was just people parking on our lot; and when I'd open in the morning, I had to take an hour just to sweep the front yard out because it was full of beer cans and everything. At least it's quiet. The only thing I object to is that fence [one built by the lodge members between the lodge and the service station]

1. The average per cent of agreement reached by two raters was 87 for classifying the interview responses as positive, neutral, or negative.

> being too high. When they had the people living here the lights used to be on at night and people walking around. Since we've been robbed the last few times, I notice how dark it is over here and how that fence blocks off everything.

The reference to being robbed involved the incident already mentioned (p. 157) in which the lodge members acted as very responsible citizens. The owner of the service station described it this way:

> That's the time I'm sure glad the [lodge] was here; because we got robbed the first of July and it was after closing hours and my boy got knifed. They stabbed him about eight times in the neck and they tied him up in the back room. Well, the kid crawled outside and gave one holler. It wasn't a very loud holler. Now this area out here is isolated after 10 o'clock; I mean it's shut down! Well, the way I understand it, one of the boys was in the mess hall, and they heard him and ran over here. One of them called the police department and the other tried first aid on him; and if it wasn't for the boys at the [lodge], that kid would have died, because no one would have seen him.

The janitorial supply salesman enjoyed very good relations with the lodge members, which are reflected in Table 9.3. He had been associated with the project from the start and had helped in the training of the members in use of equipment and supplies. He was well known to the men, who treated him as a personal friend. He found this very gratifying, as is clear from one of his responses during the interview:

> Whenever I appear on the scene—let's say, for instance, they had a job where they had to do some scrubbing on some brick—and, when I arrived on the scene, the fellows all said, "Hello, how are you! Just the man we're waiting for!" You know, this sort of thing. It makes you feel good. They have been very, very nice—all of them. Some of them are a little quieter than others, naturally, and some more aggressive than others, but all of them seem to work well and, as a matter of fact, I've never seen any of them on the job that wasn't doing something.

He was also able to comment on changes he had observed in the men at the lodge, because he had been connected with it from its early days and had been a regular weekly visitor and instructor in the use of new equipment over a fairly long period. He commented at one point on the motivational change he had observed at the lodge over time:

> I would say that, from my first contact up to the present day, that, when I meet the fellows out in the yard when I'm delivering something in the evening, why, all of them seem very happy. None of them are moroseful or that kind of thing, and they are always doing something. Once in a while I see a fellow sitting in a chair daydreaming or something, but that's a rare occasion. At first there seemed to be a little reluctance—or I shouldn't say reluctance, but some of them didn't want to learn, or it seemed that way

—when I was teaching them how to run a floor machine. They didn't want to learn. . . . Well, now that doesn't seem to happen anymore at all. . . . Everyone seems eager.

As was the case with all of the persons in contact with the lodge, he was very enthusiastic about the idea of the lodge as a rehabilitative unit. He readily grasped the implications of the research for the rehabilitation or adjustment of other groups. At one point in the study, he discussed at length with one of the research staff the problems of older persons in the society and the need for adequate programs for their care and integration into its social systems. The application of the lodge idea to this social problem had occurred to him because of the problems he was experiencing at the time in finding a suitable place for his aged mother-in-law, who was in need of support and medical care and who was largely dependent on his own modest resources.

The dairy supplies salesman was also highly positive in his attitudes toward the lodge and was probably the most enthusiastic and friendly of the regular visitors. He perceived the men as living in a very friendly and supportive environment, which he likened to the armed forces. He obviously enjoyed stopping at the lodge and was usually greeted by a number of the men with whom he was on joking terms. In discussing his relations with the lodge, he pointed out that he actually spent more time there than in any of the other places he served. A little later he said:

I stop in every morning and every evening when I come in. So I'm in there, really, twice a day. This is the only place I do stop in twice a day. Not for service, because I do deliver their products early in the morning, but I usually stop back by and holler at them; or, if I pass by and some of them are standing on the outside, I blow the horn at them, you know. Well, actually, to me—I mean, it reminds me a lot of the service, you know. Where there's a lot of guys, you know. Its very seldom you run into a group of guys like this.

It is perhaps significant that this respondent, who was black and lived in the ghetto area near the lodge, was the only one who mentioned this aspect of the lodge community with an obvious affective response, comparing it to what might have been a similar experience he had had in the service.

He was not, however, the only one to mention the friendliness at the lodge which made it a pleasant place to stop. The first dairyman who had begun service at the lodge and had handled the account for some months before being replaced, felt the same friendliness. He had described it in this way:

They are the kind of group you can sit down and talk with; and they really make you feel good after spending a few minutes with them. I just always look forward to catching this stop.

A similar feeling was shared by the salesmen for prepared meats, even though they expressed less positive overall attitudes about the lodge. This less positive overall score was produced by negative responses, although none of their negative opinions had to do with the friendliness of the men or with the value of the lodge as an institution. Also, in common with the dairyman and the janitorial supply salesman, they had the highest opinion of the abilities of Mr. Smith, who was in charge of the kitchen and commissary at the lodge. Their criticisms had to do with what they saw as the isolation of the lodge site and the possible evil effects which this might have on the members. One of them was especially strong on this point because he believed that the main bad effect of an institution like a mental hospital was the isolation of the inmates from a diverse group of people. He thought that the lodge site might inhibit the extensive social contact which he felt might have a therapeutic effect on its residents.

These two men made some of the most thoughtful comments about the experiment. They saw the value of the lodge to the members as a place which offered them an alternative to hospitalization and they considered possible difficulties which such places might have if instituted on a large scale. One difficulty they foresaw was a possible conflict with organized labor. Though union men themselves, they favored development of such alternatives as the lodge on the scale necessary to handle the social problem of chronic hospitalized patients. The realism of these concerns was shown during the experiment when the representative of another janitorial service visited the lodge and protested that it was unfair for a government-subsidized organization to compete in the private sector of the economy. He promised legal action, but ultimately no action was taken, perhaps because the lodge did not compete on a large scale for the commercial contracts which provide a good part of the revenue in this trade. It was also classed as a rehabilitative organization by local government, which avoided potential conflict with labor unions in the same field.

Relations With Local Businesses

In addition to the gasoline service station next to the lodge site, the members had continuing contact with a wide variety of local businesses in the course of operating the janitorial service and sustaining the everyday affairs of living. One of the most important of these contacts was the nearby supermarket. This store was the source of a substantial portion of the groceries bought by the kitchen manager at the lodge and an extensive set of relations developed over time between the manager of the store and the lodge representative. This relation became so friendly that on one occasion, when one of the lodge members was caught shoplifting a bottle of whiskey in the store, the management staff did not involve the police but instead telephoned the staff coordinator and released the lodge member to him without pressing charges or taking any other action.

Other regular relations evolved with a variety of businesses, including a laundromat where the lodge sent its linens and uniforms, a small, local grocery used by the members for small purchases and check-cashing, a local gardening supply store patronized by the janitorial service, and a bank near the lodge in which most of the members held checking accounts and cashed their payroll checks every week.

The various businesses just described and others in the vicinity of the lodge site were surveyed at the conclusion of the study in an attempt to measure the extent of their knowledge of the lodge as a janitorial service and to determine their attitudes toward the members and the project. The survey instrument used five subscales. They were: knowledge of the residential status of the lodge; knowledge of the janitorial service; attitudes toward the lodge organization; knowledge that the members were ex-patients; and attitudes toward the lodge members as ex-patients. The research instrument was specially developed for the study and pretested in a nearby community.

The survey revealed that there was little knowledge of the lodge among local business personnel, with many of the respondents not knowing the lodge's location or having a very clear idea of the function of the lodge. The attitudes toward the lodge as a janitorial service tended to be quite positive. Few people knew the ex-patient social status of the members, with less than one-quarter of the respondents having such knowledge. However, when the knowledge of their ex-patient status was imparted to the respondents their attitudes became even more positive. Apparently the knowledge of the former mental hospital status of the lodge members did not lower the esteem of the people surveyed.

Table 9.4 presents the matrix of correlations among the scales of the survey instrument for this sample of respondents. The table shows that those persons who knew most about the location and function of the janitorial service as a business tended to know of the ex-patient status of the members as well (*r* of scale 2 with 4). People with the most knowledge of the location and function of the janitorial service also tended to have positive attitudes toward such a business and to think of it as an asset to the community (*r* of scale 2 with 3). However, they were not particularly prone to have highly positive attitudes about the lodge after finding out the full details of the men's hospital status (*r* of scale 2 with 5).

Table 9.4 also reveals that persons who had positive attitudes about the lodge retained those attitudes after finding out that the men there were ex-mental patients (*r* of scale 3 with 5). This is consistent with the observations already made about the slight increase in approval by the respondents after information about the ex-mental patient status of lodge membership was revealed. It is also interesting that persons with high positive attitudes toward the lodge organization also tended to have more knowledge of the lodge population and living situation (*r* of scale 3 with 4). This seemed,

Table 9.4. Correlations among the Scales of the Local-business Questionnaire

Item	1. *Knowledge of the Residential Status*	2. *Knowledge of the Lodge Business*	3. *Attitudes toward the Lodge organization*	4. *Knowledge that Members were Ex-patients*	5. *Attitudes toward Members as Ex-patients*
1. Knowledge of the Residential Status		—.04	.09	.11	—.13
2. Knowledge of the Lodge Business	—.04		.39	.73	.23
3. Attitudes toward the Lodge Organization	.09	.39		.31	.39
4. Knowledge that Members were Ex-patients	.11	.73	.31		.21
5. Attitudes toward Members as Ex-patients	—.13	.23	.39	.21	

from informal observation, to be because persons with highest approval of the lodge were also those with whom many of the lodge members had friendly personal relations. Such persons naturally had more information about the lodge and the history of the men because of their personal contacts.

One example of such a respondent was the proprietor of a small bar nearby which had been adopted by a group of the members as an after-work gathering place. At the time of the survey, the men had been patronizing the bar for about three years and were well known and liked by both the owner and his wife. This was true even though there had been, on one occasion, a disturbance in the place caused by two men from the lodge, one of whom after not taking his medication had become angry with the owner over some real or imagined slight. The incident was not too distressing to the owner of the bar because, as he told the interviewer, such occurrences were almost a routine part of operating such a place in that neighborhood. Hence, he did not attribute the trouble to the ex-mental patient status of the men.

Relations Within the Lodge Neighborhood

A five-scale survey questionnaire similar to the one described for local business was also administered in the immediate vicinity of the lodge site, covering the area described in chapter 8 as the "neighborhood" (p. 133). In all, data were gathered from twenty residents who lived near the lodge site. As one might guess from the census description in chapter 8 (p. 130), the general socioeconomic level in the neighborhood was low, containing many transients who had moved into the area only out of necessity. Many could only afford low-income housing near their place of employment. Such persons did not like the neighborhood and expected to leave it in a short time; they generally would have preferred to live somewhere else. Persons in this category knew very little about the janitorial service and sometimes were even unsure of its location, although the lodge buildings were only a few doors away from where they lived. A few of these persons, however, knew a great deal about the lodge and were even on friendly terms with some of the members. This was especially true of two local residents, both living alone: one was an ex-mental patient from the same hospital as the lodge members and the other was a Hawaiian who was working with a self-help organization in the local black ghetto. The latter was well acquainted with the lodge, even though he had only been in the neighborhood for a few weeks; he was very enthusiastic about the project and believed that similar places were badly needed.

A second group of residents in the neighborhood, however, were satisfied with the location and had been living there for many years. In this group were older couples who had moved into the area by choice a long time before the study was initiated. They preferred the neighborhood to any other in spite of the changes which had occurred since they first came to live there. One of these was the "oldest inhabitant" of the neighborhood who had a local street named in his honor. A third couple were a little younger and were the parents of a large family. The husband of this family was often out of work and very short of money. For several years during the course of the study, the children had become great favorites of the kitchen manager and were friendly with some of the other members as well, although they were mainly tolerated by most of the men and were annoying to a few. In time they came to be "adopted" by the lodge and were tolerated by the members even when their antics became so annoying to some members that the executive committee had to ask the kitchen manager to assume responsibility for their behavior on the lodge grounds.

Residents in this "older" group were well informed on the lodge and very positive in their attitudes toward it. They all had been very distressed by the constant trouble in the area when the motel business had been in operation and were very pleased that the location had been taken over by a group of men whom they perceived as quiet and industrious. They knew several of the lodge members personally and liked them a good deal. They expressed absolutely no fear or uneasiness around them, even though one couple admitted that they had been uncertain at the beginning of the experiment when they first found out who the men were. Their experience with the lodge members over the three years of contact, however, had entirely reassured them, and they expressed the wish that the lodge would remain in the neighborhood indefinitely. One couple agreed the lodge was ". . . an ideal neighbor. They never make noise or cause any trouble and they keep the place in very good condition." They went on to point out how much better the roadside along one side of the lodge (and directly across the street from their house) had been maintained since the members had moved in. Their general opinion was that the lodge had definitely improved the neighborhood.

It was also plain from some of the anecdotes volunteered by this group of respondents that they had a good deal of affection for some of the men at the lodge. One couple reported that a particular member had become good friends with a pony which had been pastured in an empty lot nearby. He made frequent trips to pet and talk with the animal and often brought to it carrots and other tidbits from the lodge kitchen. He had even taken it upon himself to trim the pony's tail when it had grown so long that it was trailing in the muddy field. The pony was eventually moved and the member returned to the place for some days afterward to gaze out into the field, looking very lonely. The narrator of this story was obviously much affected by the experience and spoke movingly of the affection which the lodge member had shown to the pony.

A third and fairly large group of neighborhood residents were a number of unrelated Japanese-Americans who operated and worked in a nursery close by the lodge site. They were quite aware of the lodge as a janitorial service but knew little about the men there. Some of them knew something about the living situation in the project but had contact with the members only through the occasional business transacted between the lodge and nursery. Many of the nursery workers or their relatives were recently arrived in this country and spoke little English. They formed a fairly self-sufficient community which was isolated enough from the lodge by its location so that not much contact had occurred.

The matrix of correlations among the scales of the neighborhood survey questionnaire given to these three groups of respondents appears in Table 9.5. It shows that persons in the neighborhood who knew of the lodge as a janitorial service also tended to know of the ex-hospital status of the members (r of scale 2 with 4). It was apparent during the survey that people in the neighborhood either knew all about the lodge or else knew nothing about it at all—not even where it was located. It is plain, too, that neighborhood residents with positive attitudes toward the lodge organization also had positive attitudes toward the lodge as a rehabilitative unit—that is, they were aware that the men were ex-mental patients (r

Table 9.5. Correlations among the Scales of the Questionnaire for the Survey of the Lodge Neighborhood

Item	1. *Knowledge of the residential status*	2. *Knowledge of the lodge business*	3. *Attitudes toward the lodge organization*	4. *Knowledge that members were ex-patients*	5. *Attitudes toward members as ex-patients*
1. Knowledge of the residential status		—.17	.14	.01	.14
2. Knowledge of the lodge business	—.17		.29	.72	.34
3. Attitudes toward the lodge organization	.14	.29		.29	.77
4. Knowledge that members were ex-patients	.01	.72	.29		.47
5. Attitudes toward members as ex-patients	.14	.34	.77	.47	

of scale 3 with 5). Similarly, persons with negative attitudes toward the lodge organization retained those attitudes even when they knew of the status of the men and the nature of the lodge.

There was also a significant relationship between the knowledge of the rehabilitative role of the lodge and attitudes to that role. In general, persons who had more knowledge were more positive in attitude and *vice versa* (r of scale 4 with 5). This relationship was revealed in the experience of the interviewer on taking the survey. Persons who had not known that the men were from the hospital were often a little uneasy about the fact when it was revealed to them in the interview. They were less certain that they wished to have such a place in the neighborhood than were the persons who had known the nature of the lodge and had been satisfied by their experience that the lodge was a neighborhood asset.

Relations With the Relatives of the Lodge Members

No relative of any of the 75 lodge ex-patients was willing to provide living accomodations for him. However, during this study, a few of the relatives of the men participating in the experiment did visit the lodge and a somewhat larger number made some contact with the research staff or the men at some point in time. Those who did were almost all pleased with the project. Many were so pleased by the positive experiences lodge members related to them that they often wondered why something like the lodge had not been initiated sooner. In an attempt to get some systematic information about the attitudes of relatives, a questionnaire was sent to the closest relative of each man at the lodge who still had such contacts. The relatives were asked to express their preference for the lodge or the hospital as a treatment service and to state what they thought was the most important aspect of lodge living. Eight of the eleven relatives who completed and returned the questionnaire preferred the lodge setting; two preferred the hospital as a treatment setting; one had no opinion. They all perceived employment as the most important service provided by the lodge as they knew it. Such limited contacts with relatives as are presented here have become a characteristic feature of the returned chronic mental patient today. The paucity of data on relatives in this study only emphasizes the need for such living situations as the lodge.

10 RELATIONS WITH THE UNIVERSITY

The research reported in this book was supported by a federal grant, which is typically administered by an institution of higher education. For this study, sponsorship was undertaken by a large private university which was responsible not only for the research aspects of the project, but also for the creation and management of the community lodge itself. The assumption of these responsibilities led to a series of agreements and relations between the university, the research staff, the hospital from which lodge members came, and several community groups. This chapter will describe the relation of the university to these institutions and groups. It will illustrate the kind of administrative commitments necessary for such experiments in social innovation and it will describe the social relations which developed in carrying out these commitments.

Administrative Agreements

There were three main administrative agreements made by the university which were essential to the research project.[1] One established the legal status of the community lodge. The men at the lodge were operating a business in the community and were obliged, for that reason, to meet certain business requirements imposed by the city in which the lodge was placed. An agreement between the university and an existing nonprofit

1. A summary of all administrative agreements may be found on pp. 23–25.

"sheltered workshop" corporation defined the lodge as part of an existing organization engaged in rehabilitative therapy. This legal status solved a number of problems at once, some related to taxes, some to relations with labor and industry, and some to licensing and other local governmental regulations (pp. 23–27).

But it also raised another set of problems between the university and the nonprofit corporation. These problems arose because each party (the university and the nonprofit corporation) further delegated some of their responsibilities to the research staff when circumstances made this the most appropriate or the simplest procedure to follow. For example, the nonprofit organization was technically responsible for withholding income tax from the wages of the lodge members and for sending the appropriate reports during the year to the Internal Revenue Service. In practice, however, both these tasks were delegated to the research staff and its actions were then approved by the nonprofit organization because, under the circumstances, this was the most efficient procedure to follow. It also expressed the trust that existed between all parties involved. Such trust was an essential factor in the successful operation of the project.

The second set of administrative agreements were made between the university and the research staff itself. These were the usual ones accorded to research personnel on a federally funded grant, which gave them the status and some of the privileges of faculty members at the university. The research staff received appointments in an academic department and, though not granted all of the rights and duties of faculty status, staff members had all the privileges (such as use of the library) which were essential to carrying out the project. As a result, the principal investigator of the research project held the rank of Associate Consulting Professor and the remainder of the project staff received appointments as Research Associates. Further, as part of its commitment to support the research project, the university allowed the principal investigator to have maximum freedom in his hiring policies. This procedure permitted assembling a well-qualified staff to carry out the project.

Legal Agreements

The agreements described so far between the university and the nonprofit rehabilitative corporation presented relatively few problems. But the university also had to enter into contractual arrangements with private persons and businesses in the local community where the field research was being conducted.

One example of such a contract was the lease of a residence which could be used by the mental patients once they left the hospital. As mentioned (pp. 138–140), a motel site was chosen. Although the grant money paid for the rental of the site, it was necessary for the university to lease the motel for the duration of the experiment. An agreement with the university to do this was obtained by the research director and the university's legal officers drew up a lease with the owners of the motel. The importance of this agreement was not fully appreciated until the end of the experiment. At that time, a disagreement arose between the motel owners and the university about some of the conditions of the lease. A legal suit was initiated by the owners against the university. It was only then that the importance of the wording and intent of the lease came clearly into focus. Ultimately the university agreed to make a cash settlement which involved a moderately large sum. Since such an experience by the university may tend to inhibit it from sponsoring future field research of the kind reported in this book, it will be important to make agreements of this kind in such a way that similar problems do not occur in future community researches. This was one of the important lessons learned from the present research project.

The lawsuit also created an issue between the university and the federal granting agency which was a novel experience for both. It concerned the question of who had the responsibility to pay the settlement. Two very different points of view made the responsibility unclear. On the one hand, the legal officers of the university had drawn up the lease and could therefore be held responsible for disagreements arising from that document. This argument implied that the university should pay the settlement. On the other hand, it was possible to argue that the lawsuit arose only because the research project required that a lease be made and, therefore, the settlement cost was an expense which should be borne by the federal agency supporting the research financially. This argument implied that the federal granting agency should pay the settlement. This unclear situation illustrates an important principle: Future research of this type must be preceded by an adequate agreement between the granting agency and the grantee institution about who will pay costs (such as the legal one under consideration) which might arise from unexpected developments during the course of a community research.

Another lease agreement made by the university stands in sharp contrast to the one just described. This was the lease of the vehicles necessary for the operation of the janitorial service. In the final stages of the project, this amounted to a small fleet of two large vans and a heavy-duty pickup truck. These vehicles were all leased by the university, using grant funds, for the use of lodge members in operating their business. The arrangements in this case created no trouble at all. This was also true of the arrangements made for maintenance services for the trucks, such as the oil company credit card which was drawn in the name of the university.

Aside from legal services on specific matters such as leases, the university also provided general legal counsel for the research staff. This covered such matters as legal advice on relations arising between the community and the lodge members and on the protection of the professional staff through malpractice insurance. The latter was important, since the research staff was performing functions which were novel for persons of their training and experience. Since they might have made errors in judgment which could have resulted in an accusation of malpractice, such insurance was a necessity.

The very novelty of the innovative community situation could contain the basis for such accusations against research staff by community residents who might be offended by the behavior of lodge members. The members of the lodge daily interacted with persons in the local community who were often very sensitive to odd behavior such as that sometimes demonstrated by emotionally disturbed ex-mental patients. Although such odd behavior might be exhibited with impunity by hospital patients on leave to the community, it could not be shown by lodge members who were fully discharged patients without some danger to the existence of the lodge itself. The hospital had the advantage of being an established institution with known responsibilities and roles, and its patients—even when on leave—were protected by their continuing role as hospital patients. The lodge, however, had no such status and its members enjoyed no comparable protection. If they offended the community, their freedom was likely to be curtailed by incarceration or a demand that they be returned to the mental hospital from which they had been discharged.

The only way in which the members could derive some protection from their former hospitalization was to assume the identity of "ex-mental patients" and claim the tolerance usually accorded such persons by society. But this tactic was not open to them for two reasons: first, the object of the experiment was to make the "ex-patient" participants as independent of that role as possible; second, the tolerance of the deviant behavior sometimes displayed by "ex-mental patients" is often linked with community demands for loss of freedom which the lodge members themselves wished to avoid. Factors like these acted to reinforce the rejection by many of the lodge members of the role of "patient" as an affront to their self-respect and a threat to their autonomy. They believed that the protection of the label "ex-mental patient" was not worth the price. But the research staff had to be prepared for accusations about the lodge members' negligent responsibility even while carrying out the experimental goal of extending increasing freedom to them.

Financial Agreements

A number of special arrangements were made by the university to give lodge members the greatest possible autonomy in financial matters while still permitting the university to meet its legal responsibilities as "holder of the purse strings." The essential difficulty was that the lodge members needed the freedom to manage their financial affairs in order to create the experimental conditions of autonomy at the lodge, while at the same time the university had to maintain control over the expenditure of federal grant money. The resolution of these two needs resulted from a series of agreements, some of them ordinary ones usually associated with research grants and others especially tailored to the needs of the present experiment (p. 23).

One example of the ordinary financial agreement was the direct billing to the university of certain expenses incurred by the research project. Such expenses were paid directly out of grant funds by a university check and were handled through the purchasing department of the university. This type of transaction was legally possible only for the principal investigator of the research project. It is a typical arrangement in the administration of federal grant money. But other methods of handling money demonstrate the unusual arrangements required to meet special experimental needs. Such arrangements had to be made to facilitate the conduct of business in the community in an orderly fashion or to meet the essential experimental condition of lodge-member autonomy. Handling grant money to facilitate the conduct of business is shown by an expense account—a cash account never exceeding $500—which was established at a local bank. Items costing up to $25.00 (a limit according to grant regulations) that were often immediately needed by the work crews could be bought through this account by the research staff. This facilitated the purchase of materials such as paint brushes and floor wax which might be essential to the completion of a particular janitorial job.

Handling grant money so as to create the experimental condition of member autonomy is illustrated by the manner in which food and small items such as plates and cups were purchased for the lodge. To accomplish this, a local bank account was opened under the name "Members' Lodge," and periodic deposits of $1,200 each were made in it by the university, when requested to do so by the research staff. The lodge members themselves made the decisions about spending this money by delegating decisions to the member in charge of the kitchen and commissary duties at the lodge. He made all decisions on the purchasing of food supplies and certain other items necessary for the day-to-day operation of the lodge as a living unit. Each check written on this account was signed by both the business manager of the lodge (pp. 46, 59) and a member of the research staff. The activity in this account was recorded in a set of books which were audited by the university. This arrangement allowed the lodge members to act with some degree of autonomy in the spending of the money, but it also permitted the university, as the grantee institution, to account for the federal funds expended.

In addition to the money from the grant agency, money was also received by the members from their business venture. This produced a complex problem for the university auditors which was finally resolved by keeping two different and independent sets of financial records. One kept account of the money received from federal grant sources; the other accounted for the money derived from the operation of the business. The separate accounting became necessary because the university was responsible for administering grant funds, while the income from the business was the sole responsibility of the lodge members. The revenue from the business was allocated by means of a formula established by the lodge executive committee (pp. 58–62). Ninety per cent of the money obtained from business activity was distributed as wages to members, while the remainder was placed in a "reserve fund" that could be spent only for items agreed upon by the lodge's executive committee. Since this money was entirely independent of the funds received through the grant, the lodge members could dispose of it with no other responsibility than the usual business practice of keeping accurate record books. To keep track of this income, an account was established simply under the name "Lodge," to distinguish it from the bank account containing grant funds kept under the name "Members' Lodge."

Two separate sets of record books caused some problems for the university in relation to the lodge activity and the goals of the research staff. Since the university was directly responsible for the administration of the grant money, it assigned one of its accountants to keep a continuous audit of the project's books. Strictly speaking, this audit was supposed to be limited to accounting for the use of grant money; the task of the university auditor was therefore to audit only the set of books in which the expenditure of grant money was recorded. However, after discussions with the research staff about the bookkeeping procedures needed for the lodge, the auditor—for two reasons—gradually assumed the expanded role of consultant to the lodge on all bookkeeping and accounting procedures.

First, the auditor quickly became convinced that his job could be done more efficiently if he provided the lodge members with technical assistance for their bookkeeping procedures while monitoring the "Members' Lodge" grant funds account. To this end, he recommended and supervised changes in the organization of the books and in some of the bookkeeping procedures initially used at the lodge. He also assisted in training the lodge member who had the task of carrying out the bookkeeping operations. Second, the first auditor assigned to the lodge mistakenly believed that the university had an accounting responsibility for the money earned by the business as well as for the grant funds. This auditor contended that the university had managerial responsibility for *all* financial arrangements made in a research project sponsored by the university.

Although the idea was reasonable, a difficulty arose over the research goal of providing experimental conditions which promoted the greatest possible autonomy for lodge members. In the eyes of the research staff, an important part of that autonomy was freedom for the group to direct its own financial affairs. Thus the auditor's eagerness to meet his own responsibilities, as he perceived them, sometimes conflicted with this goal of group autonomy. Eventually, it was mutually agreed between the auditor and the research director that the university auditor would act as a consultant to the lodge members about the techniques of keeping the lodge's business books, without exercising control over the use of the money involved.

Because of his personality and his own definition of the duties of a good auditor, the first university accountant experienced difficulty in maintaining this role. Sometimes he questioned the wisdom of expenditures drawn against the business account, although such expenditures were made with the approval of the lodge's executive committee or, in some cases, of the entire membership. Nevertheless, the arrangement worked reasonably well in spite of the auditor's concern. The surveillance problem was finally resolved when a new auditor was assigned to the research project. The second auditor was more readily able to accomodate himself to the autonomy the lodge members had attained by that time in controlling their own financial affairs. He seemed much more at ease in the consulting role he had to play; during his tenure, the arrangement worked much more smoothly.

The difference between these two university accountants in their ability to work within the agreement on managing the financial affairs of the business illustrates an important point about the difficult role of "consultants" in social innovative experiments. In this case, the consultant (a university accountant) had to give the lodge members advice on the technical skills of bookkeeping while avoiding, as much as possible, any violation of the autonomy the lodge members had in making their own financial decisions. This task was accomplished by the two different auditors with varying success; the role was comfortable for one and not for the other. This interaction between personality traits and task role stresses the need for the professional consultant to *restrict* his role as an expert in behalf of autonomy for the participants in the newly created social subsystem. Hence, in his role, the "expert consultant" must be willing to tolerate what he perceives as "mistakes" in the judgment and behavior of the participants. Furthermore, the consultant must keep a tight rein on his advisory functions so that he reduces the tendency of the more passive participants to relinquish their autonomy to a person they perceive as an "expert" whom they may judge to be better qualified to make decisions, even about their own lives and welfare.

Other Agreements

Two other agreements with the university provided the lodge with material advantages in purchasing two vital and expensive commodities: food and medicine. Because of the volume purchases made by the university, it occupied a very favorable market position as a buyer of these items. The benefits of this favorable position were passed on to the lodge through special arrangements with the university's commissary and with its pharmacy in the medical school.

Under the agreement with the commissary, the lodge member who was kitchen manager (p. 48) prepared a weekly order of foodstuffs needed for the lodge that were available from the commissary. Under this arrangement, such orders were delivered to the commissary by messenger on Friday of each week; supplies ordered were picked up by the lodge's driver on the following Monday. Later, by mutual agreement, orders were sent by mail, which eliminated an extra trip to the commissary every week. The change was a suggestion of one of the member truck drivers from the lodge who broached it with the commissary business manager on his own initiative. Since it seemed likely to be more convenient for both parties, it was adopted as a regular practice.

One further adjustment was made in buying practices of the lodge at the instigation of the commissary manager. After several months of transactions, the commissary realized it was doing a lot of special purchasing in order to complete requests from the lodge because of special preferences expressed by the kitchen manager for particular types and sizes of packaged merchandise. The volume of special purchasing became so inconvenient the manager of the commissary approached the kitchen manager of the lodge to find a solution to this difficulty. In the end, the kitchen manager found a local store able to provide the special items at nearly the same savings available from the university commissary. Special orders were shifted to the local store, while regular items continued to be obtained from the university commissary. This final arrangement prevailed for the duration of the experiment. In all, the lodge purchased almost $12,500 worth of food and other supplies from the university commissary. Through this arrangement with the university, the lodge was able to buy almost 28 per cent of its food and supplies at wholesale prices.

A very significant expense in the operation of the lodge was the cost of supplying lodge members with necessary medication. Most of the lodge members needed tranquilizing medication to aid them in the control of their psychotic symptoms. Since these tranquilizing drugs were vital to the members' ability to live outside the hospital, an adequate supply of such medication was as important to the survival of the lodge as provisions for food and housing (pp. 47–48). During the course of the experiment, almost $9,000 was spent on medication for lodge members. Almost all of this medication was for the alleviation of neuropsychiatric symptoms. Because of the large volume of medicine to be bought during the study, the research staff arranged with the university to make such purchases through the outpatient pharmacy in the teaching hospital of the medical school. Obtained in this way, medicine was provided at wholesale cost plus a 10 per cent surcharge. This resulted in great savings, since almost 97 per cent of the medicine bought by lodge members came from the university's pharmacy. Arrangements to permit such medicine to be bought through the university required only a letter from the principal investigator of the research project identifying lodge members needing medication and the name of the prescribing physician who was the house physician for the lodge. As new residents entered the lodge during the course of the experiment, the university's pharmacy was routinely informed and the names of the new men needing medication were added to its prescription list.

Attitudes of University Personnel Toward the Lodge

There was essentially no contact between the university staff and lodge personnel. The physical site of the lodge was approximately four miles from the university campus, and major interactions with the university took place through the professional research staff on the project, as is usual in the administration of research grants. In general, lodge members knew far more about the university than university staff did about them. Nevertheless some university staff members did have repeated contacts with lodge members during the experiment and came to know some of the men quite well. An annual interview was held with these university staff members in order to assess their attitudes toward the lodge and its participants. They were asked to comment on the lodge as a rehabilitative unit and as a business venture; on the assets, liabilities, and future of the lodge; on changes which they noticed over time; and on the adjustment of the lodge members themselves and their own relations to these men.

The most obvious facet of interview responses by these university staff members as a group is that their overall evaluation of the lodge was primarily positive. Table 10.1 summarizes the degree to which these university employees responded positively to the lodge or to its members and the degree to which such responses indicated neutral or negative attitudes.[2] Table 10.1 also shows the pattern of responses for each of the four university staff members who were interviewed on an annual basis. Persons having the most sustained contact with the lodge members were the two university auditors who acted as consultants to the lodge and as representatives of the school's "internal audit division." They visited the lodge regularly, every two or three months, to audit the lodge's financial books. In pursuit of this, they became well acquainted with the members—espe-

2. The average per cent of agreement reached by two raters was 98 for classifying the interview responses as positive, neutral, or negative.

Table 10.1. Per Cent of Positive, Neutral, and Negative Attitudes Expressed by University Staff About the Lodge at Annual Interviews

Respondent	*Positive Responses* (%)	*Neutral Responses* (%)	*Negative Responses* (%)
All staff responses	73	17	10
First auditor	71	13	16
Second auditor	84	14	2
Legal advisor	56	29	15
Commissary business manager	85	15	0

cially those holding clerical or managerial positions in the lodge organization.

Table 10.1 shows that the first auditor was less positive than university staff members as a group, because of a higher proportion of negative responses. This person was the auditor with the least flexible attitudes in his role as a consultant (p. 172). It is not surprising to find that his negative attitudes were almost entirely related to perceived shortcomings in the lodge members' ability to perform the technical work of bookkeeping at the lodge; in effect, he was unhappy at the inability of the men at the lodge to fill the role of a typical accountant. For instance, in discussing the lodge bookkeeper, he said, "Now take Mr. Murray in his lapses of attention . . . he failed to carry out the instructions—simply did not do the work he indicated he knew how to do and was going to do, and just failed to get it done. Of course, that would not be responsible behavior."

Another attitude expressed by this auditor changed from positive to negative over time. At the beginning of the experiment he was optimistic about the business prospects of the lodge and cited its increasing revenues as evidence of this. But by the time of his replacement by another auditor for the lodge (p. 173), his opinion had changed and he felt that the lodge had been a failure as a business enterprise. Not surprisingly, he based his later opinion on the inability of the members to perform their managerial and accounting tasks with the consistency and skill which his own standards led him to expect. It is important to note, however, that his negative attitudes were not all adversely critical. He also expressed dissatisfaction with the recreation facilities located near the lodge and with the public transport available to the members because of the lodge's physical location. These attitudes reveal his concern for the welfare of the members, that welfare being quite distinct in his eyes from their skill as bookkeepers or managers of a business enterprise.

The second university auditor clearly held more positive attitudes toward the lodge than the first, primarily because he expressed fewer negative attitudes rather than decreased neutrality (Table 10.1). The second auditor seemed more at ease and more flexible in his role as consultant.

Nevertheless, he fulfilled his responsibilities as auditor with thoroughness and vigor. Basically, he appeared to have a stronger sense of the rehabilitative mission of the lodge than did the first auditor. This is clearly reflected in his attitudes, since his negative comments about the operation of the lodge were concerned with what he perceived to be an *overemphasis* on the business aspects of the lodge to the detriment of its rehabilitative function. For example, when asked what changes he might recommend in practices at the lodge, he responded:

> Well, one change. Not change, but one thing I've noticed that perhaps might be good or bad—I'm not sure . . . Mr. Edwards [the lay coordinator, p. 84], I know, is a very energetic and enthusiastic person and he's interested, I think, in making as much money as he can for the [janitorial] service; and I'm not sure if this is good because . . . I know he'd like to get another truck or two so he can have more people out and all this and I'm not sure if the end would justify the means. . . . Well, anyway, I think it would become too much concern about being a profit-making organization as opposed to—in other words, perhaps maybe pushing the men too hard or trying to get too much out of them. I don't think he'll do this, but this is a possibility so this might be a problem.

Later in the same interview, he elaborated on the same point, "Of course, I didn't explain that very well, but I think if too much is made of—you know—increasing the size, the volume, of the business, it might mean the rehabilitative aspect might be overlooked."

These views are consistent with his eagerness, compared with the first auditor, to modify his role as an accountant so that it would more realistically fit the needs of the experimental social system. It is interesting to note that the two auditors represent, to a degree, the same opposition of views which existed within the executive committee of the lodge society, namely, the members who valued the lodge as a business venture versus those who valued it as a rehabilitative unit (pp. 88–100).

The legal advisor was clearly the least positive in attitude toward the experimental project. This was accounted for not by his negative attitudes but rather because of a high percentage of neutral responses. A glance at Table 10.1 shows this very clearly. The most likely reason for this pattern of attitudes may be the infrequent personal contacts which the legal advisor actually had with lodge members. Of the four university staff members listed in Table 10.1, he was the only one who did not have prolonged, direct, personal contact with men at the lodge during the course of the experiment. His relationship to the lodge was carried out almost entirely through the professional research staff, especially the principal investigator. Because of this trained lawyer's lack of personal knowledge of the living and work situation of the lodge members, he withheld judgment on many issues raised by the interview questions about the lodge.

Support for this interpretation of the lawyer's perception of the lodge and its members may be found by analysis of the same attitudes expressed at different times during the course of the experiment. The first interview with him was conducted at a time when he had just experienced his first contact with lodge members through their operation as a janitorial service. He employed them to do a regular cleaning of his apartment and he continued that service until he moved out of the apartment. In that interview, 77 per cent of his expressed attitudes were positive and 10 per cent were negative, only 13 per cent were neutral. By the time of the second interview 12 months later, he had had no further direct contact with the lodge or its members and the percentage of his neutral attitudes rose to 30 per cent. At the same time, 25 per cent of his attitudes were negative, reflecting some recent problems with the lease of the lodge site, the remaining 45 per cent being positive. The third interview with the lawyer occurred more than 24 months after his first contact with the lodge as a customer of its janitorial service. The proportion of negative attitudes expressed then was virtually the same as at the time of the first interview, namely, 11 per cent of all responses. However, neutral attitudes now accounted for 45 per cent of his responses—more than three times the original proportion at the first interview, leaving almost the same percentage of positive responses as at the time of the second interview (44 per cent). The general pattern of all his interviews shows a gradual increase in the proportion of neutral responses over time, at the expense of positive attitudes. Negative attitudes remain relatively constant except when under the influence of a specific problem which had arisen prior to the second interview. At the time he had regular personal contact with lodge members, however, the pattern of his attitudes is very similar to that of the other university staff members, as Table 10.1 demonstrates.

The commissary business manager was unmistakably the most positive of the university staff members interviewed during the course of the research study. Although shown clearly in Table 10.1, this positiveness is more vividly found in the content of his replies during the successive interviews. In responding to a question about the lodge he said: ". . . I think it is a terrific thing. I think we are getting along—we are going to have more and more mental-type things with the stress of today's living, perhaps, and maybe this is one of the answers for it." A little later in the same interview he added, ". . . I think this problem here is probably quite similar to retired people. A feeling that they are needed. They are still useful human beings. I think this is something that we are going to have problems with more and more. I'm not trying to philosophize." But more than simply holding the attitude that the lodge was a beneficial place for handicapped people, the commissary business manager also had a high regard for the ability of the lodge members to operate as his peers in a business relationship. In an early interview he said of one of the lodge members, ". . . I've been impressed, especially, by the fellow that drives your truck that comes in here. . . . He has impressed several of us. I was talking to my storeroom man this morning and I asked, 'Gee, do you think he's a patient?' and he said, 'Yes, I think so.' But he seemed to be quite well adjusted, I thought. In fact, I sometimes wonder if we're not the ones that aren't quite well adjusted either." Asked more about this particular lodge member, he continued:

> . . . for example, [the driver] said, 'Gee, I have to bring these orders over on Friday and sometimes you're kinda busy.' So I told him to arrange to have it put in the mail so I'd have it Monday morning. So he arranged the whole thing and we've been [getting] the orders through the mail and it saved him time and actually us at the same time. So this is something: he had a problem, and he suggested it, and we helped him solve it by our cooperating too. I thought that was pretty good. I mean, it's something that showed initiative.

In a later interview during the study, the commissary business manager compared his business relations with the lodge to the relations he had with other agencies in the university community. The lodge appeared to come off best in the comparison. He first volunteered that the way in which the lodge dealt with the university commissary was "probably more responsible than some of our present cooks" working with fraternities on campus; then he elaborated:

> Well, of course . . . you're trying to compare apples and oranges a little bit, in that the fraternity group—they are a larger group—that's number one —and students dictate a change of policy so frequently that the cooks are confused by the students—who are confused—and so this is a different picture. They come down and pick up merchandise more frequently, change their orders more frequently, where the [lodge members], on the other hand, rarely change their orders at all. It comes in and we can, once a week, fill their order, and they pick it up and there's no question about it. If we are shorted on something, we tell them and they say, "Okay, next week is all right" and this has been very simple. . . . This is another factor: it's a pleasure to do business with the [lodge].

There seemed to be a change in the attitudes of this university staff member during the course of the experiment toward perceiving the lodge more as a business establishment and less as a rehabilitative unit. Two factors suggested this impression. First, with the passage of time he expressed a greater percentage of neutral attitudes. At the first interview the distribution of responses into positive, neutral, and negative attitudes was 95 per cent, 5 per cent, and 0 per cent, respectively; at the last interview the comparable proportions were 75 per cent, 25 per cent, and 0 per cent. By itself, this percentage change would be difficult to assess. There was neither variation in contact with the lodge, as was the case of the university legal advisor who showed a similar trend of attitude change, nor was there any other apparent change in the commissary manager's relations with the lodge to account for such a shift. But the annual interviews revealed a possible explanation, namely, a change in the content of expressed attitudes from the first to the last interview.

Most of the positive attitudes expressed in the first interview with the commissary business manager reflected his view of the lodge as a place for rehabilitation. He perceived the lodge to have a beneficial effect on the men and on the surrounding community. This generalized positive attitude about the value of rehabilitative services in the community was a strong component in the very high percentage of positive attitudes (95 per cent) expressed in his first interview. In some answers, this positive view induced enthusiastic responses praising the behavior of lodge members which might have gone unnoticed if observed by him in a group not labeled as ex-mental patients. By the last interview, such enthusiastic praise has dissipated and the behavior of lodge members is being assessed in comparison with other ordinary business contacts he encountered in the daily operation of the commissary. The lodge members are given credit by him when they perform well in such a comparison (for example, in comparison with the fraternity cooks just mentioned), but excessive praise and excessive concern are absent. This new perspective is evident in the last interview, when the commissary business manager responds about his contacts with the lodge. In the course of his answer he says, "Sometime I should probably make a special effort and go over [to] look at the installation again. I did that at the beginning; and there might be something that we could suggest that would be helpful and, at the same time, observe how they are maintaining, and so forth." This shift in content is revealing. For while it led to a decrease in the proportion of positive attitudes expressed by the commissary manager near the end of the study, it also testified to the appearance of a far more important gain in the status of lodge members in the eyes of the commissary staff. The lodge was apparently being viewed as the equal of other ordinary business agencies with which the university commissary dealt. As a business, the community's usual standards were being applied to it.

Attitudes of Lodge Members Toward the University

Systematic data were not obtained about the attitudes of lodge members toward the university. However, knowledge of the special relation between the school and members was so pervasive at the lodge that such data from each member probably would not have varied enough to elaborate an understanding of their attitudes toward this relationship. The most uniform perception of the university by lodge members concerned its being the source of all financial support for the lodge itself. All members knew that the lodge had an experimental status and that the research study was being conducted under the auspices of the university. They also knew that most of the professional research staff were employees of the university. This kind of information was especially well known to lodge members who held clerical or managerial positions, so that it quickly diffused through the organization when they repeated it.

This knowledge influenced the behavior of lodge members in making decisions about spending money which originated from grant funds. There was a very strong feeling among those lodge members responsible for making such decisions that they must try not to deviate from university policy. This feeling was reinforced by the research staff on occasion as a way of keeping purchases within the bounds of those that could be realistically approved by the university. This feeling also distorted lodge members' attitudes toward the university auditors when they made their regular visits to the lodge. The auditors were looked upon as important and powerful men, especially by those lodge members who held managerial positions. These leaders were themselves disposed to admire authoritative figures. The auditors were thus seen as the representatives of a powerful organization (the university) which controlled lodge financing and had the authority to make judgments about spending practices of lodge members. This was revealed particularly when the auditors raised questions about the members' spending practices with respect to their own money in the business account, which was not the responsibility of the auditors. The auditors' right to question these expenditures was never challenged by the men living at the lodge, only by the research staff. Not even those members who were most jealous of their autonomy and who sometimes resisted regulation by the research staff ever questioned the right of a university auditor to criticize the use of revenues gained from their own employment. Knowledge of where lodge funding originated would have led them to relinquish control over their own funds had not the research staff intervened.

Another more general attitude was even more pervasive at the lodge than that linked directly to financial support by the university. It concerned identification of the lodge members with the school as an educational institution. Generally, the men looked upon their relationship with the university as a source of great prestige and were not at all reluctant to identify themselves to outsiders by mentioning this connection. There seemed little doubt that some of the men in particular derived a great satisfaction from this relationship. This was especially evident at certain times of the year when several men from the lodge attended sporting events at the university and, by all accounts from the men themselves, were lusty partisans for the home team. At such times, the expression of this feeling of identification by the wearing of school symbols like hats and sweatshirts was too obvious to be missed. Equally suggestive were the long and heated discussions among the men as they relived the athletic exploits of the university team during the week following a particular sporting event. Although similar behavior is commonly observed among other social groups, such as a school's students and alumni, and even among the residents of a university town, this identification was probably even more important to lodge members who had often been deprived of many of these psychosocial satisfactions so enjoyed by other citizens in the community.

11 MEDICAL CARE FOR THE MEMBERS

Experimental social innovation differs from most other forms of social problem solution because of the responsibility which must be assumed by the researchers on a 24-hour basis for the lives and welfare of participants in the experimental subsystems. This is not the only difference (Fairweather, 1967, p. 20), but it is an important one. Both for that reason and because of legal and humane considerations, arrangements were necessary to insure the health and general medical welfare of the men at the lodge.

Since the men at the lodge volunteered for an experimental program in community living under the supervision of the research staff, its responsibility to meet their health needs was clear. The legal aspect of this responsibility arose from the relation of the researchers as mental health professionals to the men as ex-patients from a mental hospital. The direct release of men from the experimental ward in the federal hospital to the lodge emphasized that legal responsibility. The community lodge and the experimental hospital ward were directly linked by the fact that the ward served as the "feeder" to the lodge. Since the ward physician had to approve the lodge as a suitable place to which he could send his patients, he had to be confident that his medical responsibility to them would be fulfilled by the standards of medical welfare maintained by a responsible research staff for the lodge society.

This specific example of the ward physician's responsibility raises a broader issue: medical jurisdiction in rehabilitation. The domain of medicine over rehabilitative effort is part of an informal tradition in American society and is also carried into many formal and legal arrangements, such as aspects of the organization of the Veterans Administration and of the Social and Rehabilitation Administration in the Department of Health, Education, and Welfare. Much of the history of efforts to rehabilitate the physically and mentally handicapped has occurred in medical settings or with dominant medical participation, partly because of the common involvement of illness in the definition of the handicapped and partly because medical persons often are highly motivated to apply themselves to such problems. In the nineteenth century, the definition of behavior disorders as "mental illness" extended the jurisdiction of medicine to the treatment of what are now called "neuropsychiatric" patients. It has been viewed therefore as a natural part of the medical person's responsibility to society.

The experimental society described in the present study sought to decrease the reliance of the men on the sick role and, to this end, medical influence on its organization was kept at a minimum. For example, the lodge was legally formed as a nonprofit business enterprise and not as a rehabilitative unit. Thus, it was subject to all the health and other safety regulations required for business and group living. But, beyond these formal requirements of the law, tradition and ordinary prudence made some arrangements for medical consultation appropriate and necessary. The eventual organization of the lodge included special relations with the hospital from which all members came, as well as private arrangements with a physician in the community. These two aspects of medical care have already been mentioned (pp. 23–24) and will be discussed subsequently in greater detail (pp. 187–194). In this chapter it is necessary to describe the content of the research staff's medical concerns within the lodge itself.

The first concern was with ordinary medical care which any group of persons require to handle minor illness and emergencies; this was easily taken care of by arrangements with the private house physician, who also provided preventive medical services. In addition, some emergency matters were handled by special arrangement with the federal hospital, particularly expedited admission of an acutely psychotic lodge member should that be necessary.

A second and greater concern revolved around the use of tranquilizing medication by the men at the lodge. Past experience had shown that it was very important for persons leaving the hospital to continue their medication if they were to avoid being rehospitalized. Ninety-seven per cent of the men who lived at the lodge took some medicine while they were there. The mean daily dose of tranquilizers was 457 mg., converted to chlorpromazine equivalent as a common standard of measurement. With such individual dosages, it was vital that some plan be developed to insure that the men would take their medication regularly. Eventually a system evolved in which one of the lodge members (the business manager usually) occupied a "peer-nurse" role (p. 50); he dispensed the medicine, invariably taken orally in pill form, to those men who tended to forget or to resist. He was himself supervised by the coordinator in consultation with the house physician.

The peer-nurse held a position of great responsibility. When the men first moved to the lodge the staff coordinator assumed that each member was responsible for taking his own medication. When one member did not take any medicine for nine days and had to return to the hospital in a psychotic state, the incident led to more stringent supervision by the coordinator of the administration of drugs at the lodge. The arrangement ultimately allowed those members who did not resist or forget taking medicine to take it as their own responsibility, much as would be true of any citizen in society. It is apparent that the role of peer-nurse replicated many of the same behaviors required of the nurse on a hospital ward. This is only one more example of the conflict, so many times encountered by the research staff, between making the lodge members as autonomous as possible and permitting behavior which might destroy the experimental subsystem. The taking of prescribed medicine was an area in which men at the lodge had relatively little autonomy, not only because of the role of the peer-nurse but because of the supervisory behavior of the coordinator and the house physician.

The Medical Role of the Coordinator

Some of the reasons for the coordinator's responsibility in accounting for the use of medication were products of the overall medical responsibility outlined earlier in this chapter. Because of his position at the lodge and his daily contact with the men there, the coordinator became a major consultant to the house physician on the behavior of the lodge members and their response to prescribed medication. As a corollary to this role, the house physician came to rely on the coordinator for seeing that supplies of medicine were replenished when necessary and that prescriptions were followed. This kind of responsibility could be delegated only partly to the peer-nurse, since periodic checks had to be carried out by the coordinator himself.

During the time that the experiment was in progress, these arrangements seemed essential to the research staff and to the house physician. Both parties felt that such procedures were necessary to fulfill their responsibilities to the men at the lodge and, to a great extent, to protect them from some of the consequences of the behavior of those men who stopped taking their medicine regularly. Later information, informally derived from observing the autonomous operation of the lodge after the experimental phase of the project was completed and the men were no longer under research staff supervision, showed that the lodge members themselves were fully capable of handling the problems of medication in a way which would not destroy the organization. After the staff supervision stopped, one of the most capable members assumed the peer-nurse responsibility himself, though with much reluctance and misgivings (p. 50). Apparently he was successful in the role. This result is consistent with prior work in mental hospitals which shows that group members would not assume leadership responsibilities when some recognized outside authority was physically present (Lerner and Fairweather, 1963). From this later information, it now seems possible to suggest that continued supervision of medication by the staff after the lodge group was fully formed and functioning mainly suggested the staff's subjective comfort. It probably did not occur because the lodge members were objectively unable to fulfill this responsibility.

In the matter of general health and preventative medicine, there were overlapping areas of cooperation between the house physician, the federal hospital, and the staff coordinator. The responsibility of the coordinator for the supervision of medication use had a counterpart in other medical matters at the lodge in which the house physician depended on him for on-the-spot supervision of the general health of the lodge members and for reports of their behavior and response to prescribed medication. The two professionals usually acted in consultation to make and evaluate changes in tranquilizing medication and other such treatments.

But the most general role played by the coordinator in the health and welfare of the lodge members was as a resource person on a 24-hour basis. The officer of the day (p. 62) on duty at the lodge could always reach the coordinator by telephone at any hour of the day or night in case of emergency. This "on-call" responsibility was held by the coordinator directly working with lodge members, although the other members of the research staff were available for relief in case this coordinator was out of town or otherwise unavailable.

This duty was also in support of other responsibilities at the lodge which occupied the staff coordinator. He generally was the first to be contacted for the first-aid care of minor injuries and for consultation on personal problems. He was also in charge of transporting persons to the hospital if their physical or mental condition warranted such action. This aspect of the coordinator's role was seldom required, but when such action was necessary it was often vital to the existence of the lodge. This was especially true of those rare instances which involved extreme psychotic behavior by lodge members; such an incident occurred on only four or five occasions during the entire existence of the lodge experiment.

Other responsibilities for health matters falling to the coordinator were more routine. They included such things as the personal hygiene of the members and fulfilling such specific requests as the house physician made from time to time. An example of such a request was the periodic weighing of some lodge members who had medical problems associated with obesity. In some cases this was combined with serious physical conditions like diabetes, so that weight control was of the prime importance; in other cases it was simply a matter of the usual medical difficulties associated with an extreme overweight condition. Most regulated weight checks were done on orders of the house physician, but eventually other lodge members, who felt that they had the same problem but to a lesser extent, decided to participate as a means of exerting their own control over the problem.

The House Physician

Although the house physician for the lodge dealt with a population of members who had all been patients in a mental hospital, he was not a psychiatrist. His specialty was internal medicine. However, his medical experience had included working in a mental hospital, so that he was practiced in the ability to relate easily with people showing psychiatric symptoms. He was also aware of the importance of finding and holding maintenance levels of tranquilizing medication with such persons. With this basic knowledge to build on, he quickly established a successful role as the "private doctor" of the men at the lodge.

A nonpsychiatric specialty was an advantage to the house physician and to the research project in several other ways. It aided his attempt to establish the particular role required of him as the private medical consultant of the men at the lodge, and it prevented any possible feelings by the men that they were somehow still in a mental hospital setting. It was important to avoid the condition at the lodge of "regular visits to the psychiatrist," because of the possible effects this would have had in maintaining a self-concept of themselves as "mental patients." That perception, and the role which it might generate for persons holding it, was something which no part of the experimental program could support without compromising its goal of reaching the greatest degree of autonomy and positive self-regard of which the lodge members might be capable.

It was also easier for a physician who was not a psychiatrist to follow the role assigned to him in the research design. It was not a typical psychiatrist's role, since it required the suspension of many of the typical psychiatric methods devised for treating persons diagnosed as "mentally ill" on an individual basis. The object of the experiment was to let the social processes, generated partly by the men themselves, act as the "treatment method" in the program. One community psychiatrist consulted during the planning phase of the experiment stated that he believed he would be very uncomfortable in the role of house physician, as it was described to him, and thought that the same would be true of most persons in his specialty. He therefore suggested a nonpsychiatric physician for the role.

The actual physician who filled the role during the study was inclined to agree with this judgment, though he believed that his experience in working in a neuropsychiatric setting was also important. In an interview during the experiment, he was asked if he thought that a person in his medical specialty was an appropriate choice for the role of house physician in a project like the lodge study. His positive answer was qualified:

> Well, I think an internist who's had previous experience with patients of this type, who is familiar with the problem inside the hospital . . . I think somebody with previous experience and somebody who had sympathy with this type of illness would be the best type of person. Otherwise, why, you wouldn't understand exactly what [the patient's] problem was and know exactly what was going on, really.

It is probably beneficial for a physician in the position just described to have some commitment to the solution of social problems and to have or at least understand research values for discovering those solutions. Attitudes of this sort ought to make it easier for him to adopt that special research role which combines the fulfillment of his medical responsibility with the needs of the experimental project. In the present study, the house physician did have such attitudes and readily understood the need for his full participation in such an experimental role. This made it easier for him to make the necessary (and sometimes inconvenient) adjustments in his usual procedure when the experiment required it. For example, at one point in the experiment, a large supply of drugs had to be stockpiled for the use of the men at the lodge. Although this was necessary, it was inconvenient for the physician, since he had to provide storage space in his already crowded offices for the extra medicine. That he did so is only one of the many instances in which this physician made some special effort for the sake of the experiment.

The Role of the House Physician

To begin with, the house physician was the overall medical authority and consultant to the lodge in the community. His position served to protect the lodge and the research staff from those social sanctions which might be imposed on an institution like the experimental subsystem which did not have some kind of provision for professional medical supervision of the health of its members. During the study, such persons as the relatives of the men at the lodge occasionally made inquiries about the health care enjoyed by the members and were always relieved and gratified to know that a house physician was on call for emergencies and for regular medical checks. He also met the requirement for appropriate medical coverage of what could be viewed as a systematic treatment program for "ex-mental patients." Although no such situation ever arose during the study, the supervision of the health of the lodge members by a physician insured that no complaint could be lodged that the men participating in the experiment were receiving medical treatment without proper medical advice and supervision.

The house physician also provided the lodge members as well as the staff coordinator with certain feelings of security and with an authority to whom they could turn with confidence for medical treatment and advice. In addition, he was an authority figure whom the men respected when taking prescribed medicine, controlling their weight, or in other medical matters where members occasionally showed resistance. On many occasions, the willingness of the lodge members to respond to this medical advice prevented or postponed their return to the hospital.

Routine medical attention was an important part of the role of the house physician and was the core of a program of preventative medicine at the lodge. This took the form of periodic follow-up of the tranquilizing medication of each member (at first monthly and then at three-month intervals when experience showed that the longer time was adequate). Annual physical examinations for each member were also included in the preventative program. In cases where it was warranted, extra laboratory work was done to evaluate the condition of certain members who were on very large dosages of phenothiazines or who were borderline diabetics.

Emergency medical attention by the house physician was limited to those matters, such as minor surgery, which could be performed in his own consultation rooms. More serious emergencies were handled by him by taking the affected person to the nearest hospital, but this happened only rarely. Usually matters which required lengthier hospitalization were handled by an arrangement with the federal hospital to be described later in this chapter. Again, in the matter of emergency medical care, the men at the lodge and the research staff derived more psychological support from the availability of the house physician than from actual use of his care. There were only two or three cases of minor surgery during the entire three-year period of the experiment.

A number of special medical problems occupied the house physician in his role on the project. These were problems common to populations of neuropsychiatric patients and they are familiar to out-patient clinics which deal with large numbers of such persons. But they are unusual problems for the ordinary practice of an internist in the community and made special demands on his time and energy. For example, the house physician only rarely had to manage gross psychotic behavior of the lodge members; almost invariably, this sort of problem occurred at the lodge and was the concern of the lodge coordinator (p. 50). It was common, though, for him occasionally to meet minor hostilities and resistance from lodge members, especially in regard to taking their medication. This emerged as one of the continuing problems at the lodge. We should note, however, that it was not a problem unique to the experience of the house physician or even confined to populations of neuropsychiatric patients. In an interview during the study, the house physician recalled one of his experiences from the Second World War: "In the army, when they had people on [a drug], for example, over in the Mediterranean, why, you couldn't depend on the individual soldier taking his own medication. You had to give it to him; and, not only that, you had to see that he swallowed it. So people are not, in general, 100 per cent reliable about this sort of thing." He also expressed uncertainty on several occasions about the regularity with which many of his other patients took prescribed medicine and declared that the lodge situation was superior to his ordinary practice in providing him information on matters of this kind.

Another special medical problem was controlling the effects of high maintenance doses of tranquilizing drugs for many of the men participating in the study. This meant carrying out special laboratory tests, and dealing with the allergic reactions and with other side effects which sometimes accompanied such prolonged-maintenance medication regimens. Such problems were not special in the sense that they involved new or unfamiliar principles of medical practice for the house physician. Obviously, it was a part of his usual practice to attempt to control the side effects of drugs in any case where such precautions were relevant. Unusual problems only arose because he did not commonly have patients who had for many years taken daily doses of, for example, over a thousand milligrams of phenothiazine derivatives and were continuing the same regimen under his care. It meant adopting procedures outside his normal medical routine. As the study continued, much of this problem lost its special character as such special procedures became established and accepted by the lodge patients in his practice.

The high dosages of strong tranquilizers taken by many of the lodge residents created special medical problems for the house physician even in the case of minor illness. In discussing this matter during an interview, he said,

> . . . These drugs [major tranquilizers] that they are taking in high dosage are dangerous drugs, and anybody who is taking them does require supervision. Now, if they get an intercurrent illness, why, an intercurrent illness may be more of a problem when they are taking these drugs, for one reason or another. Now, for example, these people frequently get gastronomycitis—nausea, vomiting, diarrhea, that type of thing. Now, maybe they can't eat, and maybe they can't take their medication. If you suddenly stop medication on these people who are taking a lot of it, you may get into difficulties; or maybe their tolerance for it varies when they get sick. . . . This sort of thing does require medical supervision. . . .

Considerations like these had to be weighed by the house physician in dealing with the members' ills, even one which would ordinarily be treated outside a hospital.

The role of the house physician included a relationship with the coordinator which evolved out of their interaction during the course of the study. It was the relationship of colleagues with complementary skills who ended up being more effective as a team in handling the health problems at the lodge than either could have been separately. The coordinator was dependent on the physician for advice on medical matters required in order to supervise the physical health of the lodge members. The house physician was dependent on the coordinator for consultation and information on behavioral problems arising at the lodge which might be of medical relevance. An example of this is the familiar problem of medication use and resistance to taking it on the part of some lodge members. The physician discussed this during one of his interviews:

> . . . They feel that the medication is something that is very important to them and sometimes they try to get away from it. They want to take less when they really may need more. Not infrequently, minor adjustments in dosage are necessary to appease the patient. This usually works out . . . you just change something a little bit and it usually satisfies them and they go along with it. This is one thing [the coordinator] and I talk over on the phone quite a bit.

Usually the physician was dependent on the coordinator for an assessment of a member's behavior when a question arose about changing medication, whether the suggestion came from the lodge member himself or from the coordinator. The physician's own judgment was involved where the problem concerned dosage reductions of a powerful or addicting or otherwise dangerous drug being taken by a lodge member. Before any change in medication, the physician almost invariably consulted with the coordinator for an assessment of the problem, and depended on him for feedback of information about the patient's behavior after the change. In some cases, the coordinator suggested changes in medication which were often approved by the physician with good results. At the lodge, therefore, the coordinator acted as the main representative of the house physician to insure that particular directions and treatments were followed.

Attitudes of the House Physician

Annually during the study, a member of the research staff interviewed the house physician to record his views on a number of matters related to the lodge and its members. Three of these annual interviews covered the entire experimental period. The data from them show that (in terms already familiar to the reader) the overall attitudes of the physician varied from neutral to positive, with very few negative views expressed; 48 per cent of his responses were positive, 43 per cent were neutral and 9 per cent were negative.[1] These overall figures are of less value, however, than the content of his expressed views. The house physician was definitely positive about the rehabilitative value of the experimental community subsystem. He considered it an essential element in keeping persons out of the mental hospital and in the community. He clearly believed that it was a living situation superior to the hospital, describing the latter as involving a "prison-type routine." He declined to assess the lodge as a business, since he had no contact with the members as operators of a janitorial service, but he expressed positive attitudes about the lodge in all areas where he had personal knowledge. He rated it superior as a living unit to foster homes and other community living systems for ex-mental patients with which he was familiar. He considered the arrangements for medical care and supervision at the lodge to be superior to other community programs known to him. He was especially impressed by the ability of the men to derive an income from their business and by the comparatively low cost of maintaining a person in a community situation such as the lodge.

He believed that the lodge members themselves were a group of handicapped people who, although most probably permanently disabled, were benefiting greatly from their situation in the experimental living-working system. He saw limits to their abilities and did not foresee a time when they would completely lose their dependence on some kind of medical authority. But at the same time, he detected in the men a "great pride in being able to be out of the hospital . . . doing what they are doing." He observed that the men at the lodge greatly preferred living there to being in the hospital and that this showed in their behavior. In one interview, he explained: "They are leading happier lives, I think. From the standpoint of the individual . . . they appear to be much happier than they would be in the hospital, as evidenced by the fact that they resist strongly [going] back into the hospital. They resist it; and, if a major illness forces it—makes it necessary—why, they are extremely reluctant to go back in." He went on: "I am continually impressed by the severity of the psychiatric disability that these people have, by the very large amounts of medication they have to take to keep under control, and by the fact that this project seems to be working out so well as far as useful employment for them goes. Really, I think it's quite amazing."

The physician was always tremendously impressed by the lodge members' very courteous behavior and warm appreciation for anything he did for them. In these respects, he felt they were more considerate and polite than his usual patients. As he put it: ". . . a doctor sometimes gets more

1. The average per cent of agreement reached by two raters was 98 for classifying the interview responses as positive, neutral, or negative.

satisfaction out of taking care of these people than you do out of a lot of other people. Just because of the fact that they appreciate what you do for them—which may be relatively little." To a great extent, his complaints about their personal cleanliness and their tendency to distribute cigarette ashes around his consultation rooms during a visit were apparently offset by their politeness and considerate behavior. Many of the physician's attitudes reflected his awareness of the social processes at the lodge and their effect on the members. He saw the main beneficial effects of the lodge to be an increase in pride and self-esteem for the members, their increased responsibility and ability to manage their own lives, and their ability to work as a team in reaching their goals. The only negative attitudes he expressed were that he perceived the social system as continuing to maintain some dependent behavior by the members. He also indicated, however, that the amount of dependency involved was probably irreducible, given the fact that chronic psychiatric ex-patients were the persons living at the lodge.

The physician had mostly positive feelings about his own role in the experiment. The only concrete dissatisfaction expressed during the interviews concerned the sloppy appearance and habits of the men during visits to his offices, which he felt had bad effects on the rest of his practice. On the other hand, a disadvantage which he had anticipated at the beginning of the experiment did not develop: The men at the lodge did not seem to have the high incidence of illness which he had expected, and he commented at the end of the project that they had been no more trouble in that respect than any of his other patients. In all other respects he seemed satisfied with his role. He felt that he was part of the project and took an interest in the results of the experiment. He enjoyed a very good working relationship with the successive coordinators at the lodge and was especially satisfied by the confidence he felt in their medical arrangements. His assurance that the treatment he prescribed for any member would be reliably carried out at the lodge and the feedback of information on the behavior and reactions of the members in response to his treatments continuously bolstered that confidence. His role seemed to afford him a great deal of satisfaction as a working physician and as a scientist; it appealed as well to his humanitarian interest in the welfare of the men at the lodge. Considered together, these factors seemed to outweigh the inconveniences he perceived to be associated with the role.

Special Agreements with the Hospital

Throughout the study, an intimate relationship existed between the federal hospital from which the lodge members came and the research project. An experimental ward at the federal hospital acted as the feeder system for the lodge (pp. 28–30), since all members of the lodge came from that one hospital ward. Since the experimental ward was oriented around a treatment program in which the patients acted in groups, all the men going into the lodge were trained group members who had been exposed to the same set of treatment experiences (p. 28). During the experiment, the lodge held that special relation to the hospital which was enjoyed by any other community program approved as a posthospital living situation for its patients. If a patient volunteered and was assigned to the community lodge according to the research plan, he departed from the hospital on a two-week leave of absence which served as the trial period in the lodge setting. The trial period led either to a return to the hospital or to release from the hospital, usually by trial visit or discharge. These were all ordinary hospital procedures applied to the experimental situation. However, there were special arrangements made with the hospital for the experiment which fell outside usual procedures and did not extend beyond the period of the study itself. These special agreements were of two kinds: agreements for carrying out special research procedures and those related to the medical welfare of the lodge members.

During the planning phase of the experiment, negotiations among the parties to be involved in the project established a set of agreements which were designed to create the best possible conditions for carrying out the research investigation. These arrangements among the hospital, the university, the federal granting agency, and the nonprofit corporation made it possible to go through with the experimental design and its related plans (pp. 23–25). For its part, the hospital agreed to provide access to its population of patients through the experimental ward. It also agreed to allow the necessary sampling procedures which made possible the random assignment of persons to the lodge or to the control group. Without the random assignment of men to the various conditions of treatment, no meaningful comparative analysis of the experimental data could have been possible. This experimental requirement is questioned in a medical setting on the ethical ground that such a disposition of patients constitutes a denial of possibly beneficial treatment to some of the participants. It was made clear to the hospital management, however, that the relative benefits of the experimental and control conditions were unknown and that the experiment was designed precisely to find out whether the experimental treatment was better than existing practices. It was argued that it was impossible to say before the experiment which was the better treatment program, although the experimenters hypothesized that the lodge treatment program would produce more beneficial results than the control program would. The hospital management agreed with this argument. The hospital agreed also to the various testing programs carried out on the experimental ward and in other areas of the hospital as part of the project. It cooperated in allowing the discharge of patients to the community lodge as soon as possible without violating its own policies, and pledged to work cooperatively with the university and with the nonprofit corporation to complete the research project.

In support of these commitments, the hospital furnished special medical assistance to the lodge as a part of the experiment. The most important of these aids was the agreement to furnish medical care to ex-patients at the lodge. By arrangement with the chief of the psychiatric service, men living in the community subsystem could be returned to the hospital immediately in any case where the research staff judged it was necessary. This privileged access to hospital beds was primarily used for treating psychiatric problems. Still another agreement allowed the treatment of emergencies due to physical illness or injury at the hospital, either as an outpatient or by readmission to the hospital. Other aids to the medical welfare of the men at the lodge were special only in the sense that they were established hospital procedures applied in a novel way as a part of the experimental program. This included such matters as delivery of medical summary reports on lodge residents to the house physician, and an arrangement so that on the date of hospital departure each of the men going on leave of absence or trial visit received a thirty-day supply of medicine.

PART IV. COMPARISON OF THE COMMUNITY ENVIRONMENTS

12 THE COMMUNITY ADJUSTMENT OF LODGE MEMBERS

This chapter begins a transition from a description of the community experiment to its evaluation. It presents a comparison of the community adjustment of the lodge members with their matched controls who, when released from the hospital, participated in traditional community mental health programs such as outpatient treatment (p. 30). At the outset of the experiment, several hypotheses were advanced which predicted that patients who participated in the lodge program would make a more adequate community adjustment than those who did not (p. 28). Specifically, the hypotheses were:

1. A community social subsystem which provides a place of residence and work for mental patients will increase time out of the hospital, increase employment, and enhance personal self-esteem when contrasted with a program using those community facilities typically available to mental patients, such as visits to mental hygiene clinics while living at home (control condition).

2. The community social subsystem will reduce the cost of patient care.

Patients' statuses in the community were assessed systematically every 6 months subsequent to their point of eligibility for hospital departure. In this study, the durability of treatment effects was evaluated through 40 months of follow-up in an attempt to obtain more information about the relationships of early and late follow-up assessments. It was decided that follow-up forms would be completed for each participant every six months for the 2½-year period while the lodge was open. Follow-up was also continued at 4 months and 10 months after the lodge closed. This created a total follow-up period of 40 months. Since the sample was accumulated over a 3-year period, individuals entered the program at different times during the experiment. Accordingly, each individual was followed from the time he entered the sample until the discontinuation of the study. All participants in the sample were followed for at least 6 months. Table 12.1 presents the sample sizes for two comparative groups for each follow-up period.

The sample size that exists for any 6-month period is the total sample for that time period. Thus, the 35 persons at 30 months are the total number who were in the study for 30 months and are, because of the random sampling procedures employed, a representative sample of the total group. The number at each time period, therefore, should be regarded as the total number for that period and *not* as a reduction in sample due to attrition, which is displayed separately in Table 12.1.

Follow-up procedures were planned as an integral part of the research and were carried on continuously throughout its entirety for all persons in the sample. Arrangements were made at the outset to obtain assistance in completing the follow-up forms. When necessary, a variety of agencies were involved. Much of the success of the follow-up was due to the unfailing cooperation of social workers and psychologists in both California and other state hospitals, as well as in VA domiciliaries, VA hospitals, and VA regional offices throughout the country.

From the time an individual entered the sample, his movements were followed in great detail. For example, records were kept of movements from ward to ward within the research hospital, each move to the community, returns to the research hospital, as well as moves to other institutions. Dates of each move were recorded so that at each 6-month follow-up period the physical location of every subject could easily be ascertained. The 6-month follow-up date was exactly 6 months from the date the

Table 12.1. Sample Size and Attrition at Different Follow-up Periods

	Lodge Sample				*Control Sample*			
		Loss By Attrition				*Loss By Attrition*		
Follow-up Time (Months)	*Available for Comparison*	*No Data*	*Death*	*Total*	*Available for Comparison*	*No Data*	*Death*	*Total*
6	75	0	0	0	75	1	0	1
12	57	2	0	2	48	0	6	6
18	40	0	0	0	36	3	3	6
24	30	0	0	0	27	3	7	10
30	16	5	5	10	19	0	5	5

patient first entered the sample. An individual's 12-month follow-up date was 6 months from his 6-month anniversary date, and so on through the 40-month period of follow-up.

Follow-up information was acquired in two ways: through taped interviews and questionnaires. Those persons who were in the hospital on their 6-month anniversary date, whether or not they had been in the community during any part of the previous 6 months, were interviewed. The information obtained from these interviews constitutes some of the data for the detailed discussion of failing to remain in the community that is presented later in this chapter (p. 216). Also interviewed on their follow-up dates were those lodge members who resided at the lodge at that time. These interviews are the data for a later discussion of the lodge members' reactions to their community living situation (p. 232).

In addition, at each follow-up time two questionnaires were sent out for all of the subjects in the sample who were in the community, whether they resided in the lodge or in some other living situation. One questionnaire, which was usually sent directly to the person for his completion, consisted of four attitude scales, each with five items which were completed by checking one of five phrases ranging from the most positive to the least positive response. For example:

I like the place where I live
________a great deal.
________quite a bit.
________somewhat.
________only slightly.
________not at all.

One of the five scales concerned the individual's satisfaction with his living conditions, the second his satisfaction with leisure activity, the third his satisfaction with community living, and the fourth his satisfaction with the job he held. This last scale could not be used for comparative analysis, however, because most of the control group remained unemployed during the follow-up period. Each scale was scored by summing the scores of the five items comprising it. The most positive response received a score of five, the least positive a score of one.

At the same time that these scales were being completed, a respondent questionnaire was mailed to a relative with whom the subject was living or with whom he kept in contact, or to some other person, such as a foster home sponsor or friend who had sufficient knowledge of the participant's situation to complete the questionnaire. If the individual was living alone, both forms might be sent directly to him or to an agency office with the request that the forms be completed through an interview. When the person lived in the community lodge, this form was completed by the consultant to the lodge.

This form referred to as the *respondent form* is in two parts. The first part contains six items. They relate to frequency of contact with friends, verbal communication with others, appraisal of symptom behavior, drinking behavior, physical-activity level, and amount of time employed. There was also space provided for information about any hospitalizations of which the research staff might not otherwise be aware, such as a county hospitalization, and for any comments about the individual that the respondent might think would be informative.

As in the questionnaire just mentioned, each item was answered by checking the most appropriate phrase. For example:

Since leaving the hospital Mr. Smith
________gets together with many friends regularly.
________gets together with some friends regularly.
________gets together with a few friends regularly.
________gets together with one or two friends.
________is alone most of the time.

Each of these items was scored on a five-point scale.

The second part of the respondent form consisted of two scales: One was a 12-item group-living scale which measured his adjustment to other persons in his community living situation. One item was:

Mr. Smith helps with the work around the house
_____Always _____Often _____Sometimes _____Rarely _____Never

The other scale was an 18-item leisure-activity scale which contains such items as:

Mr. Smith goes to the movies
_____Always _____Often _____Sometimes _____Rarely _____Never

The items in both of these scales were again scored from one to five. Five was the score of the most active alternative.

For the individual who was hospitalized on his follow-up date, whether or not he had been in the community during part of the previous 6 months, the patient questionnaire was not completed, and only three items on the first part of the respondent questionnaire were answered by a member of the person's current ward staff. These items concerned his verbal communication, symptom behavior, and physical-activity level. Of course, any time he spent in the community or time that he was employed during the 6-month period was recorded.

All of the mailed follow-up forms were accompanied by separately typed, individually addressed letters which made the requests for information quite personal. Also enclosed were stamped, addressed return envelopes to facilitate immediate mailing of the completed questionnaires. Letters to the subjects and respondents were brief requests for information regarding the subject's community adjustment which stated that the knowledge gained from the inquiry might be helpful in improving hospital programs. Letters to other hospitals, agency offices, and the like, provided a short description of the research project, specific information regarding the completion of the forms, and other explanatory statements that might aid in their completion—especially that relating to the criteria of employment and time in the community.

Most of the forms were completed and returned very promptly, but obtaining a few required additional letters and telephone calls which, in turn, led occasionally to contacts with various institutions and outpatient departments. In one instance, eight letters and several telephone calls were required before valid information about one person's follow-up status could be obtained. There were some unsuccessful and some partially successful visits made by social workers in the various communities. In such instances, the social worker often succeeded in finding a relative or friend with whom the person had been staying briefly, only to learn that he had again moved on. Occasionally the worker could only gain a very vague description of the ex-patient's behavior and activities during his brief stay. One person, for example, was finally located in a small Oregon town where he had settled with a newly acquired wife. The field social worker who found him and his wife met with considerable resistance on his first visit but was eventually able to get the follow-up forms completed.

Besides the migrant person, accurate information was also difficult to obtain about the "hospital-hopper" whose hospitalizations in numerous institutions seldom lasted longer than a month and who typically lived for brief periods of time in different locations in several communities. Often letters or telephone calls to hospitals were required in order to get the correct dates of hospitalizations and to learn about the subject's current community living situation. In such cases, the assistance of field workers was required because these nomads usually would not voluntarily return a completed form. Even with all this help, there were a few persons about whom no information could be obtained, although presumably they were still alive. Table 12.1 shows the small number who were lost to the sample due to lack of information or death for each time period.

Comparative Evaluation

Community Tenure

In this investigation, the cumulative number of days an ex-patient remained in the community during the course of the experiment was adopted as one of the critical outcome criteria for comparing the effectiveness of the new ward-and-lodge treatment subsystem with the traditional ward-and-aftercare treatment subsystem. This single criterion is a standard against which hospital treatment is often judged. From society's point of view, the mental hospital exists as a social institution providing psychiatric care to the patient for his emotional disturbance during his time of need. It is presumed that the goal of care is amelioration of the disturbance, and that the hospital's treatment activities should result in the patient's return to the community to pick up his normal personal and social life where it was interrupted prior to his hospital stay.

How well the small-group ward-and-lodge treatment subsystem worked with respect to community tenure may be tested by comparing those who participated in the lodge with their matched controls. Patients who volunteered for the lodge experience were initially matched in pairs on age, diagnosis, and previous hospitalization, and then randomly assigned to traditional aftercare programs (volunteer-nonlodge) or to the lodge society (volunteer-lodge: pp. 30–37). Henceforth, these two groups will be referred to as the control and lodge groups, respectively.

Figure 12.1 presents the differences between the lodge and control groups on community tenure for 6 months through 40 months of follow-up assessment. This graph presents the median cumulative percentage of time in the community for the two groups. It shows that the median percentage of time spent in the community is greater for the lodge than the control group at every measurement from 6 to 40 months. Figure 12.1 also shows that a "residual effect of lodge residence" occurred in this social experiment—differential tenure in the community continued at the 34 and 40 month follow-up points which occurred *after* the lodge was closed.

To test statistically the hypothesis that the lodge treatment subsystem would reduce recidivism, median tests were used to compare the lodge and control groups on the number of persons available for comparison as presented in Figure 12.1. At 6, 12, 18, 24, and 30 months, this test yielded chi-squares with one degree of freedom of 15.36 ($p < .001$), 12.96 ($p < .001$), 11.88 ($p < .001$), 10.95 ($p < .001$), and 4.93 ($p < .05$), respectively. Median tests were also carried out for the 35 persons available at the two time periods subsequent to the closing of the "old" lodge and opening the "new" one (p. 110). These comparisons of the lodge with control group members yielded chi-squares at 34 and 40 months with one degree of freedom of 4.01 ($p < .05$), and 5.39 ($p < .05$), respectively. Consequently, time in the community is still significantly greater for the lodge than the control group, even after the original experimental conditions were altered.

Even though the scores for each 6-month interval are accumulated throughout the study and are thereby not independent, the median tests clearly show that the lodge group was living in the community a significantly greater proportion of time for any follow-up period at which the two groups might be compared. The original experimental hypothesis predicted that the small-group ward-and-lodge treatment subsystem would have a beneficial effect upon community tenure of chronic mental patients. The

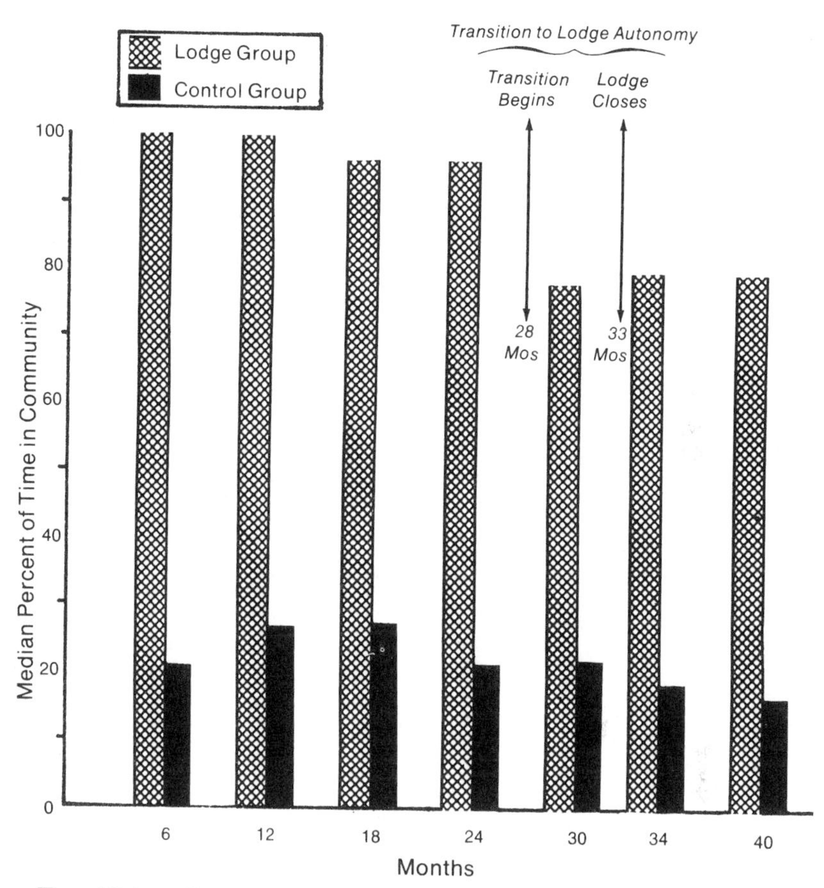

FIG. 12.1.—*Comparison of lodge and control groups on time in the community for 40 months of follow-up.*

data suggest unmistakably that the experimentally created subsystem achieved the desired effect of sustaining durable community tenure for the lodge members when compared with the tenure of those who also volunteered but did not go to the lodge.

Full-time Employment

Obtaining work and remaining employed was selected as the second critical outcome variable to be explored in this study. One intention of this investigation is to determine what changes in the employment status of chronic patients can be made when the social arrangements for his stay in the community initially place him in gainful employment.

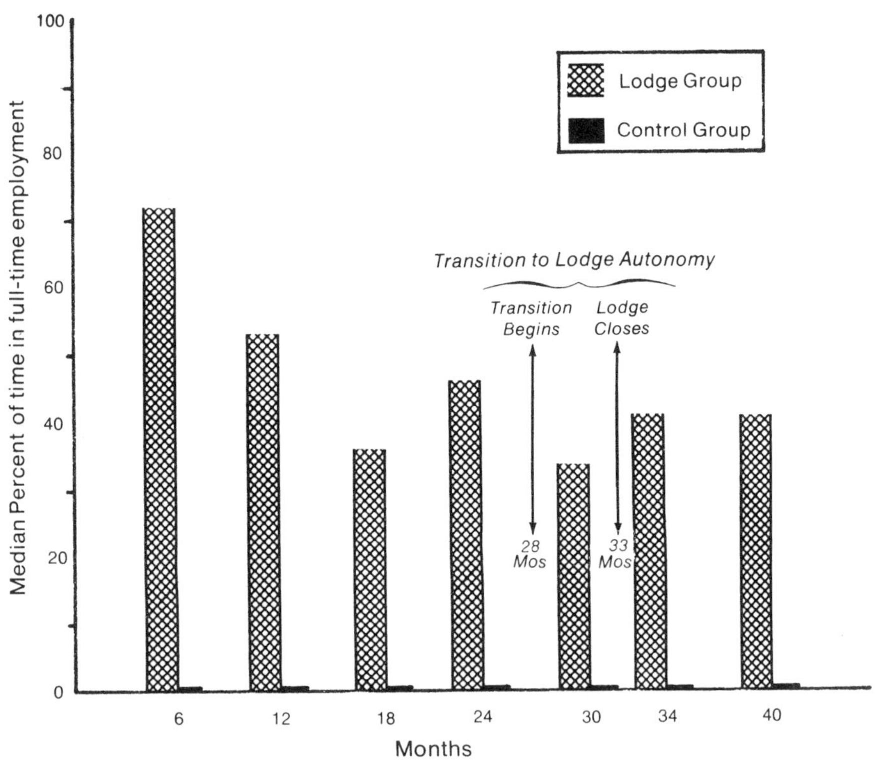

FIG. 12.2.—*Comparison of lodge and control groups on employment for 40 months of follow-up.*

The effect of the lodge upon continuing employment may be seen in Figure 12.2. The median values computed for the samples shown in Table 12.1 clearly indicate that full-time employment throughout the 30 months of the experiment is much greater for the lodge group. In fact, so few individuals were employed full time in the control group that its median score was zero, regardless of the time at which the measurement was made. Median tests comparing the employment of the lodge and control groups at 6, 12, 18, 24, and 30 months yield chi-squares with one degree of freedom of 75.00 ($p < .001$), 30.44 ($p < .001$), 15.25 ($p < .001$), 14.02 ($p < .001$), and 7.64 ($p < .01$), respectively. Median tests were also completed for the 35 persons available for comparison on follow-up information gathered after the "old" lodge was closed and the "new" one was opened (p. 110). Thirty-four- and 40-month follow-up periods yielded chi-squares with one degree of freedom of 7.13 ($p < .01$) and

7.13 ($p < .01$), respectively. As with the time-in-community variable, each 6-month interval represents accumulated data which is interrelated by definition. Nonetheless, the chi-squares show that the lodge group was employed a significantly greater proportion of the time for any follow-up period at which the two groups *might* be compared.

Since the experimental plans deliberately created a situation permitting full-time employment, it is to be expected that this opportunity for employment would be reflected in the comparison of the lodge with the control group. However, the fact that members of the lodge group remained fully employed significantly longer than the control group members does not logically warrant the conclusion that this effect was due exclusively to the lodge situation, since lodge members were free to leave the lodge at any time and secure full-time employment elsewhere in the community. Actually, of the 75 patients who went to the lodge, only five remained the full time (3 years). Thus, there were a substantial number of lodge members who could have secured employment for varying periods of time after leaving the lodge.

Employment information for lodge group members after leaving the lodge was available on 52 of the original 75 persons who were sent there. (The employment situation of the remaining 23 could be determined only with reference to their lodge residence, not beyond it.) Of this group of 52, two-thirds (35) showed no days of employment subsequent to leaving the lodge. The 17 persons who had attained post-lodge employment fared little better than the control group; their median employment time was 47 days, or little more than a month and a half during 18 months of follow-up. When lodge members were not in the "old" or "new" lodge, they resembled the control group, with a clear tendency to be unemployed if they were in the community at all.

It is clear from the results of the experiment thus far presented, then, that two of the propositions in the first experimental hypothesis with which this chapter began were actually confirmed. The lodge *did* retain patients in the community longer than the other arrangements for community tenure which control patients could make. The lodge situation also *did* provide more frequent and longer employment on a full-time basis than other employment situations which the control group members were able to locate when and if they went to the community looking for work. And lodge members were not able to secure employment once they left the lodge. Their employment record outside the lodge strongly resembled that of the control group.

Other Criteria of Community Adjustment

Community tenure and full-time employment have been termed social-change outcome criteria because they reflect aspects of behavior that the community expects from returning mental patients. Beyond these two social-change outcome criteria, however, may be found a number of other indices of successful community adjustment, any one of which could have been adopted in place of full-time employment or community tenure. In this investigation, such criteria were measured for every accessible patient each 6 months for 30 months and twice in the next 10 months through the use of follow-up questionnaires (p. 201). The chi-squares comparing the lodge and control groups on these measures are presented in Table 12.2.

What is immediately evident from this table is the striking fact that despite the very clear differences found between the lodge and control groups on time in the community and full-time employment, no such differences appear on these outcome criteria except for the difference with respect to satisfaction with living in the community for the 12-month time period. Out of 70 comparisons, only one is statistically significant. The fact that no striking differences appear on these criteria suggests the possibility that in terms of these relatively gross measurements, the two groups of patients are for all practical purposes alike. Therefore, it seems worthwhile to consider how these two groups of chronically hospitalized mental patients may be described in general terms when data about them is pooled.

Table 12.2. Chi-square Values[a] Comparing Lodge and Control Groups on Follow-up Items

	Follow-up Time (Months)						
Item	6	12	18	24	30	34[b]	40[b]
Patient Self-evaluations:							
Satisfaction with living conditions	.04	1.73	1.18	3.31	.06	.24	.06
Satisfaction with leisure activity	.04	3.56	.00	3.31	.06	.48	.63
Satisfaction with community living	.52	4.33[c]	.49	.64	.06	.04	.06
Respondent Evaluations:							
Association with friends	.01	.00	.01	.60	.06	.46	.02
Verbal communication	.06	.09	.02	.01	.00	.00	.53
Appraisal of symptom behavior	.57	.00	.51	.06	.00	1.60	.09
Drinking behavior	.70	.07	.27	.04	.06	.25	.06
Activity level	.83	.75	.03	.24	.00	.85	.53
Social responsibility	3.24	2.92	.10	1.08	.06	1.37	.63
Leisure activity	.34	1.72	.65	.28	.06	.24	.06

[a] All chi-square values have been corrected for continuity using Yates' formula, and have 1 df.
[b] 34- and 40-month measures were taken after conditions of the experiment were changed by closing the lodge 33 months from the beginning of the experiment.
[c] Significant at .05 level.

For the three follow-up assessment devices measuring ex-patients' satisfaction with their living conditions, their use of leisure time, and their preference for community versus hospital living, the score were uniformly high, with median values ranging from 18 to 22 points out of a possible 25. Thus, both groups were highly favorable toward aspects of living in the community, which probably is the result of a strong preference for community living contrasted with hospital living. This interpretation is all the more plausible when viewed from the lodge members' perspective. As shown in detailed periodic interviews with lodge members, they almost unanimously stated that they were glad to have the freedom coincident upon departure from the hospital (pp. 211–215).

Beyond the three criteria relating to satisfaction with the community living situation and the patients' reaction to it, six of the criteria deal with various aspects of social behavior as distinct from individual behavior and attitudes. These are the social-responsibility scale, the leisure-activity scale, and the scales relating to friendships, verbal communication, and drinking habits. Patients in both groups reveal themselves able to take on the responsibilities associated with group living situations such as dormitory or household membership. For the most part, they tend to indulge in the passive types of leisure activity (reading, radio listening, and TV watching) and to be well satisfied with this aspect of their community living. They spend much of their time alone or occasionally with one or two friends, not being very verbally communicative or oriented toward interaction with others. Three out of five tend to be drinkers of alcoholic beverages, but no distinct patterns of drinking are discernible from the data relating to this behavior. Many in these two groups are likely to show minor symptomatic evidence of their emotional disturbance, so that raters cannot view them as normally behaving persons in the community. Similarly, they tend to appear energetic and active, but without direction of their actions which appears indicative of a generalized motivational energy to accomplish goals.

To sum up all of this evidence, one might conclude that the major effect of the lodge situation upon those who went there was to support their stay and productivity in the community without grossly affecting their individual psychosocial adjustment. As has been indicated quite clearly in the chapters relating to the internal processes of lodge operation (pp. 45–126), the lodge group revealed themselves to be no less a disabled group, when measured in terms of commonly used adjustmental criteria such as those presented in this section, than any other group of chronic mental patients such as those with whom they were matched (the control group). Their seclusiveness, inarticulateness, eccentric behavior, and passivity in social interaction were no deterrent, however, to their capacity to remain productively occupied in the community when an appropriately designed social situation was provided for them. In the lodge, they could adopt participative social roles within their limited capacities. Whatever rewards and ego enhancement these new social roles may have provided the lodge participants, they are clearly not revealed in these comparisons of rather gross behavioral rating criteria.

Treatment Costs

The differential allocation of economic resources in complex societies represents the impact of human values upon the use of those resources. Relative expenditure expresses priorities making up a particular conception of the good life which a society's members are willing to support financially. In a society as materialistic and object-oriented as that of contemporary America, allocation of resources for the support of marginal groups within the society may always be grudging, even in an historical era when it is fashionable to assist "those in need." Much of the reluctance of the society to provide for its marginal members has revolved around the concept of "value given for value received." The assumption is that a man's worth may be defined by what he can produce, and that he should be paid accordingly.

Any new proposal for care of marginal persons which requires any financial support is typically greeted with skepticism if not outright suspicion. At the very least, any new organization of such services or programs is likely to be looked upon as potentially expensive, usually on the basis that introducing new services creates as well as meets needs. It is therefore necessary to evaluate the community lodge in financial terms if it is to be seriously considered as an alternative to mental hospitalization.

For several reasons, the problem of establishing the community lodge was made relatively easy at the outset. First, the amount of investment in materials to establish a living situation and a work organization was minimal because of the personnel and the business involved. All of the members were men, permitting joint sharing of living quarters by people accustomed to living in large hospital wards. Work tools and equipment, such as floor buffers, brooms, rakes, and the like, for a janitorial and yardwork service were relatively inexpensive to purchase. When a suitable location was found, a lease was negotiated on an annual basis with the property owners and similar lease arrangements were made with an automobile dealer who provided the vans and pickup trucks used to carry out the janitorial and yardwork services. Thus the major capital investments for this organization were contracted for on a lease-rental basis.

Once this new social institution had been created in the community, its survival depended upon the establishment of a reasonable relationship between income and outgo. To be sure, at the outset it was understood that the community lodge would be fully supported by research funds, whatever the cost. But one of the major interests in the experiment itself was the determination of exactly what it would take in the way of financial support to maintain such an institution in the community. For this reason, substantial attention was given to the maintenance of accurate records of expenditures and income in order to evaluate the economic viability of this new social institution.

First we shall compare the costs of operating a community lodge with the costs of other alternative treatments available to the chronic psychiatric patient. It must be remembered that supervision of the lodge was treated as part of the experimental investigation, and was systematically varied during the course of the experiment. In order to present accurate cost comparisons, therefore, the cost for each of the three periods of leadership —professional, untrained lay persons, and members—must be computed independently.

Figure 12.3 presents a comparison of the daily cost per person for the various types of treatments that would be available to him in the local area in which the community lodge was established. It can readily be seen that the least expensive hospital alternative (state hospital) is almost twice as expensive as the lodge organization when professional supervision is used and when work income is *not* employed to defray expenses of its operation. When member supervision is used and work income is employed to defray costs (the most inexpensive treatment setting), the daily cost per person is only $3.35 in the community lodge. Any other alternative, including Veterans Administration hospitalization, is clearly substantially more expensive. Any administrator solely concerned with the most inexpensive method of housing chronically hospitalized psychiatric patients can hardly avoid considering a social system which *decreases* by at least *one-half* his cost per patient day. Combined with the control over their own destiny and the opportunity for productive and moderately remunerative work, its financial feasibility recommends it favorably as a viable solution to the social problem of the chronically hospitalized mental patient.

The Lodge Members' View of Their Subsociety

To the individual lodge resident, however, financial feasibility is naturally not a primary concern. The existence of the lodge in the community potentially expanded the number of socially feasible alternatives available to him, and it would undoubtedly be this type of feasibility that would mean the most to him. No evaluation of this experiment would be complete without some consideration for the lodge member's own view of the special world which had been devised for him and which he ultimately operated himself. Information of this sort was gained from the lodge members primarily through structured interviews conducted every six months.

The questions were designed to cover systematically such topical areas as the lodge member's view of his own role at the lodge; the contrast be-

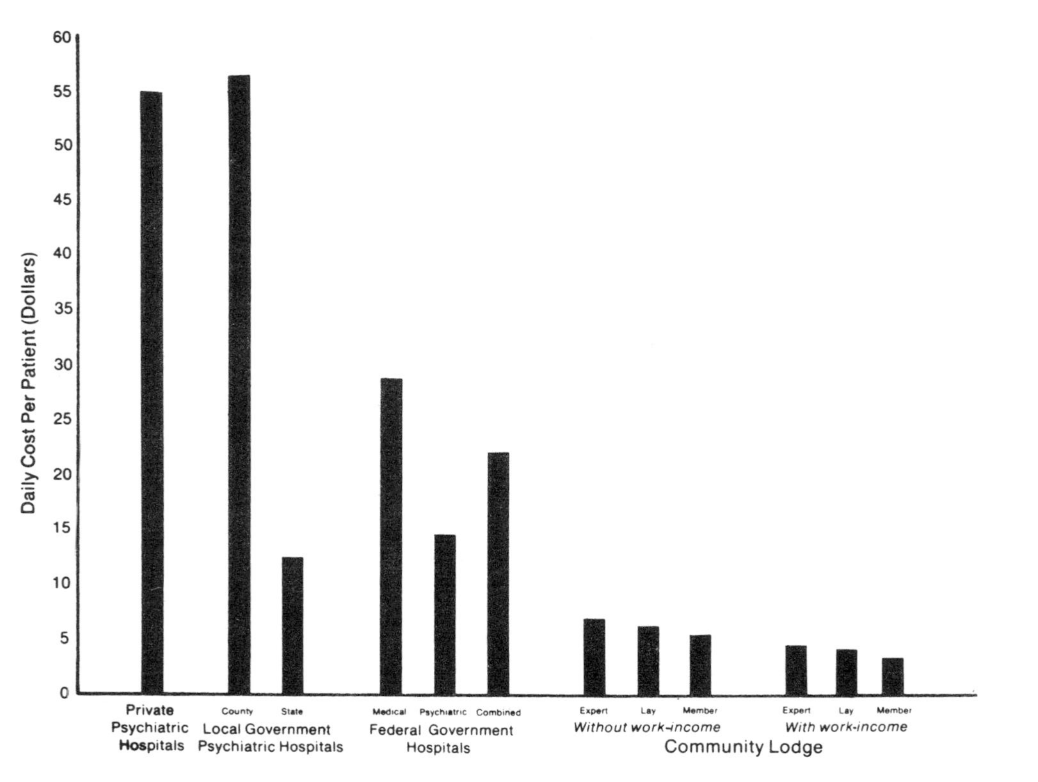

FIG. 12.3.—*Mean daily cost per person for alternative treatment settings in California Bay Area, 1964–66.*

tween the type of responsibility he was asked to undertake as a lodge member compared with the degree of responsibility required of him as a resident in the mental hospital from which he came; his own evaluation of the work he performed at the lodge and the expectations he held concerning that work; his use of leisure time; the advantages and disadvantages he saw in living at the lodge; the ways in which he felt the lodge might be improved as a living-working situation in the community; the differences he saw between what he expected the lodge to be like and how he found it after living there at least six months; the relations between the lodge, its business customers, and the surrounding neighborhood; and the effect of living at the lodge upon his self-concept as a "mentally ill" person. All questions were asked in an open-ended format, giving the respondent a free range of expression for his reaction to the topic being covered, to be followed by additional probing about the how's and why's of his reaction. Seventy-four questions were asked on each occasion, two examples of which are: "What have been your problems since coming to the lodge?" and "Do you expect to leave the lodge at any time? If so, where would you go and what would you do?"

Responses to these questions were tape-recorded at the lodge on each occasion, using lodge supervisory personnel as trained interviewers. The tape recordings were subsequently abstracted into abbreviated written form. Reliability of this abstracting process was examined by having two judges abstract from the same interviews 140 pairs of responses, for which there was 91 per cent agreement. Once abstraction from the tape recordings was completed, all responses for each item were ranked by assigning the highest rank to the most positive response. Ranking reliability yielded a rho of .87. The rank position for each item then became a score for the person located in that rank position. A correlation matrix of the relationship between these ranks on 49 items abstracted from the interviews was computed, and an electronic computer was used to examine the clusters that the correlations formed (Tryon and Bailey, 1965).

The cluster analysis yielded seven relatively independent domains of expression by lodge residents in viewing the subsociety in which they lived. The average interrelationship between clusters is .13; the median correlation is .09. Each of the seven clusters was given a label to reflect the common theme underlying the items clustered, as follows:

Cluster 1—Satisfaction with Living-Working Conditions. This cluster groups items related to likes and dislikes about living and working at the lodge, including relationships between lodge members and with customers of their business.

Cluster 2—Acceptance of Lodge Society. This grouping of items concerns the willingness of lodge members to live in the lodge according to its rules, rewards, and work assignments.

Cluster 3—First-Class Citizenship as an Unexpected Lodge Benefit.

This cluster concerns the sometimes amazed revelation by lodge members that living at the lodge is like living in the normal community, something they failed to anticipate at all.

Cluster 4—Preference for Communal Life. This item grouping reflects the personal freedom and responsible role each lodge member must assume as part of the conditions for his living there, a substantial contrast for him to hospital living.

Cluster 5—Rejection of Hospital Norms. This cluster of items reflects the opportunity for normal community living which so strikingly contrasts with the minimally demanding hospital environment in the lodge members' view.

Cluster 6—Denial of Psychiatric Disability. This cluster concerns both indirect admissions of disability (isolation from others living at the lodge), plus a self-concept which reflects feelings of normal community relationships and confidence in remaining in the community were the lodge to close.

Cluster 7—Confidence in Worker Status. This item grouping reflects the confident outlook toward his prospects which the lodge member derives from his status as a worker at the lodge.

Were there any aspects of the lodge members' attitudes toward living at the lodge that significantly differed from other aspects? To answer this question, cluster scores were assigned to each lodge member for each occasion on which he was interviewed. These were converted to standard scores with a mean of 50, a standard deviation of 10, and a range from 1 to 100. The means for each group interviewed at each time period (6 months through 30 months) were computed, and a simple rank test of significance applied. No significant difference between clusters obtained, suggesting that the seven clusters were about equally valued by lodge members. The mean for all clusters was 50.08, resting at the very center of the normalized distributions of scores.

The further question now arises as to whether or not significant differences in attitude may be found with regard to specific subgroups of lodge residents. Two factors are of special interest in evaluating the lodge members' view of their world. First, since the social status of the worker at the lodge was particularly important to its members as a sign that they "belonged" (pp. 88–100), it is appropriate to ask whether there were any significant differences between members in their attitudes toward lodge living when their social position within the lodge is taken into account. Second, lodge members can be classified in terms of their ultimate fate in the community. It would also be informative to inquire whether there are significant differences in attitude between lodge members who remained in the community compared to those who were known to have returned to the mental hospital.

The organization of the lodge society contained the social statuses of crew chief, worker, and marginal worker (p. 59). Accordingly, all 75 persons who lived at the lodge were classified into one of these three categories by two consultants who were intimately acquainted with each person's daily work. These two consultants reached 76 per cent agreement. After these lodge members were grouped into the three worker categories, mean cluster scores of 207.4, 196.9, and 198.7 were obtained for the crew chiefs, workers, and marginal workers, respectively. A Friedman rank test for the significance of the difference between these means yielded a χ_r^2 of 6.0 (2 df), which is significant beyond the .05 level. The means show that crew chiefs were the most satisfied with their work status, the marginal workers, who did minimal work, were the next most satisfied group, and the least satisfied group were those who were steady workers but did not attain supervisory work status. None of the three groups showed any differential emphasis upon one or another of the seven clusters of attitudes about living and working at the lodge.

Similar effects were observed for a comparison of those who did and those who did not return to the mental hospital. Of the 36 persons interviewed at the lodge at the end of 6-months' residence, 27 ultimately did not return to the hospital, while 9 did during the course of the next two years. A rank test revealed both groups to have substantially similar attitudes toward lodge life, with no particular cluster of attitudes being stressed by either group compared with any other cluster.

The finding of the relationship between worker status and personal happiness in a social situation may well be a common phenomenon in societies. Those who had the most positive attitudes toward living at the lodge were the crew chiefs. They were the leaders of the lodge society who had the decision-making powers in the organization. If they aspired to leadership positions, their aspirations must have been realized. The marginal worker, on the other hand, often appeared to be satisfied with having a recognized social position in the group—something he had not achieved in the past. He perceived his role as important to the group's operation. He too had aspired and, at least in part, achieved. The worker, on the other hand, often seemed to aspire to the crew chief's social position but he did not attain it. Thus he was the only member of the lodge that did not in large measure fulfill his expectations.

Those at the top of the social structure perceived their role as the most responsible, while those at the bottom perceived their role as contributing to the overall effort as long as the rest of the group were able to tolerate their presence (pp. 58–64). The extent to which this theme interwove the deliberations of the executive committee of the lodge, leading to the "business" and "rehabilitation" factions, and to the worker's "revolt," is presented elsewhere (pp. 96–100). Generally, it is critical that marginal persons perceive themselves as having a personally meaningful role in the social structure.

The Lives of Those "Failing" In Two Different Community Situations

Reasons for Hospital Reentry

Pursuing the theme of the need for a meaningful status in the social structure, it will be instructive to examine the perceptions of those who failed to remain in the community, whether at the lodge or elsewhere. These two different social situations (lodge and general community) for returning mental patients are undoubtedly stressful in different ways, since they place different demands on the individual. In order to obtain an understanding of life in the community for hospital returnees, whether from the lodge or elsewhere, each was interviewed as soon as feasible after he reentered the hospital. This period never exceeded two weeks, and normally the interview took place within 24 hours after he reentered the hospital.

Each of the returnee interviews was tape-recorded and responses were abstracted from these recordings. The abstracted responses were then placed in coded categories for analysis. Two raters reached 93 per cent agreement on abstracting the responses and 75 per cent agreement on the content of the responses. Reliabilities were also established for coding these responses by using the same two judges. For the lodge interviews, 82 per cent agreement was reached, and for the nonlodge group agreement on 86 per cent of the classifications was attained. Only the interviews conducted upon the patient's first return to the hospital were used. For the nonlodge group of interviews, those who had volunteered to go from the hospital to the lodge and who functioned as the control group in the experiment were combined with those who did not volunteer. This pooling of the volunteer and nonvolunteer nonlodge samples of interviews was decided upon because both groups returned to the same community programs and no essential differences between these two groups existed either in community tenure or length of employment (pp. 242-245).

Because the actual social situation in the community was markedly different for the two groups, the returnee interview content varies somewhat. However, both groups were queried concerning their reasons for reentry into the hospital and their future plans now that they had returned to the hospital.

Table 12.3 presents the reasons for returning to the hospital for both the lodge and nonlodge groups. Inspection of the table shows that significant differences exist between the lodge and the nonlodge community situation. By far the greatest proportion of those in the lodge group returned because of personal reactions, such as feelings of discomfort, to living in the community lodge situation. And the fewest number returned because of pressure from individuals with whom they lived. Those who

Table 12.3. Reasons for Hospital Reentry

Reason	Lodge (N)	Lodge (%)	Nonlodge (N)	Nonlodge (%)
Personal reactions to living situation	24	80	53	55
Disruptive interpersonal relations	5	17	4	4
Pressure to return from those with whom he lived	1	3	40	41
Total	30	100	97	100

$\chi^2 = 17.71^a$ (2 df)

[a] Significant at .001 level.

returned to nonlodge community living situations also had a high percentage of returnees because of personal reactions to their living situation, but 41 per cent of that group returned to the hospital because of pressure from relatives or friends. In comparing the lodge and nonlodge groups on their future plans, however, no significant differences were obtained ($\chi^2 = 4.41$, 2 df).

Typifying the resignation of the returning nonlodge group member was this comment: "I don't know. Guess I'll always be in the hospital as my wife won't have me back home and I can't get a job and lead a normal life." The fact that the proportion of lodge returnees who mentioned difficult interpersonal relationships as influencing their return to the hospital more frequently than did nonlodge group members suggests that the group living-working situation at the lodge placed a greater premium upon competence in this area. But here it is important to note that lodge members most often perceived their return as a result of their own discomfort. This is congruent with an earlier finding of the acceptance of deviant behavior by lodge members (pp. 63–64).

Living Conditions in the General Community

What do we know of the living conditions for those returning to the community as described by them when they returned to the hospital? Figure 12.4 shows that 52 per cent of the nonlodge group located themselves in residential areas of cities or towns, 37 per cent sought out the central city area where inexpensive hotels and rooming houses are available, and 11 per cent headed for some kind of rural location. Figure 12.5 shows that the largest proportion of the group lived in houses (47 per cent), one-third found hotel rooms, residence clubs, and rooming houses for shelters (33 per cent), while 17 per cent spent most of their time in apartments or trailers. Figure 12.6 shows that during this time, one-third (33 per cent) of the group lived alone, 38 per cent lived primarily with relatives, while 15 per cent and 14 per cent, respectively, lived either with their immediate family (wives and/or children) or with friends and

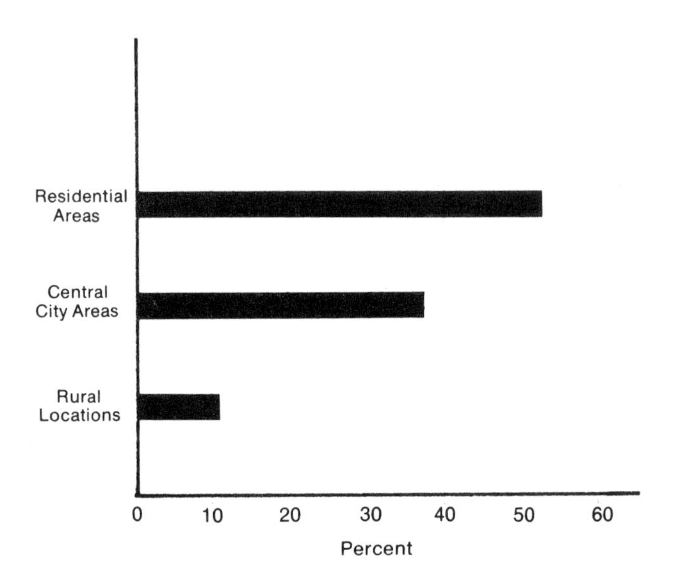

FIG. 12.4.—*Initial residence location.*

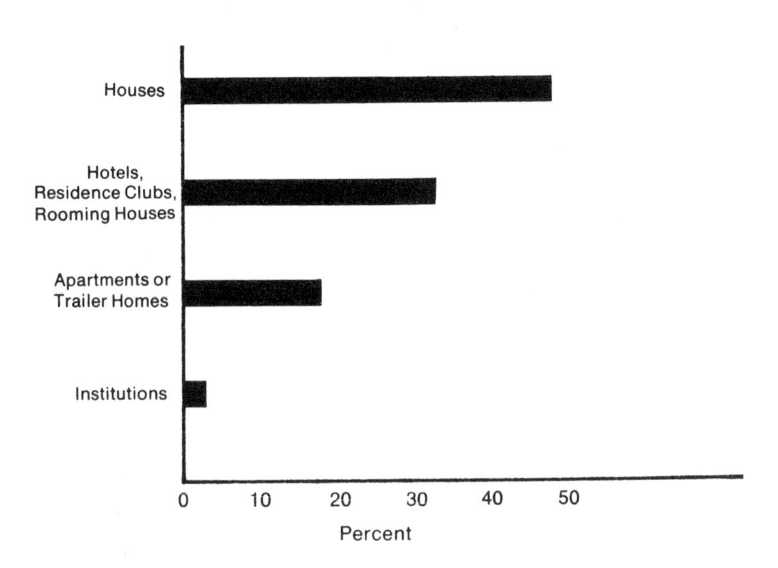

FIG. 12.5.—*Type of dwelling.*

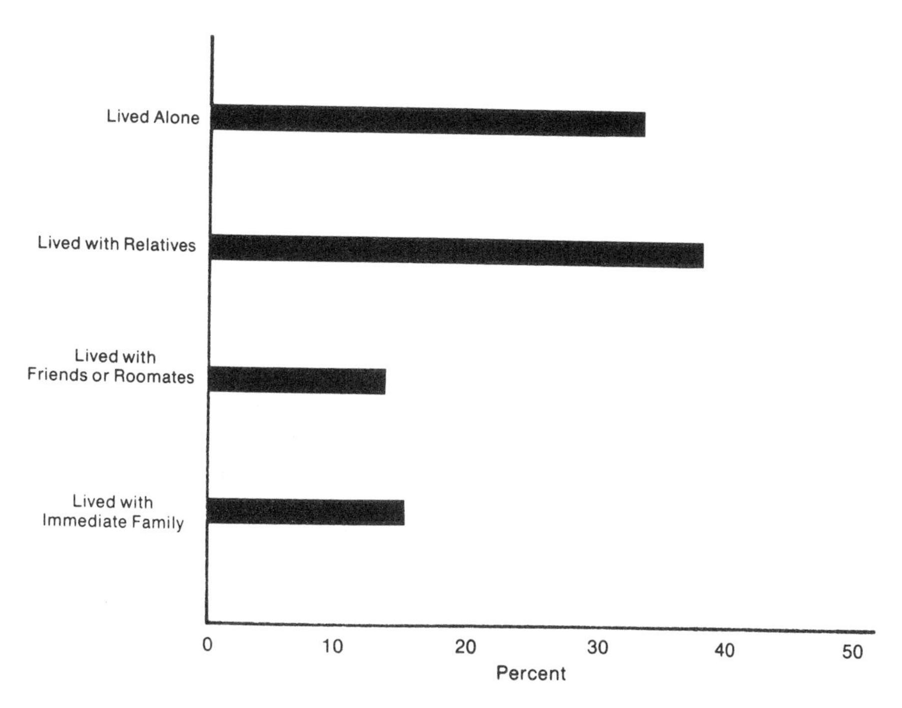

FIG. 12.6.—*Living arrangements.*

roommates. Thus, the major burden of community tenure for four-fifths of this group was delegated to relatives. Figure 12.7 shows that of those not living alone, 40 per cent remained in the same community situation from one to three months and 21 per cent lived up to one month, while 21 per cent stayed more than six months. Eighteen per cent of the group remained in the same situation from three to six months. Thus, 79 per cent of the group not living alone did not remain in the same community situation for more than half a year, a relatively short time for attaining an adjustment to community living, especially with this heavy dependence upon relatives.

Several aspects of this adjustment were explored with returning non-lodge group members in the interview. Among them were their friendships, their recreational activity, their feelings of loneliness, and their use of medications while in the community. Figure 12.8 shows that almost one-third (32 per cent) reported they had no friends while out of the hospital. The other 68 per cent of the group varied in their friendship patterns. Half of the group met new friends they had not known before leaving the hospital, 10 per cent reported contacts only with relatives or neighbors or persons they previously knew in the hospital, while 7 per cent of the group

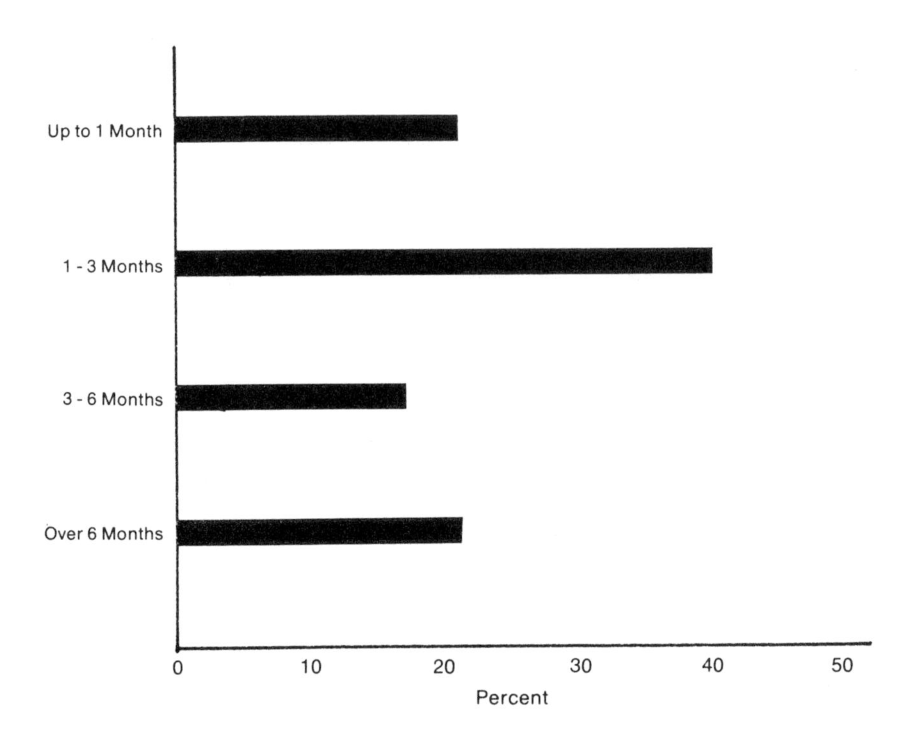

FIG. 12.7.—*Duration of stay with others.*

saw only persons they had known during their previous hospitalization. Figure 12.9 reveals that one-quarter of this group contacting others dealt only with male friends, 41 per cent of the total group saw both male and female friends, and a mere 3 per cent reported sole acquaintanceship with female friends. And Figure 12.10 shows that almost two-thirds (65 per cent) of the group reported only a few friends, while the remaining 35 per cent reported seeing numerous friends.

When asked how they would describe their recreational activities or the use of their own leisure time, nonlodge group members revealed themselves in general to be relatively inactive. Figure 12.11 reveals that 6 per cent of the group merely stayed around their residence doing nothing in particular, while 61 per cent engaged in passive, solitary games and amusements such as TV watching, radio listening, reading, sitting around, or walking alone in the neighborhood, making a total of two-thirds of the group. In relative proportion (Fig. 12.12), almost half of these activities took place where the persons were staying (48 per cent), an identical proportion did go out in public, and the remaining 4 per cent carried out leisure-time activity at other people's houses. As suggested by this data,

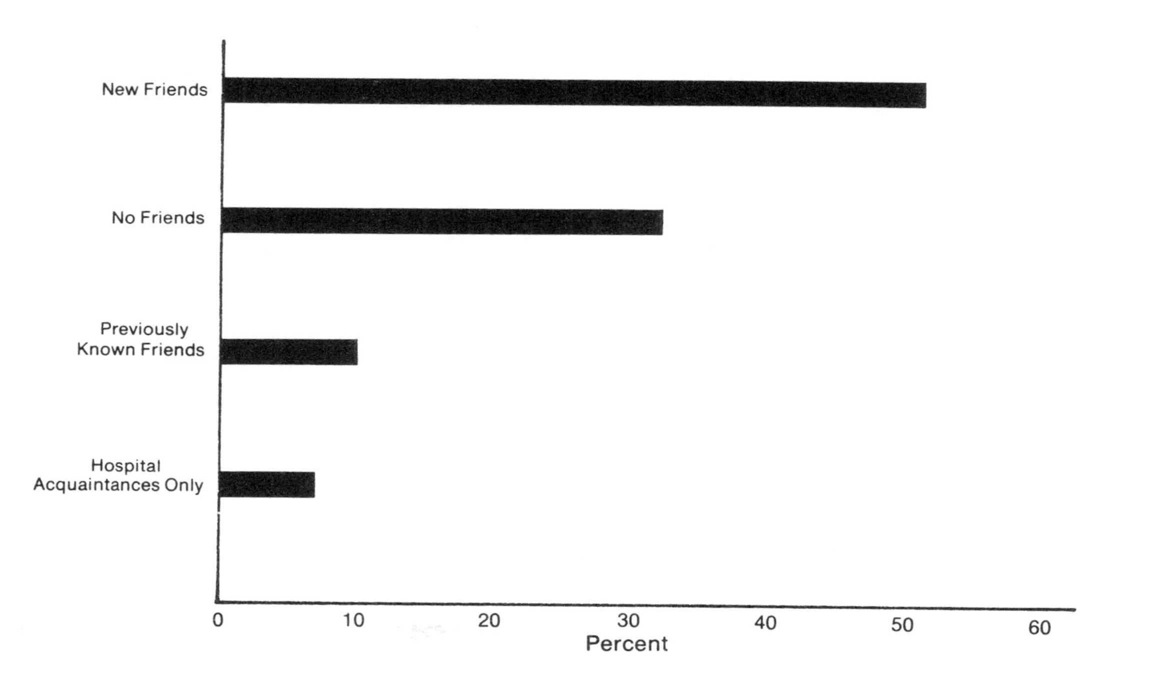

FIG. 12.8.—*Friendships in the community.*

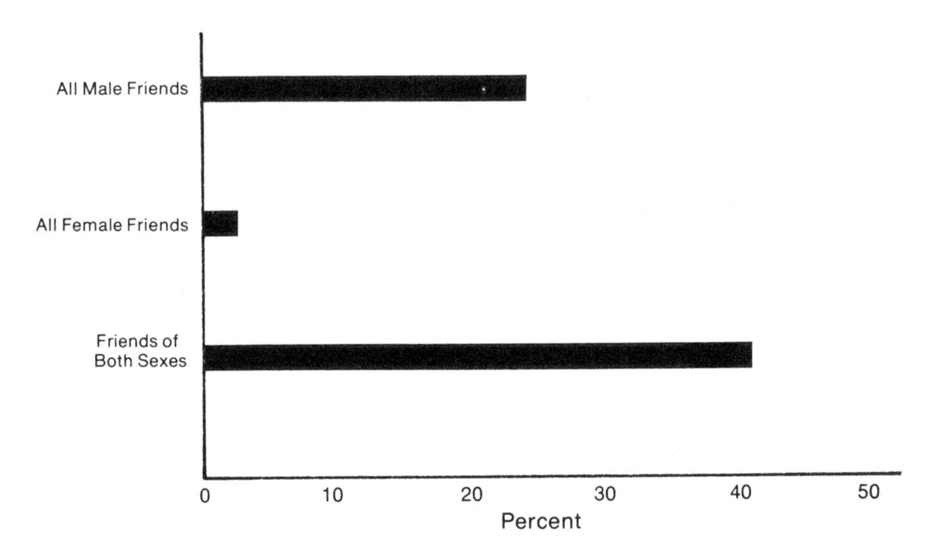

FIG. 12.9.—*Sex of friends in the community.*

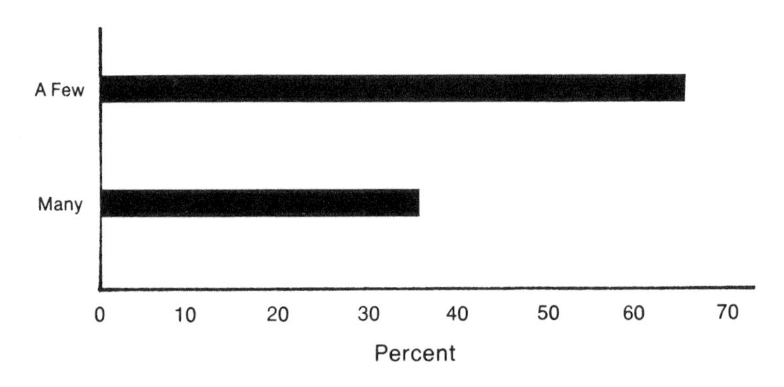

FIG. 12.10.—*Number of friends in the community.*

Fig. 12.13 shows that 59 per cent of the group spent this type of time alone, almost one-quarter (24 per cent) spent it with relatives, and 17 per cent spent it with friends.

It is not surprising then that almost half of the group (44 per cent) reported some degree of loneliness while in the community (Fig. 12.14). They were also asked if they missed associating with the hospital ward small group to which they had belonged (Fig. 12.15). Fifteen per cent

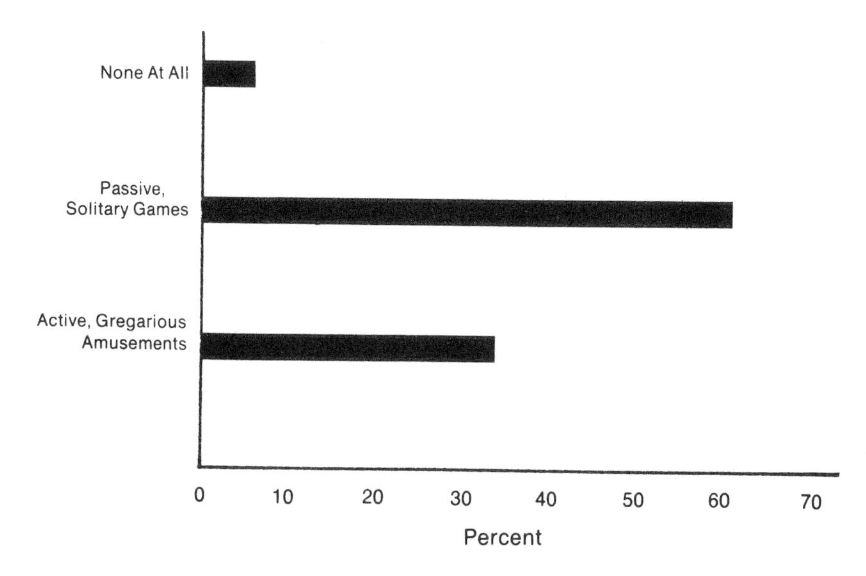

FIG. 12.11.—*Type of recreation in the community.*

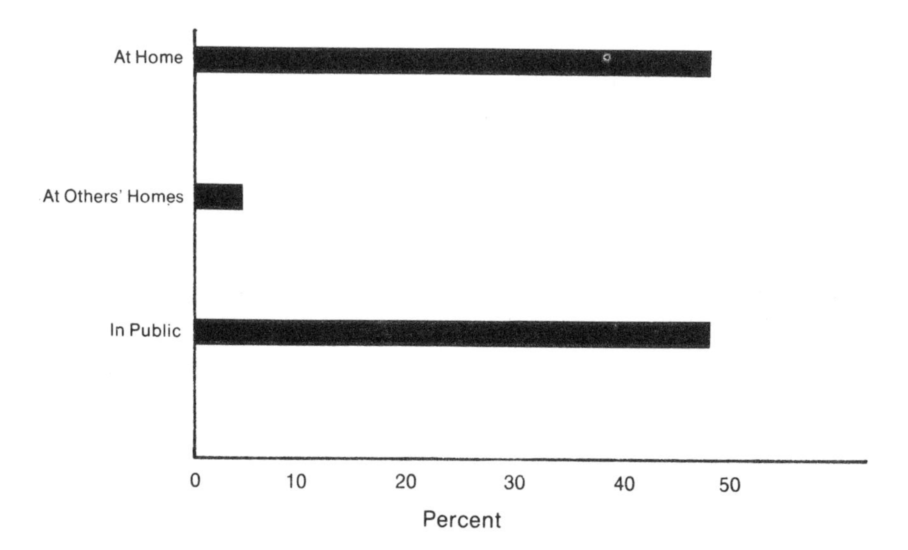

FIG. 12.12.—*Location of recreation.*

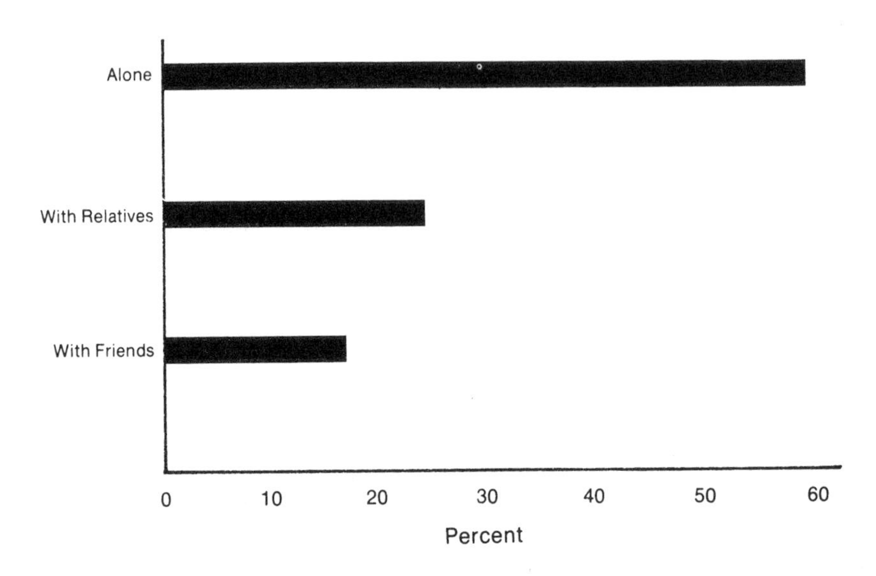

FIG. 12.13.—*Recreational companionship.*

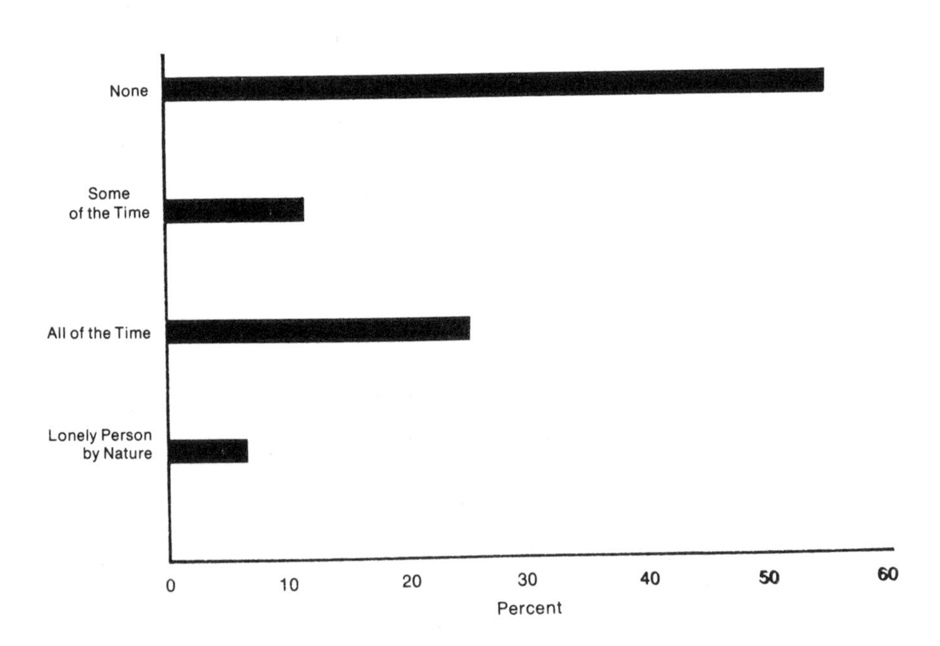

FIG. 12.14.—*Feelings of loneliness in the community.*

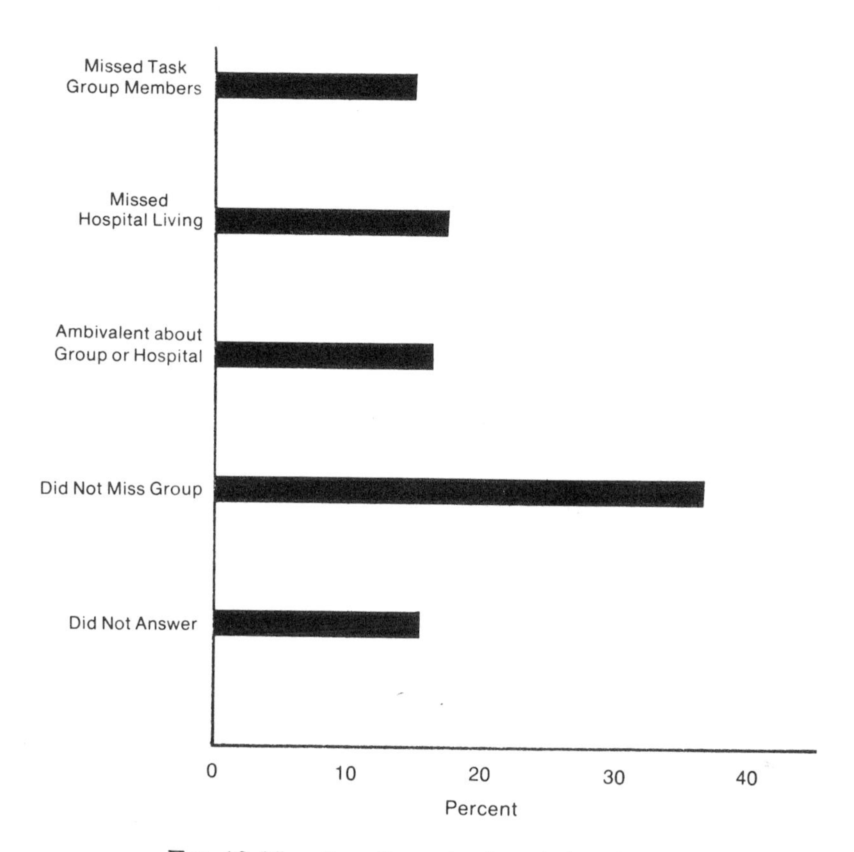

FIG. 12.15.—*Loneliness for hospital task group.*

disavowed recalling such associations, while an equal proportion admitted to missing them. Almost an equal percentage were ambivalent in their feelings about this issue (16 per cent), while 17 per cent clearly missed being in the hospital, although not necessarily being in the small group to which they were assigned before discharge. The remaining 36 per cent denied such feelings.

Before turning to the employment experiences which the returning patient had while in the community, it is instructive to contrast the nonlodge group's use of medication with the situation which prevailed at the lodge. In the lodge, a system for effective management of medication was evolved (pp. 50–51). Under this condition of medication management, no lodge member was returned to the hospital under conditions of failing to take medication after the first few weeks of the lodge's existence.

Now let us examine the returning nonlodge patients' reports of their experience in this area (Fig. 12.16). Of the 98 persons involved, 12 per

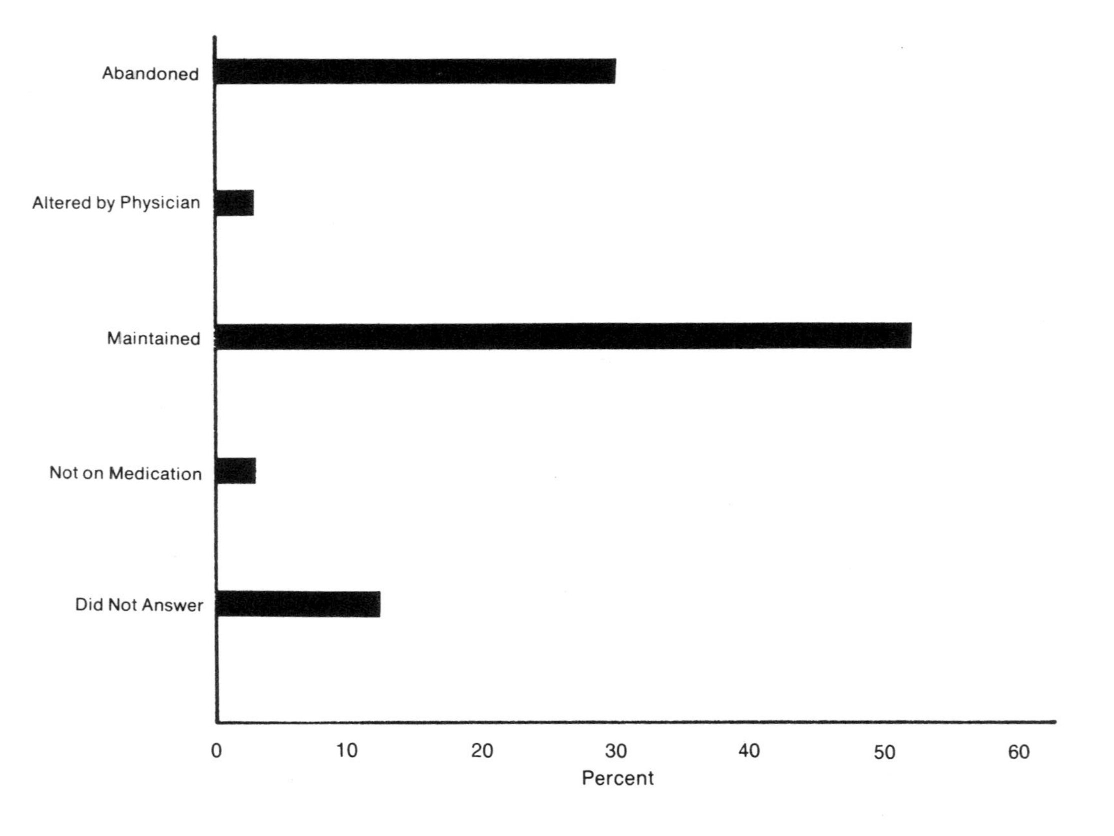

FIG. 12.16.—*Use of medication in the community.*

cent did not reply to the question concerning medication use, while 3 per cent of the group were either not on prescribed medications while in the community or were only provided medications to be used as they felt the need for them. In the remaining 85 per cent of the group, 30 per cent mismanaged their use either by altering or abandoning prescribed dosages or by not renewing prescriptions when they were exhausted (which often was associated by these respondents with inability to pay for a refilled prescription). The remaining 52 per cent of the group reported they continued their usage according to the instructions given them upon leaving the hospital or according to alterations in dosage prescribed by a supervising physician in the community. In sum, approximately half of the group were able to keep up a successful conformity with medical advice about their use of medications while in the community, whereas at least three in ten returning patients clearly did not do so. The extent to which this laxity contributed to their hospital return cannot be estimated from the information gained from the returning nonlodge patients.

The nature and effects of stress upon employment in the lodge society have been discussed elsewhere (pp. 55–58). Specific employment experiences of the nonlodge group will provide a more thorough understanding of the typical work situation for persons leaving mental hospitals.

The first area of interest concerns work-seeking experiences. Of the 98 persons, 45 per cent admitted to looking for work after their hospital departure, but about half of these either gave up the search quickly or did not follow through on opportunities which became known to them (Fig. 12.17). One-quarter of the group readily admitted that they did not bother to look for work at all, while 3 per cent planned to enter another institution without seeking work. Another 12 per cent felt no need to look for work since they considered themselves retired or technically disabled or medically unable to undertake the rigors of employment. Finally, 15 per cent assured the interviewer that they already had a job secured prior to their hospital departure.

Fifty of the 98 persons shared information with the interviewer about where they sought work (Fig. 12.18) and the type of work they were looking for during their stay in the community. Almost half of this group (46 per cent) sought work in companies or businesses, 26 per cent tried the route of employment offices, typically those operated by the state government in urban areas or the farm labor offices in the rural areas to which they went. The same percentage (6 per cent) used two other types of facilities to get work: One group sought out other governmental agencies such as vocational rehabilitation agencies or postal facilities; the other went to union hiring halls. Only 2 per cent indicated they depended upon newspaper advertisements or telephone calls in seeking work, while 14 per cent sought to secure work through personal contacts with others they knew in the community.

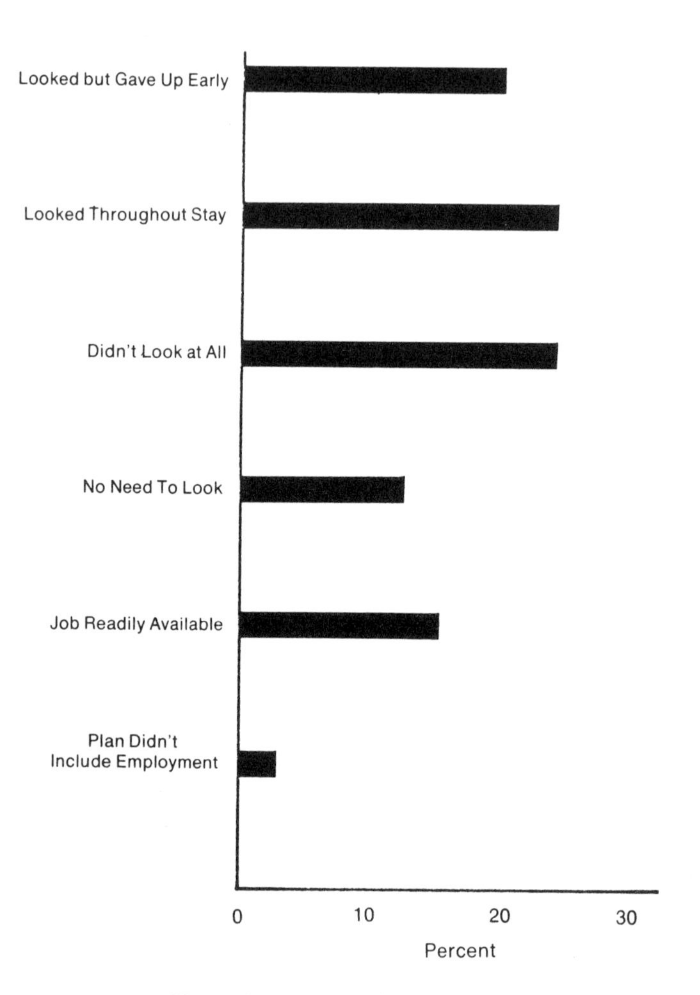

FIG. 12.17.—*Work seeking.*

In considering the kind of work which these 50 persons sought, it is worthwhile to compare the same categories of jobs with the proportions of those 31 persons who actually admitted holding employment during their stay in the community (Fig. 12.19). For example, exactly half of the group of 50 indicated they had sought common-labor or sheltered-workshop (aside from farm work) employment after leaving the hospital; only 17 per cent of the 31 persons admitted getting work of this type. Almost one-quarter (24 per cent) of the 50 sought relatively skilled blue-collar or low-level white-collar employment such as clerking or waiting tables; only 8 per cent of the 31 holding jobs actually got work of this type. Sixteen per cent of the 50 persons seeking work looked for salesman's or office

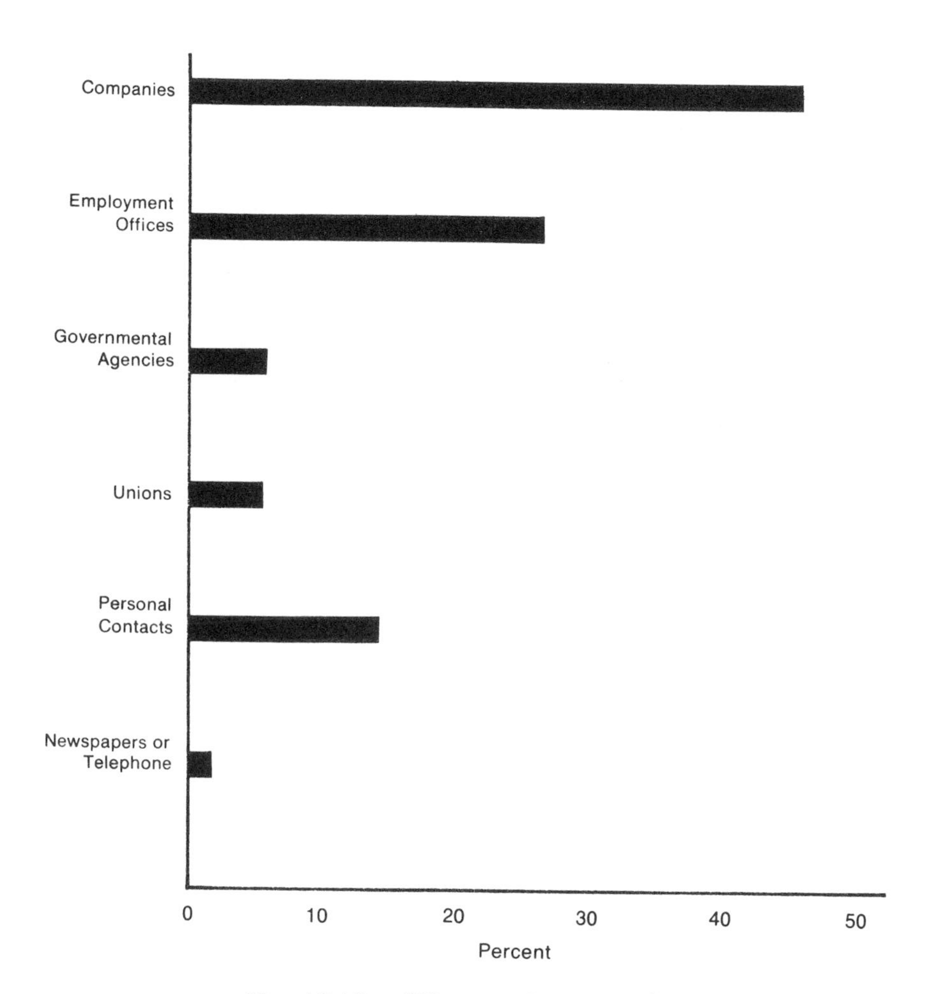

FIG. 12.18.—*Where work was sought.*

jobs; 3 per cent of the 31 were able to secure this kind of employment. Eight per cent of the 50 looked for farm labor jobs; 2 per cent of the 31 actually held this kind of work. One person of this group of 50 nonlodge persons sought executive or professional types of work; one person of the 31 held this kind of work. Overall, 67 persons, or 68 per cent of the 98 nonlodge group members returning to the hospital, failed to secure or did not look for employment after leaving the hospital.

Looking further into the experiences of the 31 persons who actually held jobs (Fig. 12.20), we find that almost one-third (32 per cent) held their jobs no more than one week. Another 36 per cent held their jobs up

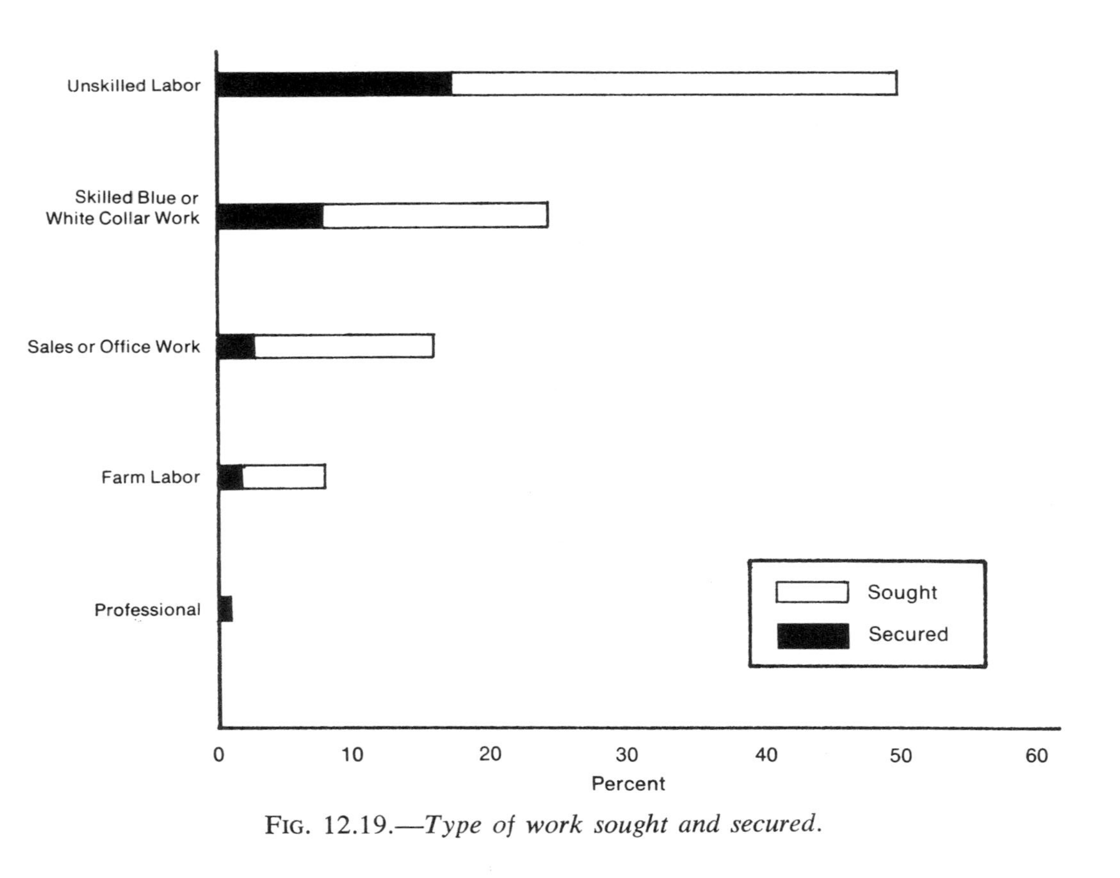

FIG. 12.19.—*Type of work sought and secured.*

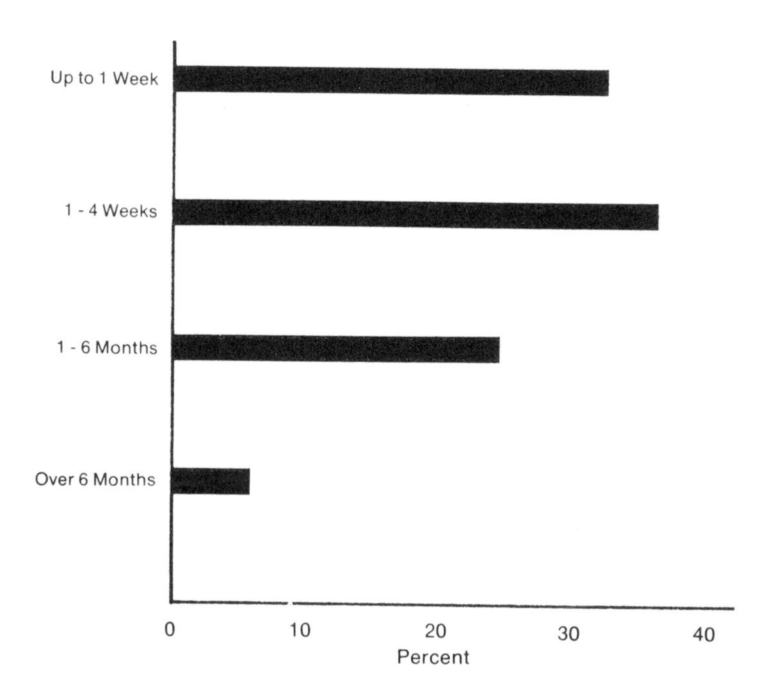

FIG. 12.20.—*Length of time jobs held.*

to one month; another one-quarter held their jobs between one and six months. Six per cent held their jobs over six months; this percentage refers to 2 persons in this employed group of 31. No estimate of their earnings was secured from 6 of these 31 persons; the median *total* estimated earnings for the other 25 was $182. Fifty-eight per cent of the group earned up to $500 during their stay out of the hospital; another fifth earned between $500 and $2,000, and one person (3 per cent) earned more than $2,000 while outside the institution. As a group, they earned a total of $13,400, or $536 per person on the average for all of the time the 31 were outside the hospital. Thus, even the third of the returning nonlodge group able to secure employment displayed poor ability to hold a job or command enough earnings to finance a stay in the community from this source of income, their own labor.

It is worthwhile to note the kinds of employers who were actually willing to give these 31 patients jobs. Seven per cent secured work with former employers; 16 per cent worked for friends, relatives, or neighbors; 13 per cent were self-employed. Nearly a third (32 per cent) worked for a company or business, while another 3 per cent got their work through the auspices of a union. Sixteen per cent found work in some kind of sheltering institution such as the Salvation Army, Goodwill Industries, or a sheltered workshop operated under the state vocational rehabilitation agency. Ten per cent found work with a local, state, or federal governmental agency, while one person found work in an educational institution. Thus, about one-third of the group depended upon their own devices or upon friends, relatives, and neighbors (36 per cent), another third found work with some kind of business firm (32 per cent), and the remaining third found some kind of institutional employment where hiring policies are likely to tolerate the "risks" that might be encountered in employing discharged mental patients.

Speculation about whether or not the experiences of this particular group of former mental patients who attempted some kind of adjustment to living in the community and failed are representative of those generally encountered can only be ended by a careful effort to carry out an investigation which has representativeness as its deliberate intention. What may be said from the material presented here about nonlodge group members is that trying to reestablish previous supports in the community or to construct them anew appears to be terribly difficult, particularly for the patient with long periods of previous psychiatric hospitalization.

Living Conditions in the Lodge

Earlier chapters have detailed the developing identification with the lodge society and the concern which came to be expressed by all for the continued success of the janitorial and yardwork business. At this point it seems appropriate to consider the views of lodge living conditions which those returning to the hospital reported immediately after their readmission. Figure 12.21 shows that in terms of relationships with other lodge residents, 67 per cent of this group indicated that they felt they had gotten along satisfactorily. Twenty-three per cent felt their experience was more differentiated, with some residents liking them while others did not. The final 10 per cent felt they couldn't get along in the lodge social situation.

In discussing at this time what these returnees felt were their major adjustmental problems while living at the lodge, almost one quarter (23 per cent) declined to provide information in this area (Fig. 12.22), while another 7 percent felt they had no problems while there, despite the fact that some kind of impetus related to lodge living led to their readmission to the hospital. A sizeable proportion of this group (36 per cent) admitted to having major problems either with the working conditions at the lodge (13 per cent) or with respect to violating what they felt to be unreasonable regulations upheld by the lodge organization (23 per cent). The former ranged all the way from comments about the lack of work to the view that there was too much work or too long work hours, and the latter were mainly concerned with fines for not working or with drinking behavior or

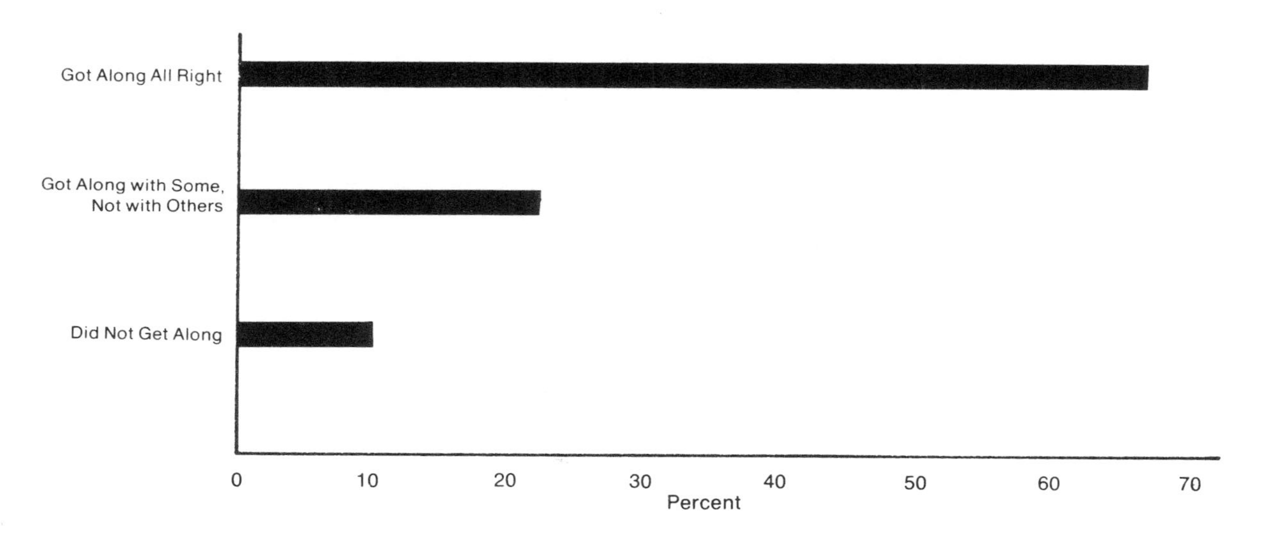

FIG. 12.21.—*Relations with lodge members.*

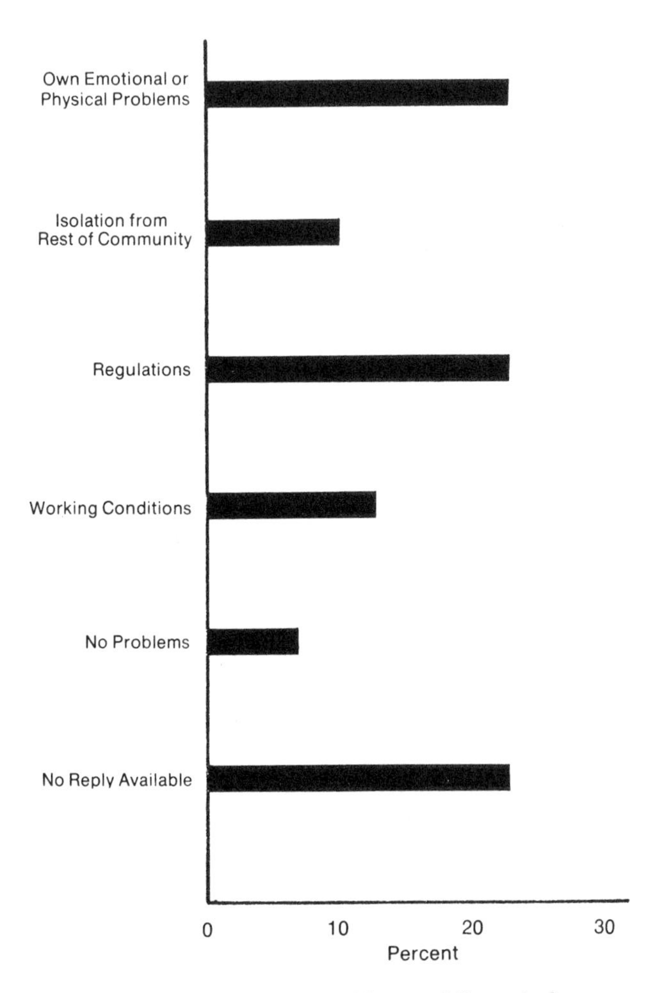

FIG. 12.22.—*Major problems while at lodge.*

personal hygiene violations. Only one person complained about physical difficulties in living at the lodge, mainly related to his sleeping and medication use, and one-fifth of the group felt their own emotional difficulties made it hard to live at the lodge, while 10 per cent admitted to feeling isolated from the rest of the community while living there. Thus, something more than one-third of the failures (36 per cent) found it diffiicult to adjust to the conditions of living at the lodge, another 30 per cent either did not answer the question or denied having adjustmental difficulties while living there.

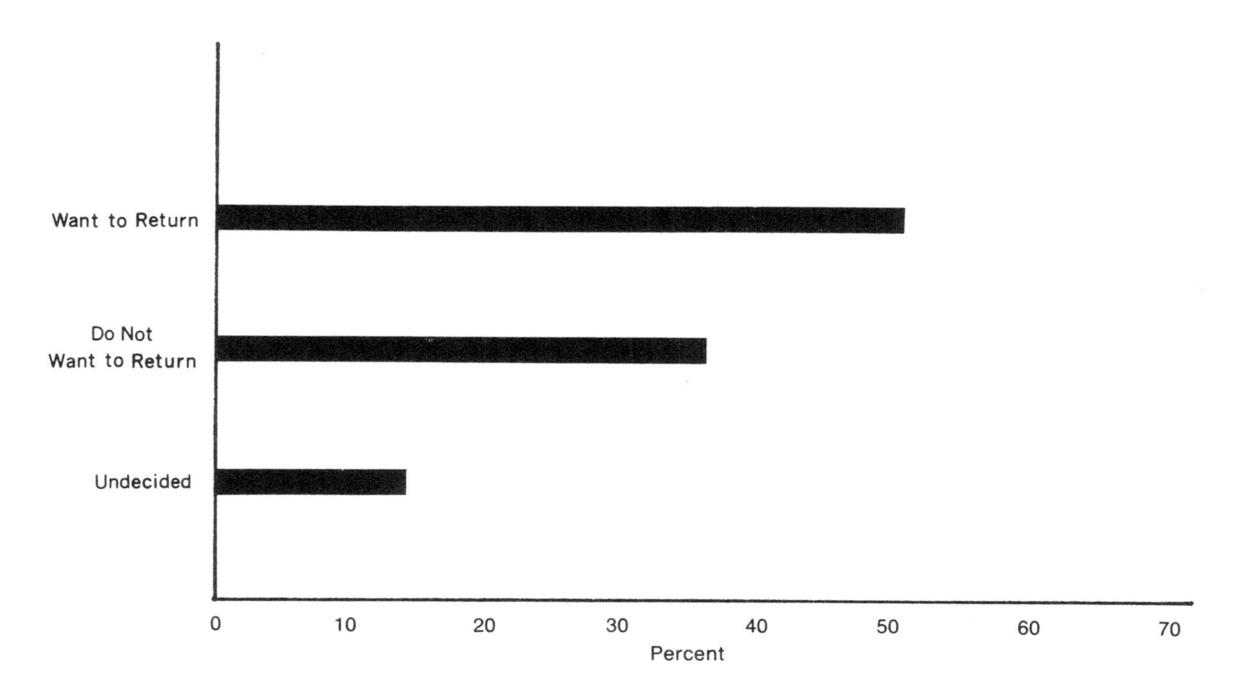

FIG. 12.23.—*Willingness to return to lodge.*

It is of particular interest to determine from those who "failed" the extent to which they would be willing to return to the lodge. When asked this question, a majority (51 per cent) of the group, many of whom later returned to the lodge, indicated their willingness to do so (Fig. 12.23). Within this group, 27 per cent replied unconditionally, 7 per cent said they would return provided lodge residents permitted them to do so, and 17 per cent suggested that they would be interested in doing so were certain changes in the lodge environment more to their liking to come about. A third of the group indicated their unwillingness to return, 20 per cent emphatically stating their abhorrence of the idea and the remaining 13 per cent doubting they would be interested. One person replied that he already had other plans in mind than returning to the lodge, and 13 per cent could not decide whether or not they would be willing to return.

Finally, those who indicated some interest in returning to the lodge were asked to consider whether or not they felt they could solve what they considered to be their major adjustmental problems as an accompaniment to reestablished lodge residence. Of the 14 persons who indicated interest, 64 per cent stated they would be willing to work at solving or altering their adjustmental problems if they return to the lodge. Twenty-eight per cent of this group replied either that they would not change their adjustmental status upon returning to the lodge (14 per cent) or that they could not do so (14 per cent), while 6 per cent doubted it would make any difference even if they did change their status in this regard. Thus, almost two-thirds of the group willing to give the lodge another try were also willing to make some effort on their part to establish a better adjustment to lodge living, while approximately a third doubted such a change was possible for them for a variety of reasons. Despite its newness to them and the fact they had to reenter the hospital, it would appear that the lodge social situation was still attractive to them as a viable means of leaving the hospital. Moreover, these patients above all others were aware that they would return with the expectation of support in the community in precisely those areas where as individuals they were most vulnerable, namely, securing employment and tolerant social support of their efforts to work out a successful and even participative role in the social life of the community.

The Lodge as Social Problem Solution

This chapter has been concerned with evaluating the effects of a newly designed social system upon its participants. The statistical comparisons reveal that lodge residents remained longer in the community, and were employed for a longer time than their matched counterparts. The social situation did not appear to have a noticeable effect upon their individual attitudes or behaviors. To a substantial degree, the lodge treatment subsystem was less expensive than any other existing alternatives. Lodge members seemed to be more satisfied with having a place in a tolerant society than an opportunity to engage in productive work.

Those who failed to adapt to lodge living conditions did so because of personal problems or disrupted relationships with other lodge members, not because a decision to return to the hospital was made for them as was the case with many of those who returned from other community settings. Nonlodge group members depended primarily on personal contacts, friends, and relatives for both shelter and employment. A majority lived in isolation from others in the community. For lodge members, despite failure, vague guesses about the future were most often replaced by intentions to return to the lodge and make a renewed effort at adjustment there. When comparing the two social situations in the community—one where the individual returning patient can depend upon and become a member of his own social group and the other where the individual must try to make his way as best he can without such peer group supports—the lodge situation clearly has the upper hand.

A moral issue is raised by the discussion of treatment costs. This is the problem of relating financial values to human values. Few, if any, of the alternative treatment arrangements available to the mental patient aside from the lodge have been directed overtly toward abolishing the subordinate social status of the psychiatric patient in this society. None, except the community lodge, has been specifically created with supportive social conditions under which a former patient has a major role in working out his own destiny in the community. Since establishing a lodge for chronically hospitalized mental patients is substantially less expensive than the costs to the community of incarceration and treatment in a large mental hospital, the only meaningful requirement for its adoption by society is a commitment by a community to provide new social institutions for its members which permit personal autonomy and growth.

13 THE EFFECT OF VOLUNTEERING AND CHRONICITY ON COMMUNITY ADJUSTMENT

The first chapter in this section was concerned with evaluating the effects of the innovated subsociety upon the length of stay, full-time employment, and the psychological and social adjustment of those who participated in it. It is now appropriate to turn our attention to two other important variables that were suspected from the outset as factors likely to have a marked effect upon the community adjustment of persons in the study—volunteering and chronicity. From previous studies, it seemed most probable that the more chronic patients would make a poorer adjustment in the community except for those in the lodge subsystem who had specific aid in helping them adjust (Fairweather, 1960, 1964; Fairweather and Simon, 1963). Since the sample was almost entirely a chronically hospitalized group (p. 32), it also seemed highly probable that many individuals would not volunteer because they might fear leaving the hospital. Those who refused to volunteer might be similar individuals to the volunteers and would not therefore adjust any better in the community. This assessment of the possible effects of chronicity and volunteering led to the formulation of the following two specific hypotheses (p. 28).

1. Patients who do not volunteer to live in the community subsystem will demonstrate no better personal and social adjustment than patients who do volunteer but cannot live in the subsystem (control condition).

2. The community social subsystem will have its most beneficial effect upon the most chronic patients.

The initial research design was established to test these two hypotheses in addition to those formulated in the preceding chapter. The design characteristic permitting a test for the effect of chronicity was presented in Table 3.2 (p. 30). That table shows that the sample of volunteers and nonvolunteers were stratified into three groups, namely, nonpsychotics, psychotics with 0–4 years of previous hospitalization, and psychotics with more than 4 years' previous hospitalization. A comparison of the community adjustment of these three groups constitutes the test for the hypothesis concerning differences that might obtain as a result of chronicity.

The design characteristic that permits testing the hypothesis about volunteering can also be seen in Table 3.3 (p. 30). Here it can be readily seen that the volunteer-nonlodge group and the nonvolunteer-nonlodge group differ only in the act of volunteering itself. Thus, a comparison of these two groups permits a test of the hypothesis concerning volunteering. Before this comparison can be made, however, it must be determined that both samples are equivalent in all other regards, so that extraneous variables will not affect statistical evaluation of the volunteering variable.

An exploration of Table 3.6 shows that the volunteer- and nonvolunteer-nonlodge groups were significantly different on three variables. The nonvolunteers had spent significantly less time in mental hospitals; they more often held lower middle-class and upper lower-class employment, that is, employment of a higher social class level; and they were more frequently social drinkers. In order to compare for the effects of volunteering alone, both groups must be equated on these historial adjustmental variables so that sample differences do not affect comparisons designed to assess the effect of the act of volunteering itself. This can be accomplished by a matching process whereby 75 participants in the nonlodge-nonvolunteer group are matched on age, diagnosis, and length of hospitalization with the 75 persons from the volunteer-nonlodge group. It has already been shown in previous studies that matching on these characteristics equates patient groups on other demographic characteristics, a matter discussed earlier in this investigation (pp. 30–37).

Accordingly, each member of the volunteer-nonlodge group was matched with a member of the accumulated pool of 183 persons in the nonvolunteer-nonlodge group on age (within 2 years) and chronicity (exactly, in terms of membership in the three diagnostic subgroupings). Where more than one person in the pool of nonvolunteers could be matched with a volunteer, the person selected for matching purposes was chosen at random. In this way, two groups of 75 persons each were formed. Since only age was permitted in the matching process to vary within two years of the age being matched, a statistical evaluation of age was required. A chi-square test revealed no significant difference between the newly matched groups with respect to age ($\chi^2 = 0.00$, 1 df). Both groups had a median age of 43 years. Table 13.1 shows no significant differences on 18 other personal background characteristics after matching of the two groups. These two matched groups now differ only in the major characteristic that members of one group, when asked, volunteered to go to the lodge situation (and did not) and the other group, when asked, did not volunteer. Hereafter in this chapter, this latter group will be referred to as the nonvolunteers and the former as the volunteers.

The Act of Volunteering

Willingness to enter a treatment program on the part of patients is an issue that typically does not arise within the context of the American medical community. When a person enters the sick role (p. 10), he abrogates a number of his rights and privileges, chief among them being control over the treatment to be accorded him. It is assumed that he places his trust and confidence in the ministering healer, and whatever that person decides is presumed to be for his own welfare. Within the mental hospital, as in every hospital, these norms also prevail. But the situation changes when the patient's return to the community is under consideration. A new treatment program in this social arena may depend upon the individual's willingness to participate in such a program, since he has regained his "normal" rights and privileges.

Regardless of whether or not the person does enter a treatment program, however, his willingness to do so also raises the broader issue of how important such a motivational indicator is to his ultimate fate. The question which must be answered thus becomes: Are there any essential differences between persons who indicate such willingness and those who do not, with respect to their adjustment in the community? To answer this question in comparative terms, the matched volunteer and nonvolunteer groups will be contrasted with respect to the same criteria used in evaluating the differences between those who entered the lodge situation and those who did not. This will constitute the statistical test of the first hypothesis mentioned earlier (p. 238).

Table 13.2 presents the available nonlodge samples for a period of 30 months from the point of eligibility to depart the hospital. The number of matched persons used for the comparisons ranged from 150 at 6 months to 27 at 30 months. The reduction in the size of the samples at various points in time exists because patients in the study were accumulated over time, a sampling procedure discussed elsewhere (pp. 30–37). The important point here is that the decrease in sample size by time period is not due to attrition but is instead the total representative sample available at that time. In fact, there was some minimal attrition in both groups due to death and failure to complete questionnaires, as shown in Table 13.2. Since the sample is accumulated, the statistical comparisons for each of the five time periods (6, 12, 18, 24, and 30 months) are inter-related and do not logically con-

Table 13.1. Comparison of Volunteers and Nonvolunteers on Demographic Characteristics after Matching

Variable	*Volunteers* (*N* = 75)	*Nonvolunteers* (*N* = 75)	*df*	χ^2
Median Age	43	43	1	0.00
Race, %:				
White	80	79	1	0.00
Other	20	21		
Military Service, %:				
Service-connected pension	53	60	1	0.43
No service-connected pension	47	40		
Military service, 0–131 weeks	51	49	1	0.01
Military service, 132 weeks and over	49	51		
Military rank, buck private or PFC	57	53	1	0.06
Military rank, higher than PFC	43	47		
Neuropsychiatric Hospitalization:				
Median age at first hospitalization	29	30	1	0.67
Median number prior hospitalizations	2	2	1	0.11
Median weeks prior hospitalizations	286	251	1	0.03
Type of Hospital Admission, %:				
Voluntary	45	41	1	0.11
Commitment	55	59		
Parents' Marital Status, %:				
Married and living	81	81	1	0.04
Other	19	19		
Brought up by, %:				
Both parents	56	60	1	0.11
Other	44	40		
Days since Last Contact with Relatives, %:				
0–16 days	51	49	1	0.03
17 days and over	49	51		
Employment:				
Social classification of last job, %:				
Lower middle class and upper lower class	30	48	1	3.64
Lower lower class	70	52		
Median number of jobs held in last 10 years	2	3	1	2.68
Median Highest Grade Completed	12	12	1	0.44
Drinking Behavior, %:				
Heavy drinkers	27	32		
Social drinkers	46	49	2	1.48
Nondrinkers	27	19		
Police Arrests, %:				
One or more	55	57	1	0.00
None	44	43		
Marital Status, %:				
Single and never married	55	45	1	0.96
Other	45	55		
Current Monthly Income while Hospitalized, %:				
0–$124	49	51	1	0.01
$125 and over	51	49		

Table 13.2. Nonlodge Subsample Sizes and Attrition Losses at Different Time Periods Before Matching

	Volunteer Samples				*Nonvolunteer Samples*			
		Loss by Attrition				*Loss by Attrition*		
Follow-up Time (Months)	*Available for Comparison*	*No Data*	*Death*	*Total*	*Available for Comparison*	*No Data*	*Death*	*Total*
6	75	1	0	1	181	2	0	2
12	48	0	6	6	123	5	0	5
18	36	3	3	6	75	8	4	12
24	27	3	7	10	48	4	0	4
30	19	0	5	5	21	12	4	16

Table 13.3. Chi-square Values[a] Comparing Volunteers and Nonvolunteers on Follow-up Items[b]

	Follow-up Time (Months)				
Item	6	12	18	24	30
Social Change Outcome Criteria:					
Cumulative days in community	.43	.14	.06	.00	.09
Full-time employment	1.25	3.70	1.95	.18	.02
Respondent Evaluations:					
Association with friends	1.03	.65	.02	.04	.18
Verbal communication	.26	.88	.03	1.07	.30
Appraisal of symptom behavior	.11	3.93[c]	.06	.15	.02
Drinking behavior	1.01	.04	.02	.04	.32
Activity level	.03	.03	.58	.02	.64
Group living scale	.06	.29	.02	.15	.02
Leisure activity scale	1.56	2.17	.19	.04	.00
Residential status	.10	.01	.00	2.24	.27
Patient Self-evaluation:					
Satisfaction with living conditions	3.46	.97	.01	.27	.97
Satisfaction with leisure activity	.02	3.79	.47	.83	.02
Satisfaction with community living	4.43[c]	6.74[d]	.02	.02	.36

[a] All chi-square values have been corrected for continuity using Yates' formula, and have 1 df.
[b] Hypotheses for this table are nondirectional, since no significant differences in community adjustment are expected between the two nonlodge groups of volunteers and nonvolunteers.
[c] Significant at .05 level.
[d] Significant at .01 level.

stitute independent comparisons. They are presented by time periods, however, so that it is clear what results would obtain should the experimenter arbitrarily choose any particular time period for his comparison.

Table 13.3 shows that three significant differences obtain on the 13 criteria successively measured for 30 months. In regard to the first of these significant differences, nonvolunteers are perceived by respondents as being more emotionally disturbed than are volunteers at the 12-month time period. The remaining two significant differences are represented by the 6- and 12-month significant chi-squares concerning satisfaction with community living. These results present a rather paradoxical situation. In the first six months, the nonvolunteers are significantly more satisfied with their community living situation than are volunteers; however, by the end of 12 months, the volunteers are significantly more satisfied with their community living situation than the nonvolunteers. The data do not suggest any ready interpretation of this reversal.

Generally speaking, volunteers remain no longer in the community than nonvolunteers and have no more time in full-time employment. Figure 13.1 displays graphically community tenure at different points in time. The bars in the graph represent the median percentage of time in the community for each group over 2½ years of follow-up investigation. The plots show the similarity between the groups in length of community tenure. And both groups are equally unsuccessful in their employment experience.

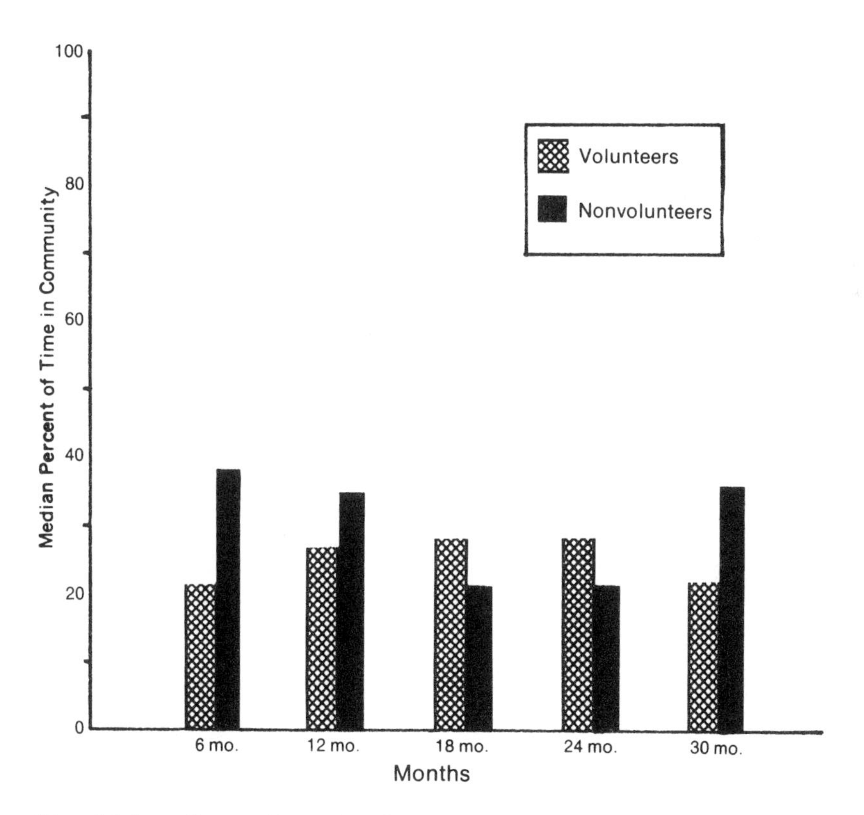

FIG. 13.1.—*Comparison of volunteers and nonvolunteers on time in the community for 30 months of follow-up.*

Most typically, both volunteers and nonvolunteers remain unemployed, even when they do get to the community where they can secure employment. Median percentage of time spent in full-time community employment is zero for both groups at all five follow-up points. Willingness or unwillingness to leave the hospital and to enter a new community-based treatment program does not itself seem to have any significant relationship to posthospital community tenure or actual employment.

Reference to Table 13.3 shows that the other outcome criteria tell substantially the same story about the community experience of volunteers and nonvolunteers. Residential status in the community (variable 10 in Table 13.3) for both groups at 6 months tends to involve living alone or with relatives, while the succeeding three follow-up assessment periods reveal a stronger tendency to be living in institutional situations (including reentry into the mental hospital). More than one-third of the respondents at 6, 12, and 18 months, and 29 per cent at 24 months of evaluation reported the patients in both groups whom they knew were back in a mental hospital. By the 24-month assessment, a third of those from both groups were to be found in some sort of dependent, institutional situation in the community itself. Throughout the follow-up period of the study, approximately half were typically reported to be living alone or with relatives, and half in an institutionally supervised situation, either in the community or in the mental hospital. This experience does not differ from previous reports on the living situations of chronically hospitalized mental patients. It is not a history of successful and independent community adjustment.

In general, both groups were particularly pleased to be living in the community. Although the patients' own evaluations of their community living situation reveal them to be rather satisfied with it, respondents' evaluations reveal that in individual behavior this was not an adjustment to normal community living (pp. 216–232). Patients were seen as more than willing to undertake the responsibilities of group living, given a dependent living situation, but they appeared to make only moderate use of their leisure time. They apparently were seen as communicating when necessary with others, but not going out of their way to do so, and they were seldom seen to relate to their friends. Typically, they were seen as nondrinkers, or infrequent drinkers, socially inactive, and displaying symptoms which could be related by respondents to emotional disturbance.

One important area which has not yet been explored that might differentiate volunteers from nonvolunteers concerns their expectancies about the future. It might very well be that nonvolunteers expected quite a different future in the community than volunteers did and, therefore, did not volunteer because of these different expectancies. However, Table 13.4 shows that this was not the case. No significant differences obtained between the volunteer and nonvolunteer groups concerning their expectations about future community living conditions, leisure activity, job conditions, and

Table 13.4. Comparison of Volunteers and Nonvolunteers on Expectations about Community Living

	Volunteer Group		Nonvolunteer Group		
Type of Expectation	*(N)*	*(%)*	*(N)*	*(%)*	χ^{2*}
Living Conditions:					
Above median	26	46	28	55	.59
Below median	31	54	23	45	
Leisure Activity:					
Above median	22	39	21	41	.01
Below median	35	61	30	59	
Job Conditions:					
Above median	25	45	21	40	.06
Below median	31	55	31	60	
Satisfaction with Community Living:					
Above median	26	46	21	40	.19
Below median	30	54	31	60	

* All chi-square values have been corrected for continuity using Yates' formula and are based on 1 df.

general satisfaction with life outside the hospital. Thus, not only did volunteers generally not differ significantly from nonvolunteers in actual community adjustment, they did not differ on expectancies about the future even at the time in the hospital when they were asked to volunteer for the community lodge.

The Act of Not Volunteering

Slightly more than 50 per cent of the chronic mental patients whose realistic future contained the prospect that they might remain in the hospital did not volunteer to accept a full-time job and living situation at the community lodge, even when it was offered. It might be that such individuals did not volunteer because they did, in fact, have a community situation to which they could return that they believed to be more desirable than living in the lodge society. Because of this possibility, when a person did not volunteer, he was also asked his reason for being unwilling to go to the lodge.

Table 13.5 presents the four major reasons for not volunteering for the community program. Almost half of the nonvolunteering group felt they generally had better employment prospects in the offing compared with the alternative offered them. Another two-fifths of the group expressed interest in living conditions different from those they imagined might exist under the proposed community lodge situation. About one-tenth of the group declared their lack of interest in that situation without elaboration. One per cent of the group saw vocational preparation as of higher priority than immediately leaving the hospital for a living and working situation.

Among these 81 persons who believed they had better job prospects, several different kinds of reasons were offered. Thirty-one persons stated

Table 13.5. Reasons Given for Refusal to Volunteer for New Community Treatment Program

Reason	Total Group* (N)	(%)
Have better employment prospects	81	46
Want different living conditions	72	41
Refusal—no reason given	22	12
Want education or training before employment	2	1
	—	—
Total	177	100

* Of the original nonvolunteer nonlodge sample of 183 persons, this information was not available for 6 of them, reducing the sample to 177 persons.

they wanted a different kind of work or a different location from that offered at the lodge. Typical comments were: "I want to get a job as a shipping clerk or a printer if I can," or "I'll look for a job in the city in sales work." Another 20 persons mentioned that they were unmotivated for full-time work. Typical comments were: "Why, that sounds like a regular 8-hour-a-day job," or "When it comes to working, I'm too nervous. . . . I want to go with my father and retire." Almost the same number (17 persons) saw their need for better working conditions than were offered, especially with respect to pay. Thus, they commented typically: "I couldn't make it with the money they earn there. I've got to support my family." Another typical comment in this group was: "I feel I won't have any trouble finding work and so I don't want to step down to doing janitorial work." Eleven others stated that they planned to return to the same work they held before entering the mental hospital. Some comments were: "I'd rather go back to my teamster's job," and "I think I will bypass it and get back to a Civil Service job where I can earn $100 a week." The remaining two persons in this group of 81 with better employment prospects felt they had work already secured, only awaiting their departure from the hospital. They said: "I already have a job in a restaurant in the city that I can start any time," and "I have several contract jobs waiting for me when I get back."

With all of these varied reasons for not volunteering to go to the community lodge, how did these persons fare? Sixteen persons never left the hospital at all. The median time the remaining 65 persons spent in the community, taking into account the maximum days recorded during the period in which each could be followed, was just over seven months. They generally failed to secure employment. The median time employed was 0 days. Two-thirds of this group were continuously unemployed. Thus, only 34 per cent of the group actually secured jobs in the community. Clearly, these hospitalized psychiatric patients' belief in better employment prospects than the one provided by the lodge had little relationship to their actual experience when they returned to the community.

Two different reasons were given by the 72 patients who turned down the lodge offer because they indicated a desire for different living conditions. Twelve, nine of them long-term psychotics, showed a preference for some kind of institutional, supervised living situation different from the lodge. Five of these never left the hospital and the other seven spent a median time of 45 days in the community. Six of these seven remained unemployed in the community. Of these seven, five returned to the hospital but two, true to their expressed preferences, were in institutional, supervised living situations. One was working as a dishwasher in the cafeteria of a Veterans Administration domiciliary; the other was living in a private home licensed for the care of mental patients. Thus, all 12 patients who based their refusal of the lodge offer on their preference for institutional living actually succeeded in achieving their goal.

But what of the other 60 patients who wanted different living conditions? All 60 indicated that they preferred a living situation which did not involve living with other mental patients. Typical comments were: "I don't think so; I would rather live at home," ". . . I feel that living with ex-mental patients lowers your position in the community." Nine of these patients never left the mental hospital during the time they were followed by the research staff. The 51 persons who did reenter the community spent a median time there of 205 days, just over six months. The median employment time for this group wanting a nonpatient environment was zero days. Two-thirds were continuously unemployed for the time they were followed—very similar to the group believing they had better employment prospects. The last respondent evaluation secured for each person in this group revealed that 49 per cent were in the mental hospital again, 20 per cent were living alone, 16 per cent were living with relatives or friends, 9 per cent were living in a marital situation, and 6 per cent were in some form of institutional residence.

Table 13.5 shows that two persons planned to obtain additional education before they considered employment. One had done college-level work five years before entering the mental hospital. He planned to get his college degree. Equipped with a pass from hospital authorities, he actually joined a registration line for admission to a nearby university, but became overwhelmed with anxiety and immediately reentered the hospital. Thus, he actually never left the hospital. The second person spent a total of 70 days in the community over the two years he was followed, all of them unemployed. He first left the hospital for two weeks, living alone in a hotel the first week and with relatives the second week before reentering the hospital for another year's stay. His final stay in the community of about two months entailed living with another relative until his return to the hospital. During all of this time, he was not employed in the community nor did he pursue further education as he indicated he would in refusing the offer to go to the community lodge.

Twelve per cent of the total group of nonvolunteers refused the lodge offer without explaining why. Of these 22 persons, 6 never left the hospital during the time they were followed. The residual group of 16 who did enter the community spent a median time there of 230 days, much like the other groups already discussed, but with a higher percentage remaining unemployed (79 per cent). At the last time a respondent was asked to evaluate their residential status, 38 per cent had returned to the hospital, none were living in a different institutional setting, one-quarter were living alone, a third were with relatives or friends, and 4 per cent were living in a marital situation. In this case, a majority (10 out of 16) were still in the community, unlike the residential status of the other groups already considered.

From these results, it seems quite clear that very often reasons given for not volunteering were either not the actual reasons, or that the reasons given were relatively unrelated to what happened to the individual. Such information raises a moral issue about the responsiblity of treatment programmers when dealing with chronic mental patients. Perhaps the most important issue concerns the point in time where their responsibility terminates. Does it terminate at the hospital gate quite without regard to what happens to the individual once he has left the hospital? Or should responsibility continue until the individual has demonstrated his ability to make an adequate adjustment in the community without need for extraneous support?

Chronicity as a Determinant in Community Adjustment

Previous studies (Fairweather, 1960, 1964) have shown that the more chronic patients make poorer community adjustments than the less chronic patients. This study was also designed to test whether or not such results would occur with this sample. To test the effect of chronicity, the experimental hypothesis stated: "The community social subsystem will have its most beneficial effect upon the most chronic members." Since the beneficial effects upon community tenure and employment derived from living in the lodge society contrasted with the general community have been amply demonstrated, the effects of chronicity will have to be explored independently for the sample that participated in the lodge and for those who did not reside there.

Comparison of Diagnostic Groups in the Nonlodge Community Situation

For the comparisons to be presented in this section, the persons who volunteered to go to the lodge but did not, were combined with those who did not volunteer to go, since there are no significant differences between them in their adjustment to the community situation which they had in common (p. 242). With respect to the social-change outcome criteria, this combination led to a maximum group for follow-up assessment from 256 persons at 6 months to 40 persons at 30 months. With regard to respondent evaluations, the numbers of patients in the successive available samples ranged from 243 at 6 months to 17 in the 30-month sample. For patient attitudes, the range in available sample members extended from 121 persons in the 6-month sample to 18 persons in the 30-month sample. Again, it should be clear that these smaller sample sizes from 12 months on are not due to attrition rates but rather represent the total random sample available for that time period (p. 242).

Table 13.6 presents the diagnostic comparisons for those not living in the lodge society. It is clear that for the three follow-up periods from 6 through 18 months, membership in a particular diagnostic grouping affected both the length of time spent in the community and full-time employment.

Figure 13.2 displays these differences in graphical form, showing the consistently greater community tenure of the short-term psychotics. Although Table 13.6 reveals that the differences between the diagnostic groups did not reach the .05 level of significance at 24 and 30 months, Figure 13.2 shows the trend of more community tenure by the short-termers continued. The reduced sample size was probably influential in lowering the chi-square value.

Table 13.6 shows that similar results prevailed for full-time employment in the community. Since few persons were employed in the nonlodge condition (pp. 242–244), Figure 13.3 presents the results as percentages

Table 13.6. Diagnostic Group Comparisons[a] for Nonlodge Living Groups on Follow-up Items

Item	*Follow-up Time Periods (Months)* 6	12	18	24	30
Social Change Outcome Criteria:					
Cumulative days in community	18.70[d]	12.08[c]	10.50[c]	4.93	4.28
Full-time employment	14.53[d]	7.30[b]	6.40[b]	3.17	3.38
Respondent Evaluations:					
Association with friends	.78	.37	.21	2.04	2.38
Verbal communication	2.03	.76	1.02	1.09	2.45
Appraisal of symptom behavior	10.97[c]	.52	.90	5.29	1.09
Drinking behavior	1.81	2.97	.12	1.27	6.48[b]
Activity level	.63	2.37	1.62	2.77	.06
Social responsibility	1.04	.47	4.94	1.12	.55
Leisure activity	2.62	.48	.66	1.12	3.22
Patient Evaluations:					
Satisfaction with living conditions	3.97	2.13	3.43	1.72	.25
Satisfaction with leisure activity	2.94	.07	1.98	2.05	.76
Satisfaction with community living	5.82	.06	3.66	3.96	3.62

[a] All chi-square values have 2 df.
[b] Significant at .05 level.
[c] Significant at .01 level.
[d] Significant at .001 level.

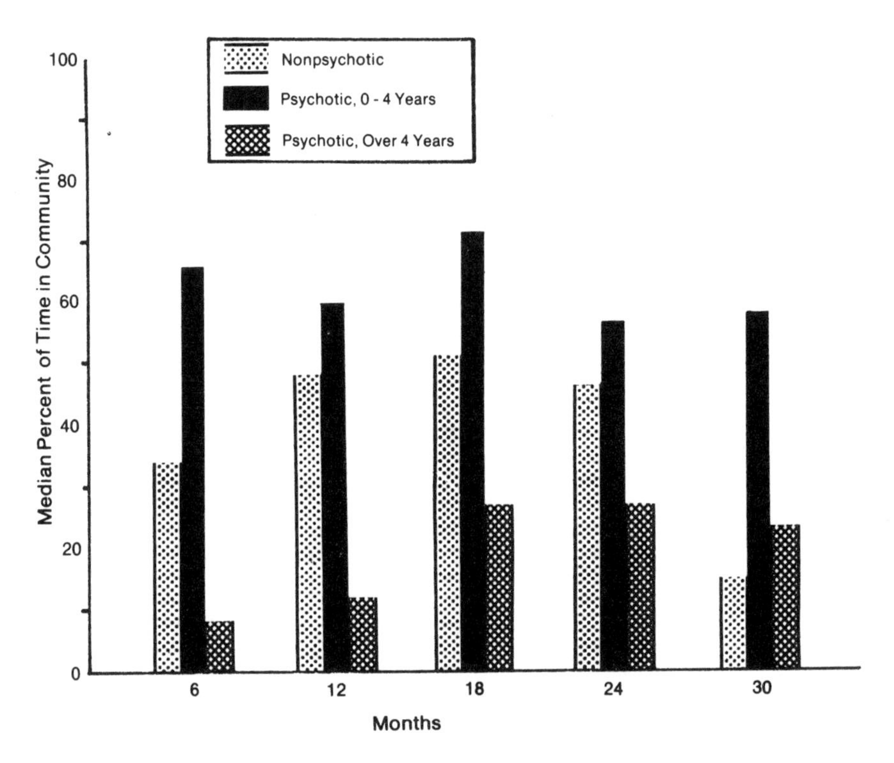

FIG. 13.2.—*Comparison of nonlodge diagnostic groups for 30 months of follow-up.*

of *unemployment*. The figure shows that short-term psychotics consistently had a smaller percentage of unemployed persons than the other two groups. At 6 months 75 per cent were unemployed, at 12 months 68 per cent, and at 18 months 51 per cent. In contrast, the nonpsychotic percentages for these periods were 88 per cent, 83 per cent, and 68 per cent, respectively, and for the long-term chronic patients, these percentages were, respectively, 93 per cent, 87 per cent, and 77 per cent. The same relative order obtained for employment as for time in the community—the short-term psychotics consistently fared better than the nonpsychotics and the more chronic psychotics. However, employment after 18 months of follow-up assessment did not reach the .05 level of significance. As with community tenure, the diagnostic groups retained their respective ranks but the sample size decreased. Thus the reduction in available sample may account for the smaller chi-square value.

No significant differences between diagnostic groups were detected with regard to the patients' own attitudes toward their community living situa-

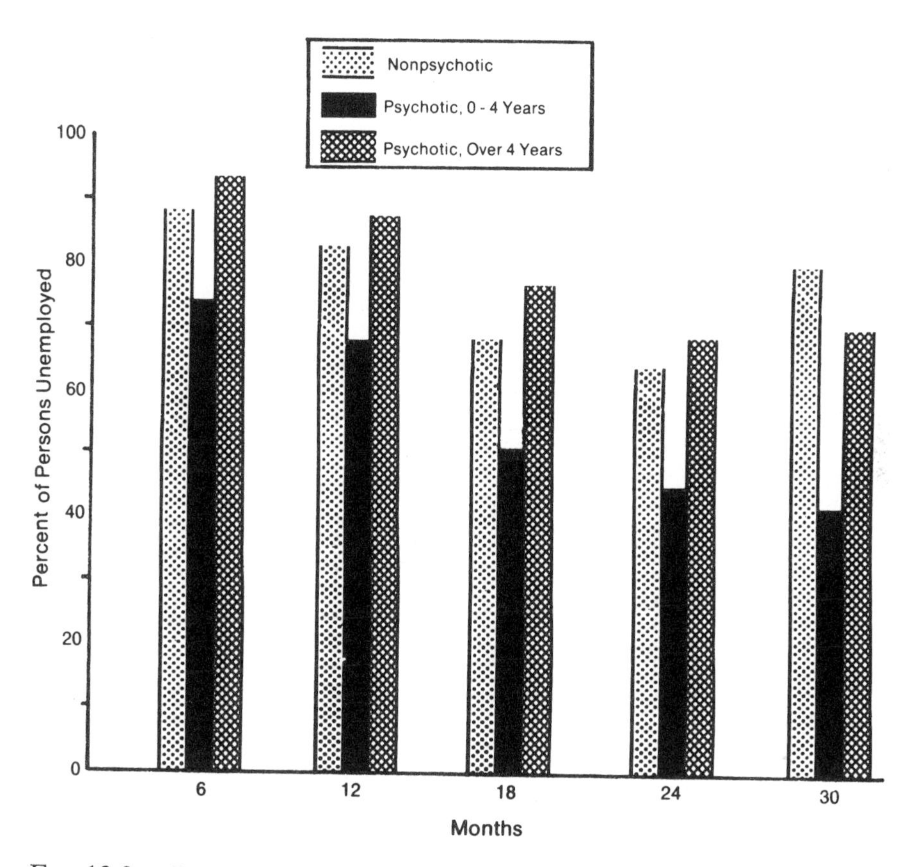

FIG. 13.3.—*Percent of persons in nonlodge diagnostic groups unemployed for 30 months of follow-up.*

tions. However, at the 6-month follow-up period, respondents judged non-psychotics and short-term psychotics to display few if any symptoms in their behavior indicative of emotional disturbance, while two-thirds of the long-term psychotics were reported to show such symptomatic behavior. Subsequent comparison between the three diagnostic groups revealed no significant differences in this aspect of their behavior. At the 30-month assessment point, both nonpsychotics and short-term psychotics were seen to be nondrinkers, while over 60 per cent of the long-term psychotics were observed to be drinking at least once in a while. No great store should be placed in this finding, however, since the numbers of persons in each of the three diagnostic groups were small and this trend was not detected in any previous follow-up period. The results just discussed appear in these tables to confirm the results of earlier studies (Fairweather, et al., 1960; Fairweather and Simon, 1963; Fairweather, 1964). At least for the first 18 months of follow-up assessment, the chronicity of the ordinary patient is a major factor in determining his ultimate success in remaining in the typical community situation available to ex-mental patients.

Comparison of Diagnostic Groups in the Lodge Community Situation

Table 13.7 presents diagnostic group comparisons for lodge members. Looking first at the two social-change outcome criteria, time in the community and time fully employed in the community, no significant differences between diagnostic groups appear. The diagnostic group comparison here shows that all diagnostic groups (nonpsychotic, short-term, and long-term psychotic) achieved about equal community tenure and employment from participation in the new community living and working situation. The initial hypothesis stated at the outset of this discussion of chronicity has been confirmed; namely, "the community social subsystem will have its most beneficial effect upon the most chronic patients." The long-term chronic patient has clearly been helped most in community tenure and full-time employment by participation in lodge living, in contrast with their poorer community adjustment under nonlodge living conditions described in the last section.

Persons living in the lodge situation, although they did not differ in tenure or employment when separated according to diagnostic group membership, did reveal significant differences on other criteria of com-

Table 13.7. Diagnostic Group Comparisons[a] for the Lodge Group on Follow-up Items

	Follow-up Time Periods (Months)				
Item	*6*	*12*	*18*	*24*	*30*
Social Change Outcome Criteria:					
Cumulative days in community	2.96	2.07	.76	.62	1.04
Full-time employment	2.98	.62	1.16	.04	.60
Respondent Evaluations:					
Association with friends	12.27[c]	2.39	1.34	3.22	.03
Verbal communication	7.49[b]	3.91	13.25[c]	7.18[b]	1.74
Appraisal of symptom behavior	6.41[b]	5.40	3.60	2.78	2.33
Drinking behavior	2.71	3.74	2.22	3.22	.00
Activity level	3.25	4.60	7.20[b]	3.56	4.27
Social responsibility	3.03	.27	.74	2.57	.00
Leisure activity	1.12	2.82	1.56	4.11	.00
Patient Evaluations:					
Satisfaction with living conditions	1.34	1.19	2.66	6.75[b]	.00
Satisfaction with leisure activity	3.50	.13	1.36	4.66	.00
Satisfaction with community living	3.60	.26	1.34	6.75[b]	.00

[a] All chi-square values have 2 df.
[b] Significant at .05 level.
[c] Significant at .01 level.

munity adjustment used in this investigation. Referring again to Table 13.7, the reader will note that respondents saw members of diagnostic groups differently on four such criteria: association with friends at 6 months; verbal communication at 6, 18, and 24 months; symptom behavior at 6 months; and activity level at 18 months. Although some of these findings may have come about as a result of chance variation, the verbal communication result bears some discussion because of its persistent occurrence in differentiating the diagnostic groups.

Nonpsychotics are rated as the most talkative, even tending to seek out others; short-term psychotics are seen as less so; and long-term psychotics display this behavior the least. Respondents for the lodge living group were the coordinators, both professional and lay (pp. 45–100), who worked closely with or supervised the work of the lodge members. Verbal communication after the 6-month evaluation changes at 18 and 24 months into a statistically significant diagnostic group difference between the psychotic and nonpsychotic patients, with the nonpsychotics being rated as the most talkative. Association with friends at the 6-month point is seen by respondents as a difference between nonpsychotics (with the strongest tendencies to get together with friends) and the psychotic patients with more solitary propensities. In contrast, evidence of emotional disturbance at 6 months and activity level at 18 months are differences between the nonpsychotics and short-term psychotics (the most active) and the long-term psychotics (clearly the least active group). Generally speaking, then, chronicity places a damper on friendship relations, verbal contact, activity level and the freedom from symptoms of emotional disturbance. Such differences, however, may tend to disappear with the passage of a great deal of time, as shown at the 30-month follow-up point.

The less chronic and nonpsychotic persons behaved more adequately in the lodge living and working situation where demands for communication with each other and with the public were a part of the social situation. Nonpsychotics functioned most adequately, according to this evidence. For example, leadership in the lodge, which required the most responsible behavior in that situation, was mainly held by nonpsychotic persons. Thus, 45 per cent of the nonpsychotic lodge members were leaders, while only 15 per cent of the psychotic persons (regardless of their being classified as long-term or short-term) assumed leadership responsibilities in the lodge situation. Members in these diagnostic groups did not differ significantly in the length of time they spent at the lodge; the median percentage of time was 35 per cent of the total time they might have been there. Thus, leadership was not related to the length of time lodge members lived in that situation but rather to how able a person was to carry out the communicative and organizing tasks in spite of his emotional disabilities.

Table 13.7 reveals that ex-patients' reactions to their lodge living situation in the community shows few diagnostic differences. Those that emerged (satisfaction with their living conditions at 24 months) may have been the result of chance variation. If not, both results indicate the same process; chronic members living at the lodge were most satisfied with their situation, the short-term psychotics next, and the nonpsychotic patients were least satisfied. This finding is certainly consistent with the fact that long-term psychotics succeeded equally as well as others in the lodge society—a result probably above their own expectations from past failure experiences.

Typically, patients in a mental hospital are not offered programmed alternatives in the community. Instead, a variety of separate activities in which some dischargees may engage and others may not are made available as discharge plans, depending upon each returning patient's personal situation, the counsel of hospital staff responsible for his treatment progress, and existing community contacts developed by patient and staff. The concept of "readiness" to leave the hospital is often expressed there as one criterion by which a patient is enabled to reenter the community. Nonlodge patients returning to the community generally failed to remain in the community and to become employed. Nonpsychotic and long-term psychotic patients fared the worst. However, the effect of living in the lodge social subsystem effectively counteracted the typical outcome of recidivism associated with continued hospitalization. The lack of differences in other criteria of community performance, regardless of whether a returnee lives in the lodge or some other community situation is striking. The differences which do appear relate to the greater emotional instability of the more chronic patients, and, by contrast, to the better performance of the less chronic.

Remaining Hospitalized as a Way of Life

Some patients with consistently unrewarding experiences in trying to get along in a society made the personal decision to remain in the hospital without chancing the risk of further pain. It is this group of patients to which attention is now turned. These persons were all members of the nonlodge group who, even though eligible, never left the hospital. In a sense, these patients are total failures since they are the residual group of psychiatric patients for whom return to the community could not be accomplished. The classic term "chronic patient" may be most appropriately applied to this group. As such, they may provide information about a sample of persons for whom no treatment programs in the hospital can be considered effective if restoring patients to the community is considered the primary goal. In this section we will attempt to discover some answers which may explain why this residual group adopted the hospital as their domicile throughout the course of the study.

The proportion of the nonlodge group at each follow-up point who ultimately became members of the consecutively hospitalized proportion of the total nonlodge sample varied from 16 per cent at 18 and 24 months to 26 per cent at 6 months. Table 13.8 presents in tabular form the numbers of such persons who were interviewed at each point in time. A specially-constructed interview was conducted with them on the hospital wards. These interviews were tape-recorded. Table 13.8 shows that the sample progressively decreases. Thus, at the 6-month point, 66 persons were available for interview, 35 of whom were destined to leave the hospital during the ensuing 6 months. At 12 months, 31 persons were available for interview. Thirteen persons had left the hospital after at least 12 months of consecutive hospitalization, leaving 18 persons available in the hospital for interview at the 18-month point. Six persons left during the next 6 months, leaving 12 consecutively hospitalized persons available for interview at 24 months. By the time an interview with persons consecutively hospitalized for 30 months arrived, only 9 persons remained, the other three having left in the intervening 6 months. The focus of the discussion will be upon the attitudes held by that group of persons who at each assessment point in time had a history of remaining hospitalized without a break from the time they first became approved for departure from the hospital. Neither the interviewer nor the patient himself at the time of the interview knew whether or not the patient would be available for interview 6 months later.

Table 13.8. Available Samples of Consecutively Hospitalized Nonlodge Patients for Five Follow-up Interviews

Months	6	12	18	24	30
Sample	66	31	18	12	9

The attitudes expressed in each interview are those conditioned by the history of hospitalization for each individual. This perspective on the data allows consideration of shifts in attitude on the same topic with increasing, continued hospitalization. Within the limits of the information actually elicited, it will thus be possible to explore the process of chronicity in microscopic form as successive increments of hospital residence accrue. In the statistical sense, these samples are not independent, since each sample contains some individuals included in previous samples.

Once the interviews with these hospital patients were recorded, responses to interview questions were abstracted by trained interviewers. Two abstracters attained 91 per cent agreement on the extracted responses. Subsequently, the abstracted responses were coded into descriptive categories. Two judges coded a sample of these responses and attained 88 per cent agreement.

The interview itself is focused around five topical areas pertinent to remaining hospitalized as a way of life. Plans for hospital departure, past and present, were discussed with each respondent, in addition to his attitude about securing employment, the kind of living situation he foresaw for himself in the community, his view of living in the mental hospital, and his subjective estimate of his own psychological well-being and its possible change in the future with continued hospitalization. This sequence of topics in the standardized interview focused the patient's attention upon hospital departure. Questioning began with: "Six months ago [omitted in the initial interview], what was your posthospital plan?" As the consecutive months of hospitalization mounted, a decreasing proportion of respondents could recall having made definite plans 6 months before. The 70 per cent at 6 months reduced to less than half the group at 12 months, and ended at 30 months with no respondent recalling what his earlier plan had been. Throughout the 30-month span, from one-third to one-half gave no reasons for failure to implement their plans, although one-quarter of the group said they had tried and abandoned them. An increasing proportion expressed the notion their earlier plans had not worked because they were not ready to leave the hospital, they were too sick to leave, or their emotional problems were not yet resolved. About one-third of the group at 6 months announced that events outside their control which had to occur before they could leave had not eventuated. Patients referred to events such as the right opportunity opening up in the community, or family relations improving.

When asked what plans they currently held for leaving the hospital, from one-fifth at 6 months to a high of one-half at 24 months indicated they had no plans. Between 15 and 20 per cent of the group indicated either vague plans or clearly psychotic, delusional intentions about leaving the hospital. In reference to concrete steps to enter the community, these patients had little interest in leaving the hospital, and this interest diminished with the passage of time in the hospital.

Patients were asked if they intended to seek work, and the type to be sought, as well as the work-seeking experience the patient had had previously. The largest percentage indicated they intended to seek unskilled work after leaving the hospital, from 55 per cent at 6 months to 22 per cent at 30 months. Overall, 79 per cent of the group answered affirmatively to this question, 10 to 25 per cent of the group even indicating an intention to seek executive or professional work when discharged. One-fifth of the group overall said they did not intend to seek work, and an increasing proportion of these respondents stated that they were too sick to work (reaching 22 per cent at 30 months). When asked about previous experience in seeking work, a continuously increasing proportion of the group replied that they had not had previous experience. This proportion began at 68 per cent at 6 months and increased to 100 per cent of the group at 30 months. Only one-third of the group at most had sought work before their admission to the hospital. And those who admitted to previous experience in this area, or at least an intention to do so, generally set their sights (perhaps realistically) on securing unskilled labor positions should they leave the hospital.

When asked to choose the kind of living situation they might consider the most desirable, a decreasing proportion over time indicated a house or apartment as the best form of shelter, 10–15 per cent indicated hotels or rooming houses, and an increasing proportion simply said they would wait and see what happened in the hospital (from 15 per cent at 6 months to 33 per cent at 30 months). Without any clear idea of how they wanted to live in the community, they were equally vague about relationships with others in the community. The most substantial proportions of each sample indicated the intention to live alone, ranging from a low of 33 per cent to a high of 77 per cent. No more than a quarter of the sample at any one time indicated the intention to stay with relatives or family, and no more than a fifth of the group said they would plan to stay with their wives or children. These patients with consecutively longer periods of hospitalization viewed life in the community as essentially isolated from others. A decreasing proportion of each sample indicated they would depend on work for their own support, while an increasing proportion stated their disability pension income would be their main source of financial support in the community. About 10 per cent of the group consistently over time were not at all sure what their financial sources of support would be while they were in the community.

When asked to imagine aspects of their living situation in the community, these consecutively hospitalized patients clearly had little ability to do so. Community life became less and less a realistic prospect with the passage of time in the hospital. Only about 10 per cent saw hotel life as a possiblity. Most believed they would be living alone, or otherwise depending upon relatives for providing a living situation.

Without a clear idea of what life was or would be like in the community, it is possible that the person who remained hospitalized would have clear perceptions about hospital living. This was the third major area explored by the interviewer: the feelings and attitudes about hospital living as it was progressively accrued by this type of patient. This area began in the interview with the question: "How do you feel about having remained in the hospital for the past 6 months?" The largest proportion of each sample was consistently satisfied with being in the hospital, varying from 41 per cent at 6 months to 33 per cent at both 18 and 30 months. They referred to the hospital as the preferred residence, as better than "outside," and one said, "It's the place I call home." About equal proportions of each sample indicated either that they realized it was necessary for them to be in the hospital, or that being there was thoroughly unpleasant experience.

This group varied from 16 per cent to 20 per cent at different points in time. About 10 per cent of the group at each point in time indicated indifference to their last 6 months of hospitalization.

When asked how long they estimated their stay would be, about 40 per cent of each sample indicated inability to guess the length of time, and this proportion increased to two-thirds of the group at 24 months. No more than 30 per cent of the group actually gave a time estimate, which generally ranged under 6 months. From one-quarter to 39 per cent of the group either felt there was still a reason for keeping them in the hospital or that to make an estimate would be hopeless.

At this point in the interview, the patient's attention was turned to the benefits he perceived to arise from his psychiatric hospitalization. The largest proportion of each sample, ranging from 22 per cent to 33 per cent, stated that treatment and medication which "calmed [their] nerves" was the main benefit they had secured. Smaller proportions indicated simply that its main benefit was as a place to receive bed and board. Few indicated that some kind of purposeful activity was the benefit which first occurred to them, or that it was a congenial environment facilitating relationships with others. Something over 10 per cent of each sample indicated it was a nonbeneficial experience, and this percentage rose to 22 per cent at 30 months. About a fifth of each sample were vague about the benefits of hospitalization, not being able to express any particular concrete notion of benefits received.

When their attention was then turned to the *expected* benefits of hospitalization, the patients were similarly vague. From 25 per cent to 66 per cent of each sample either had no idea of future benefits to be gained from hospitalization, could not imagine what they could be, or felt they would be little. Two other groups of answers were elicited by this question. From 14 per cent to 33 per cent of each sample, in an increasing proportion with the passage of time, suggested that securing concrete help to leave the hospital could be a future benefit. But a larger percentage, ranging from 32 per cent at 6 months to a low of 20 per cent at 18 months, indicated they wanted the hospital to take care of them, mostly in a custodial fashion. When asked to consider what treatment had been most beneficial, the largest proportions of each sample indicated medication was the most helpful. This proportion ranged from 35 per cent to 39 per cent in the first three time periods, to 50 per cent at 24 months, and dropped to 22 per cent at 30 months. From 17 per cent to 33 per cent of the samples could not give a specific answer to this question, and the percentage increased consistently over time. From 14 per cent to 29 per cent of the samples selected some kind of activity which kept a person busy as most beneficial, while a fluctuating percentage pointed to some kind of psychiatric treatment (ranging from 8 per cent at 24 months to 26 per cent at 6 months).

In general, the continuously hospitalized patient's perception of what the hospital had done and can do for him was inarticulate and confused. Most wanted medication to control symptomatic discomfort; few wanted concrete assistance in returning to the community. At best, they seemed relatively content with their present situation and showed no great concern for their past or future. It is no wonder that they are relatively impervious to psychiatric treatment oriented toward discharge from the hospital, or that the passage of increasing months in the mental hospital has little significance for them. This group appears to have rather effectively abrogated responsibility for their future, and passed it into the hands of others.

Finally, the patient's subjective estimate of his own well-being in psychiatric terms was sought. The question opening this area of the interview was, "Do you feel you are mentally ill?" Consistently in all samples, about half replied affirmatively and the other half negatively. Of those who answered in the affirmative, a decreasing proportion over time suggested they felt ill, were fearful, weak, nervous, or not normal. This proprotion ranged from one-third of the sample at 6 months to 22 per cent at 30 months. Of those who replied in the negative, an increasing percentage denied that their problems concerned mental illness. Rather, they suggested that they were hospitalized for physical illness, or simple confusion, or that they were no longer emotionally disturbed. The proportion increased to one-third of the sample at 30 months. A small percentage answered that simply being in the hospital was evidence that they were mentally ill, and this proportion of each sample (6 per cent to 8 per cent) persisted for the first four time periods. Combined, this evidence suggests that psychiatric symptomatology, in the view of the patients themselves, less and less served as sufficient justification for hospitalization, and that perhaps a more pertinent reason as the passage of time took place was the extent to which a satisfactory adjustment to hospital living resulted.

The last question asked in the interview concerned the patient's subjective estimate of improvement or decrement in his own condition. The question was: "Do you feel you are better now than you were 6 or 12 months ago?" A consistently large percentage of each sample answered that they felt improved, and this proportion increased over time, from 51 per cent at 6 months to 78 per cent at 30 months. At the beginning and end of these assessments, a substantially smaller percentage replied they did not feel improved, but during the three middle periods—at 12, 18, and 24 months—the proportions feeling unimproved were 22, 40, and 33 per cent, respectively. Between 6 and 11 per cent of each sample indicated they felt about the same as they had previously. Of those who felt better, the general tendency was to describe their condition (if they offered any further information) as "a bit better" than previously. Between 21 and 67 per cent of the samples expressed these feelings. The same kind of modest estimate prevailed for those who did not feel improved. An almost equal proportion, in the three middle assessment periods, indicated they felt the same or "a bit worse" than previously, ranging around 5 per cent to 15 per cent of the total samples at each point in time. At the extremes, for example, 17 per cent of the group at 24 months said they were feeling "much worse," while one-quarter of the group indicated they were feeling "much better." The general import of this information is that psychiatric symptoms decrease in importance for the patient in accounting for his residence in the hospital. On the other hand, those who express estimates of their condition in greater detail than simple agreement or disagreement with the interview questions suggest a growing tendency toward stabilization of symptoms.

From these interviews with persons as they progressively accrued longer and longer periods of residence in the mental hospital, the general impression emerges of a group for whom community living recedes ever farther from view. The hospital itself appears to take on a positive significance, and the significance of the process of institutionalization becomes apparent. Less and less concern seems evident for past or future events; less striving is apparent, and patients appear to become somewhat unwilling members of a society which they increasingly do not know how to leave. In such a way, the acutely disturbed patient becomes a "chronic."

The Significance of Participant Variables for Community Adjustment

The design of the experimental community treatment program for chronically hospitalized mental patients required the comparison of the newly created subsystem with existing practices in order that a meaningful decision could be made as to its relative effectiveness. At the same time, however, certain participant variables were recognized as potentially influencing such a comparison. Accordingly, the effects of chronicity and volunteering were evaluated as part of the experimental plan for this study.

It is clear from the evidence that participant characteristics which might have had an adverse effect upon the successful community adjustment of the participants in this experiment did not do so in the newly created social situation. The effect of living in the lodge society seems to have made irrelevant the length of time a patient had previously spent in the mental hospital. Nor did persons who volunteered to go to the lodge, when carefully matched with those unwilling to go there, achieve a substantially better community adjustment than the nonvolunteers.

Those refusing to volunteer to go to the lodge displayed a considerable discrepancy between their expectations of what would happen to them when they returned to the community and what happened when they actually got there. Similarly, those who remained hospitalized for increasingly longer periods of time became more and more institutionalized and unable to visualize for themselves the nature and detail of their own community return. The characteristics which made up their personality, their motivational strivings, and their expectations failed to provide them with sufficient support to reenter the community and stay there successfully. Only when facilitative social conditions are made available to marginal persons such as these, do they attain a successful community adjustment after a lengthy psychiatric hospitalization.

14 THE RELATIONSHIP BETWEEN THE SOCIAL SITUATION AND TREATMENT CRITERIA

Earlier researches (Fairweather, 1960, 1964) strongly suggest that the relationship among measures is influenced by the social situation in which they are completed. These studies led to the following experimental hypothesis:

"The community social subsystem (lodge) and the control condition will yield different relationships among the treatment criteria" (p. 28). Similarities and differences in the relationships generated by the two types of community social settings will be explored in this chapter.

The previous two chapters in this section have presented a comparison of the treatment effectiveness of the lodge and nonlodge social situations, as well as an evaluation of some characteristics of the experimental sample. To accomplish this, a wide range of measures were taken both during the patient's stay in the mental hospital and during the follow-up phase of the study (pp. 37–39). These measures concerned the individual patient's personal history, his attitudes, the evaluations of his fellow patients and staff personnel on his ward, his attitudes in the community, and the evaluations of others close to him there during successive six-month intervals.

A large proportion of these measures were repeatedly given to each person during the course of the study, depending upon how long each person could be followed. Thus, in the computer processing of the data, 72 per cent of the 111 variables represent the same 16 variables measured at five points in time, a total of 80 variables. Of the remaining 31 variables used in this analysis, 19 represent background facts in the personal history of the patient and 12 are scores about each patient prior to the time when he became eligible to leave the small group ward.

Since each set of social conditions in the community was likely to produce different relationships among the same variables, two separate cluster analyses were carried out. Each analysis thus encompasses the relationships between the measures within a single social subsystem, one for the lodge situation and one for the nonlodge community situation. In the case of the lodge situation, measures from 75 lodge residents were used; in the nonlodge situation, measures from 259 nonlodge community residents were used. In both cases, 73 of the original 111 variables were selected for constructing the cluster analyses. The other 38 variables were considered likely to produce extremely unstable correlations because of the small number of pairs of scores available for computation. However, these 38 variables were not simply discarded. Once the key groupings of variables were established by the operation of the program generating the interrelationships among the 73 initial variables, these omitted variables were then assigned to the cluster of variables with which they had the strongest relationship. The cluster program automatically rejected 13 variables in the analysis of the lodge situation measures, and 12 variables in the nonlodge analysis, accepting the remainder as assignable to clusters. Thus, by the automatic operation of the computer program, 98 variables were clustered in the lodge analysis, and 99 in the nonlodge analysis. The establishment of the clusters within the two different social subsystems was accomplished through factoring by the key cluster method developed by Tryon (1959, 1964) and his associates (Tryon and Bailey, 1965).

Overview of the Two Cluster Analyses

The cluster analysis method is fundamentally an associative technique for finding the strength of the relationships among a number of different measurements and then condensing them into a small number of dimensions. Although the clustering of measures in the two separate analyses involved the same variables, different configurations resulted in each case. Relationships among measures derived from lodge residents generated six clusters; those in the nonlodge situation resulted in the formation of eight clusters. Final selection and assignment of variables to these clusters was carried out as a rational procedure. This procedure for further eliminating unreliable variables involved essentially two rules of thumb. First, each variable was typically required to have a cluster loading of no less than .50, except where cluster meaning was enhanced. In the two analyses, eleven variables with cluster loadings from .41 to .49 were included.

Second, variables assigned to a cluster had to have both mathematical and logical coherence. By these procedures, 74 variables were finally assigned to six lodge clusters and 65 variables to eight nonlodge clusters.

Table 14.1 presents the results of these two cluster analyses in abbreviated form. The names which have been assigned to each cluster represent the sense of the general domain of measurement which is involved in each. The clusters are presented in the order in which they were generated by the computer program, which automatically selects as the first cluster of variables those with the highest level of mutual relationship, moving on to those with the next, and so forth, until the total amount of shared variation is essentially exhausted according to a predetermined criterion for terminating factoring of the matrix. Beside each of the cluster names, the number of variables finally selected for inclusion in the cluster is shown in parentheses. In a separate column, a numerical value indicates the proportionate share which each cluster has of the total amount of estimated variation included in the correlation matrix of interrelationships between the variables. This value functions as an index of the relative "importance" of each cluster in relation to all other clusters generated in the analysis. Thus, in both analyses the second cluster claimed the largest proportion of the total variation, but in the lodge analysis the first cluster was a close second, while in the nonlodge analysis the third cluster claimed second place.

Relationships among the clusters may be evaluated by using the correlation coefficient. Its magnitude provides the reader with an estimate of the

Table 14.1. Clustered Measures in the Two Community Situations

Lodge Situation		*Nonlodge Situation*	
Cluster[a]	*Shared Variation (%)*	*Cluster*[a]	*Shared Variation (%)*
1. Community Tenure and Employment (10)	21	1. Community Tenure and Residential Status (8)	12
2. Individual Satisfaction with Hospital and Community Living (25)	25	2. Community Social Behavior (19)	38
3. Community Employment Level and Residential Status (6)	16	3. Individual Satisfaction with Community Living (17)	17
4. Alcoholic Conviviality in the Community (10)	16	4. The Older Psychiatric Patient (2)	5
5. Community Social Behavior (18)	14	5. In-Hospital Attitudes toward Ward and Community Living (8)	11
6. Community Leisure Activity (4)	8	6. Community Employment (7)	7
		7. Prior Military Service (2)	5
		8. Service-Connected Disability Income (2)	5

[a] The number in parentheses after each cluster name represents the number of variables included in that cluster.

relative independence of each cluster from every other cluster in the analysis. Table 14.2 presents these coefficients for both the lodge and the nonlodge analyses.

In general, the clusters are independent of each other, suggesting distinct dimensions in each social situation. There are, however, a few interdependent relations in each situation worthy of comment. In the lodge situation, cluster 1 (community tenure and employment) is moderately related to measures of nonfamily group living situation in the community (cluster 3, r = .43), and to measures of social behavioral adjustment in the community (cluster 5, r = .37). In this community situation, measures of leisure activity in the community (cluster 6) are mildly related to patient attitudes relating hospital living to community living (cluster 2, r = .22) and inversely to the previously mentioned measures of nonfamily group living situation in the community (cluster 3, r = −.26).

In the case of the nonlodge situation, moderate relationships prevail between social behavior (cluster 2) and attitude measures while the patient

Table 14.2. Correlations Between Clustered Measurement Domains

	Lodge Situation					
Clusters	1	2	3	4	5	6
1. Community Tenure and Employment		—.05	.43	—.06	.37	.06
2. Individual Satisfaction with Hospital and Community Living	—.05		—.15	.14	.14	.22
3. Nonfamily Group Living Situation	.43	—.15		.11	—.02	—.26
4. Alcoholic Conviviality in the Community	—.06	.14	.11		—.09	—.01
5. Community Social Behavior	.37	.14	—.02	—.09		.30
6. Community Leisure Activity	.06	.22	—.26	—.01	.30	

	Nonlodge Situation							
Clusters	1	2	3	4	5	6	7	8
1. Community Tenure and Residential Status		.06	—.06	—.12	—.08	.29	.24	.22
2. Community Social Behavior	.06		.25	—.18	.34	.41	.00	.07
3. Individual Satisfaction with Community Living	—.06	.25		—.04	.40	.12	—.08	—.06
4. The Older Psychiatric Patient	—.12	—.18	—.04		—.06	—.09	.20	—.22
5. In-Hospital Attitudes toward Ward and Community Living	—.08	.34	.40	—.06		.07	—.06	—.07
6. Community Employment	.29	.41	.12	—.09	.07		.08	—.04
7. Prior Military Service	.24	.00	—.08	.20	—.06	.08		.17
8. Service-Connected Disability Income	.22	.07	—.06	—.22	—.07	—.04	.17	

Table 14.3. The Six Clusters in the Lodge Community Situation

Cluster	*Loading*
Cluster 1. Community Tenure and Employment	
1. Remains fully employed:	
a. at 12 months	.97
b. at 18 months	.97
c. at 24 months	.94
d. at 6 months	.93
e. at 30 months	.89
2. Remains in the community:	
a. at 18 months	.89
b. at 30 months	.89
c. at 24 months	.88
d. at 12 months	.88
e. at 6 months	.85
Cluster 2. Individual Satisfaction with Hospital and Community Living	
1. Has high morale in the hospital small-group treatment program	.66
2. Has high expectations about living in the community lodge	.61
3. Has high expectations about being in the community	.61
4. Is highly attracted to his hospital ward task group	.57
5. Is highly satisfied with his hospital task group leader	.52
6. Has high expectations about his job in the community	.48
7. Has high expectations about his living conditions in the community	.46
8. Has high expectations about his leisure activities in the community	.46
9. Is highly satisfied with being in the community:	
a. at 6 months	.96
b. at 12 months	.80
c. at 18 months	.80
d. at 24 months	.59
10. Is highly satisfied with his living conditions in the community:	
a. at 6 months	.83
b. at 18 months	.76
c. at 30 months	.73
d. at 12 months	.68
e. at 24 months	.49
11. Is highly satisfied with his leisure activities in the community:	
a. at 6 months	.84
b. at 18 months	.72
c. at 12 months	.72
12. Is highly satisfied with his work in the community:	
a. at 18 months	.80
b. at 6 months	.78
c. at 12 months	.59
d. at 24 months	.49
13. Contacted relatives at point of discharge eligibility:	.50
Cluster 3. Nonfamily Group Living Situation	
1. Has nonfamily group living situation:	
a. at 18 months	.82
b. at 30 months	.82
c. at 24 months	.82
d. at 12 months	.67
e. at 6 months	.56

Table 14.3. Continued

Cluster	*Loading*
2. Is highly satisfied with his leisure activities in community at 24 months:	.51
Cluster 4. Alcoholic Conviviality in the Community	
1. Drinks a lot:	
a. at 12 months	.84
b. at 6 months	.73
c. at 18 months	.66
d. at 24 months	.62
2. Sees many friends regularly:	
a. at 18 months	.78
b. at 12 months	.75
c. at 24 months	.68
d. at 6 months	.54
3. Has been a heavy drinker prior to hospitalization	.72
4. Is usually married	.51
Cluster 5. Community Social Behavior	
1. Is energetic, active, and ambitious:	
a. at 6 months	.80
b. at 18 months	.59
c. at 24 months	.50
d. at 12 months	.47
2. Talks freely with others:	
a. at 30 months	.85
b. at 6 months	.80
c. at 12 months	.54
d. at 18 months	.41
3. Carries out social responsibilities:	
a. at 6 months	.80
b. at 18 months	.61
c. at 12 months	.53
4. Shows few symptoms of emotional illness:	
a. at 6 months	.74
b. at 24 months	.63
c. at 12 months	.46
5. Has higher social status jobs:	
a. at 12 months	.55
b. at 6 months	.52
c. at 18 months	.51
6. Shows initiative in ward task group	.46
Cluster 6. Community Leisure Activity	
1. Makes active use of leisure time:	
a. at 6 months	.89
b. at 18 months	.89
c. at 24 months	.52
d. at 12 months	.52

is still in the hospital (cluster 5, $r = .34$) and between that behavior and employment in the community (cluster 6, $r = .41$). Satisfaction with living in the community (cluster 3) shows a similar strength of relationship to clusters involving in-hospital attitudes (cluster 5, $r = .40$). A mild set of relationships seems to prevail with respect to the older psychiatric patient (cluster 4) and the patient who tends to have had longer prior military service (cluster 7, $r = .20$), but a smaller disability income (cluster 8, $r = -.22$).

With respect to both social situations, however, it is well to keep in mind that these relationships are not very strong. The conclusion may be drawn that the clusters are fairly well-defined independent dimensions or domains of measurement in both situations.

The Lodge Clusters

Cluster 1 is entitled "community tenure and employment" because of the presence in it of these two social-change criterion variables. Not only are both the variables represented, all five assessment points in time are included. Clearly this cluster reflects the effect upon community adjustment of the living situation to which patients were sent from the mental hospital. The length of time the patient remains fully employed is unequivocally linked to the length of time he remains in the community. Furthermore, the longer he is employed full time, the longer he will have been in the community. Thus, in the lodge social situation, knowing the patient's status in regard to community tenure and full-time employment after six months in the community is sufficient for reliably estimating his status as much as two years later.

Cluster 2 is labeled "individual satisfaction with hospital and community living." In this cluster are included 24 attitudinal measures taken while the patient was in the hospital and after he went to the community. The 25th measure involves the recency of the patient's contact with his relatives immediately prior to his discharge. Generally speaking, this appears to be an optimism-pessimism dimension in patient attitudes, which are consistently maintained in and out of the mental hospital. At one end of the attitude continuum, one would encounter the patient who was highly satisfied with his ward program and held high expectations about living in the community. While in the community, this hypothetical patient would express great satisfaction with his living conditions, his leisure activities, and his work. In fact, he would be pleased just to be in the community. Finally, he would typically be a person who had been contacted by his relatives just prior to his entrance into the community, a factor which is strongly associated with his satisfaction while there. The other end of the dimension is equally pertinent, and involves the patient who is miserable as far as his satisfaction with his situation is concerned, in or out of the hospital, and who left the hospital without recent contact with his relatives. This attitudinal dimension stands apart from the length of time the patient remained in the community or remained employed there, as shown in Table 14.2.

Cluster 3 bears the title "nonfamily group living situation." Its strong relationship to the criterion measures of cluster 1 ($r = .43$) is understandable in view of the fact that the lodge was one kind of nonfamily living situation. This cluster also shows that persons who live in group situations at six months are likely to remain in this type of situation rather than becoming members of families.

Cluster 4 is labeled "alcoholic conviviality in the community," because of the strong relationship between active association with friends and heavy drinking in the community, at one end of the dimension, and solitary abstinence at the other. Associated too in this cluster are two personal history measures: One relates to the presence of a prior history of drinking behavior and the other to the patient's marital status at the time of the study. The tendency to be a "drinking buddy" while in the community is associated both with a prior history of drinking and with being married.

Cluster 5 is titled "community social behavior." This cluster involves behavioral ratings of patient adjustment while in the community. It includes a high energy level, much talkativeness, a high level of social responsibility, and a minimal tendency to display symptoms of emotional disturbance. Associated with these variables is the higher social status of the jobs these lodge residents held while in the community. This relationship suggests that the more highly rated was the patient's social behavior in the community, the higher was the social status of the job he held. Concomitantly, of course, the lower the rating of such observed behavior, the lower the social status of the job involved. Leadership in the ward task group is associated with these variables, suggesting behavioral transfer of skills exercised in the hospital to the lodge situation. This possibility was discussed more thoroughly in chapter 12 (pp. 199–237).

Least important of all is cluster 6, entitled "community leisure activity." What use the patient makes of his leisure time is unrelated to any other measured aspect of his behavior in the hospital or in the community lodge situation. It is clear, however, that the patient who invests a high degree of activity in leisure pursuits for six months of follow-up also has a high level of leisure activity for at least the next year and one-half.

The Nonlodge Clusters

The title given to cluster 1 signals one of the first and most significant differences between the relationships of the criterion measures in the lodge and nonlodge situations: "community tenure and residential status." The cluster suggests that knowledge of the six-month community tenure and residential status of a patient provide a reliable estimate of his status in this regard as much as two years later. When in the community, he is likely to be living with immediate family or relatives.

Table 14.4. The Eight Clusters in the Nonlodge Community Situation

Cluster	*Loading*
Cluster 1. Community Tenure and Residential Status	
1. Remains in the community:	
a. at 12 months	1.00
b. at 18 months	1.00
c. at 24 months	.92
d. at 30 months	.82
e. at 6 months	.77
2. Lives with relatives:	
a. at 6 months	.59
b. at 18 months	.56
c. at 12 months	.46
Cluster 2. Community Social Behavior	
1. Makes active use of leisure time:	
a. at 12 months	.86
b. at 18 months	.72
c. at 30 months	.68
d. at 24 months	.53
2. Sees friends regularly:	
a. at 30 months	.85
b. at 12 months	.83
c. at 18 months	.65
3. Carries out social responsibilities:	
a. at 12 months	.81
b. at 18 months	.64
c. at 30 months	.50
4. Is energetic, active, and ambitious:	
a. at 12 months	.74
b. at 30 months	.57
c. at 18 months	.52
5. Talks freely:	
a. at 12 months	.71
b. at 18 months	.57
6. Behaves normally:	
a. at 12 months	.64
b. at 30 months	.58
c. at 18 months	.51
7. Is highly satisfied with being in the community at 30 months:	.85
Cluster 3. Individual Satisfaction with Community Living	
1. Is highly satisfied with his leisure activities in the community:	
a. at 6 months	.87
b. at 18 months	.83

Table 14.4. Continued

Cluster	*Loading*
c. at 30 months	.72
d. at 24 months	.64
e. at 12 months	.61
2. Is highly satisfied with being in the community:	
a. at 18 months	.83
b. at 6 months	.74
c. at 12 months	.71
d. at 24 months	.67
e. at 30 months	.53
3. Is highly satisfied with his living conditions in the community:	
a. at 18 months	.81
b. at 6 months	.74
c. at 12 months	.71
4. Enjoys his work in the community:	
a. at 12 months	.81
b. at 6 months	.65
5. Makes active use of leisure time at 30 months:	.81
6. Sees many friends regularly at 6 months:	.59
Cluster 4. The Older Psychiatric Patient	
1. Is older at first NP hospitalization:	.88
2. Is older now:	.74
Cluster 5. In-Hospital Attitudes Toward Ward and Community Living	
1. Positive attitude to ward program	.92
2. Strong attraction to ward task group	.86
3. High satisfaction with ward task group leader	.79
4. High expectations regarding community recreation	.70
5. High expectations for lodge program	.70
6. High expectations regarding community living	.67
7. High expectations regarding community living situation	.61
8. High expectations regarding community employment	.61
Cluster 6. Community Employment	
1. Remains fully employed:	
a. at 18 months	.91
b. at 12 months	.84
c. at 6 months	.82
d. at 24 months	.68
e. at 30 months	.44
2. Job has a high social status:	
a. at 12 months	.58
b. at 6 months	.45
Cluster 7. Prior Military Service	
1. Tends to have had higher military rank at discharge	.79
2. Tends to have had longer military service	.77
Cluster 8. Service-Connected Disability Income	
1. Is service-connected for disability	.77
2. Has higher monthly income	.64

Cluster 2, which claimed the largest proportion of the total shared variation of the correlation matrix from which the clusters are derived, is labeled "community social behavior." These observer ratings relate to the active use of leisure time, frequent association with friends while in the community, capable assumption of social responsibilities there, high energy level, high talkativeness, and minimal expression of symptoms of emotional disturbance. Strongly associated with these measures of social adjustment in the community is one other type of measure: strong patient satisfaction with being in the community at 30 months of follow-up.

Cluster 3 is titled "individual satisfaction with community living." Its defining variables refer to the patient's strong satisfaction with his living conditions, with his use of leisure time, and with his presence in the community. Strongly related to these patients' attitudes are observer ratings of the patient's active use of leisure time and active association with friends.

Cluster 4 has highly specific referents, containing only two variables derived from the personal history of the patient. It is labeled "the older psychiatric patient," since one measure relates to the patient's age when first hospitalized for psychiatric reasons and the other to his chronological age itself. This independent dimension appropriately reflects the aging character of the chronically hospitalized residual psychotic patient population of the mental hospital, under typical conditions of hospital and community care.

Cluster 5 is labeled "in-hospital attitudes toward ward and community living." This attitudinal grouping of variables shows that positive patient attitudes toward the ward treatment program tend to be associated with high expectations about living in the community.

Cluster 6 bears the title "community employment," since it relates only to that aspect of the patient's situation in the community subsequent to leaving the hospital ward.

Cluster 7 involves another two-variable dimension entitled "prior military service." It is derived, like cluster 4, from the personal history of the patient and concerns two factors: the military rank he held upon discharge from the service and the length of that service. Not unexpectedly, the dimension shows that those with longer military service held higher rank upon discharge.

Cluster 8, labeled "service-connected disability income," deals with a third pair of variables drawn from the patient's personal history. This doublet reflects the fact that veterans who have established a connection between their military service and their psychiatric disablement also have higher total monthly incomes. Since gainful employment of patients in the nonlodge situation is not substantial, one important source of income upon which they can rely is their disability compensation. It is also important to note here that this cluster is correlated only .22 with remaining in the community. The commonly held notion that the possession of funds is the single most important factor in permitting a chronic mental patient to return to the community is not justified by this information.

Elaborating the Outcome and Other Criteria in the Two Treatment Situations

In this experiment, major attention has been directed to following patients in the community. Most of the measurement effort was devoted to obtaining a variety of indices about their community status. This allocation of research resources was undertaken for several reasons. First and foremost, evaluation of psychiatric treatment programs has in the past predominantly focused upon measures of the patient's behavioral, attitudinal, and perceptual status within the hospital where treatment programs have typically been initiated. Such evaluations often lack an adequate external criterion for judging the effectiveness of the program effort, since treatment planners often believe hospital behavior is highly related to community behavior. Such commonsense relationships have not been found to exist in previous studies (Fairweather, 1964, pp. 273–82; Fairweather and Simon, 1963; Forsyth and Fairweather, 1961). This situation has led to a strong recommendation for adopting the behavioral adjustment of the returned patient in the community as the most useful criterion for judging the effectiveness of psychiatric treatment.

During the planning phase of this investigation, it was decided that three criteria would be adopted to judge the effectiveness of the treatment subsystems being compared in this social innovative experiment. The predecessor of this experiment (Fairweather, 1964) demonstrated that the posthospital adjustments of patients who returned to the community were related to being employed and living in a socially supportive situation. It was decided, therefore, that the effectiveness of the treatment subsystems used in this experiment should be judged in terms of the extent to which recidivism was reduced and employment maintained in the community. But it was also felt that a socially acceptable solution to the problem of rehabilitating chronic psychiatric patients could not be evaluated adequately without the introduction of a third criterion, namely, a person's subjective sense of satisfaction with participation in community life, a kind of morale measure. This criterion was adopted primarily on humanistic grounds. For evaluation of the current experiment and the planning of future treatment programs, therefore, knowledge about the relationships between these three measures (community tenure, full-time employment in the community, and patient satisfaction) was considered essential (pp. 37–39). With respect to these objective social-change outcome criteria, what is immediately evident from Tables 14.3 and 14.4 is that the two different social conditions produced different relationships between them. The correlation between cluster 1 (tenure) and cluster 6 (employment) in the nonlodge situation is .29 (Table 14.2). In contrast, these two measures are so highly related in the lodge situation they are members of the same cluster. This linkage between community tenure and employment is found in the lodge situation alone.

Equally important, the same variables are included at every point in time for both the lodge and nonlodge situations. Although the reasons for this relationship may be different in each social situation, such behavior is apparently predictable regardless of the social situation in which it is measured. Knowledge that the community tenure and employment status of patients at six months is sufficient for predicting his status two years subsequent to that follow-up assessment point is extremely important for future experiments. It should allow experimenters to have more confidence in evaluating psychiatric treatments by using shorter follow-up periods of time. The nonlodge situation presented in Table 14.4 offers a striking contrast. No variables unrelated to employment appear in cluster 6. On the other hand, cluster 1 shows that residential status in the community is associated positively only with days in the community and living with his immediate family or relatives or friends. Thus, tenure in the community for the nonlodge patient clearly depends *not* upon being employed but upon the living arrangements he is able to work out with others.

Measures of patients' subjective reactions to community life are also of importance, since they constituted the third criterion for evaluating the effectiveness of the treatment subsystems. Table 14.3 and 14.4 show clearly that individual satisfaction with the treatment programs in the hospital and in the community is not related to community tenure or employment. In the lodge situation, it is evident that attitudes toward the hospital treatment program and expectations about living in the community are positively associated with measures of individual satisfaction with various aspects of being in the community (cluster 2). In the nonlodge social situation, however, such attitudes not only are unrelated to community tenure and employment, they are situationally specific. As Table 14.4 shows, attitudes in the hospital are located in one cluster (cluster 5), while attitudes reflecting individual satisfaction in the community are located in another (cluster 3).

Aside from relationships among the three outcome criteria (community tenure, employment, and satisfaction) there were other areas of measurement in the experiment. The first of these is social behavior in the community. As Table 14.3 shows, in the lodge situation, measurements of such behavior are classified into three rather independent clusters (clusters 4, 5, and 6). Behavior related to drinking and friendship tended to separate from general adjustment in the community and from the patient's level of leisure activity there. Cluster 5 contains some suggestive evidence of behavioral similarity between the hospital and community-lodge social situations. The cluster links behavioral initiative in ward-task groups with energetic and responsible behavior in the lodge setting. The relationships among these variables only partially exist in the nonlodge situation, as shown in Table 14.4. Behavioral adjustment of the social kind in the community was segregated to one cluster (cluster 2), except for activity with friends at six months and use of leisure time at 30 months.

Another major difference between the two social situations is that in the lodge only three variables relating to the personal history of the patient appeared in any of the six clusters. One was related to satisfaction and two were related to social drinking in the community. On the other hand, in the nonlodge situation three clusters of personal history variables appeared which were relatively independent of any of the others, as the correlations for clusters 4, 7, and 8 show in Table 14.2.

The Problem of Treatment Programming for the Hospitalized Psychiatric Patient

Persons responsible for planning treatment programs for hospitalized psychiatric patients, particularly those patients who have had extensive periods of hospitalization, must consider several facts emanating from the cluster analyses just presented. The study of the relationships between measures in three different social situations (the hospital ward, and two different social situations in the community) carry several implications for the program planner. Certain conclusions seem inevitable.

1. *Some measures of attitude and behavior are situationally specific.* In a previous study (Fairweather, 1964) it was learned that measures evaluating the behavior and attitudes of program participants were specific to the hospital or to the community. In the current experiment, it was learned that the relationships between the three selected criteria of community adjustment (tenure, employment, and satisfaction) were different depending on the social situation in which they were measured. Tenure and employment were related in the lodge situation, but not in the nonlodge situation. Satisfaction in the hospital was related to satisfaction in the lodge situation, but not in the nonlodge situation. Certain kinds of behavior (social adjustment and employment) in the lodge situation were unrelated, but they were related in the nonlodge situation. Personal history was related to specific behavior in the community nonlodge situation, but was unrelated to any hospital or community behavior or attitudes. Such items of personal background, on the other hand, were related in a different way to behavior and attitudes in the lodge situation.

2. *Attitudes and behavior are unrelated in any situation.* Satisfaction in both the lodge and nonlodge situations was generally unrelated to certain measures of individual performance such as tenure and employment in the community. Knowledge, available from previous studies of such patients (Fairweather, 1964; Forsyth and Fairweather, 1961) was

again confirmed in this experiment. Only in a few cases were attitudes associated with behaviors, for example, cluster 3 (Table 14.4) has two behavioral variables. Otherwise, attitudes segregated into clusters separate from clusters involving behavioral measures.

3. *The same attitudes or behaviors are correlated over time.* In both the lodge and the nonlodge situations, measurement over time, regardless of whether attitudes or behavior are involved, are related. Only the extensive degree to which following the patient in the community was undertaken could have revealed this finding. But such knowledge represents a major advance in the refined understanding of treatment criteria, quite apart from awareness of the ways in which they are related in different social situations. Shorter periods of follow-up for such patients as part of treatment evaluation seems feasible; in most cases, as has been previously recommended (Forsyth and Fairweather, 1961), six months seems sufficient.

How do these conclusions relate to the work of the treatment programmer? First of all, it is clear that the evaluation of treatment program effectiveness requires *multivariate* criteria, because of the lack of relationship between some variables and because the situational specificity of measurement yields different relationships among the criteria, depending upon the situation in which the measurement takes place. Several examples should serve to highlight this need. The evidence in Tables 14.3 and 14.4 clearly shows that even though participants are satisfied with a community program, one should not at the same time expect them to exhibit a high level of performance, at least in terms of reduced recidivism and sustained employment. Both in the lodge and nonlodge situations, patients expressed gratification at being in the community, but these attitudes were unrelated to whether or not they remain there or were employed. This difference between benefit defined in terms of patient satisfaction with a treatment program and benefit defined in terms of the accomplishment of certain performance goals for program participants is nowhere more clearly demonstrated than in regard to expectations about employment. Having high expectations about community prospects with regard to living conditions and employment is unrelated to tenure and employment in the community, regardless of whether it is in a community lodge or elsewhere. In a previous study (Fairweather, 1964), job expectancies were related to the patients' having held jobs prior to hospitalization, not to securing employment when the patient went to the community from the hospital. Hence, these recurring relationships and distinctions between the patients' reaction to a treatment program and the goals which the treatment institution might expect the program to serve must always be an integral part of decision-making with respect to implementing such programs. Only by adopting multiple evaluative criteria can the treatment programmer hedge against the implications of these varying relationships just outlined.

If the goal of adopting a new treatment program is to improve the community tenure and employment of the chronic psychotic patients, what the patient does or feels in the hospital or in the community will probably be unrelated to this goal. If programs for such patients are to stress both individual performance (such as tenure and employment) and humanitarian considerations, criteria of effectiveness must be adopted which include both types of measures. In such a case, treatment would only be effective when *both* the patients' behavior and feelings of self-enhancement had been achieved.

15 GROUP PROCESSES IN THE HOSPITAL AND COMMUNITY SOCIAL SUBSYSTEMS

In the study of the small-group ward treatment program conducted in 1964 and described earlier (pp. 28–29), only a limited investigation was made of the dimensions of group structure and process in patient groups; the information gained was incomplete and dealt with only a few of the many possible variables (Fairweather, 1964). But the completion of that experiment did not signal the end of interest in more detailed study of group processes on the experimental ward. Interest persisted for several reasons—the ordinary scientific curiosity about a little-known subject, the continued interest in the social system (i.e., the experimental small-group program) which provided the participants in the experimental groups for this study (pp. 29–30), and the opportunity provided by the current research project to make a comparative study of such group processes in the two different settings which together comprised the innovative treatment subsystem described in this book, namely, the hospital ward and the community lodge. The rapid turnover of group membership in the hospital setting offered a further opportunity to observe such processes as they were affected by changing group membership. It seemed to the research staff especially important to discover how stable the group processes would be with changing group members and how a complete change in membership might affect these processes. Finally, information could be obtained on the development of a group from its birth, so that it offered the possibility of studying some of the processes that occur in the evolution of groups. To satisfy all these interests, data for a longitudinal analysis of group processes both in the hospital program and in the community social subsystem were collected. The results of these analyses will be presented in two segments: an account of group processes in the hospital setting will be presented first; then a description of the same processes as they occurred in the community setting will conclude this chapter.

Group Processes in the Hospital

From the beginning, one of the goals of the present experiment was to collect data which would permit the analyses of real-life group processes. In order to accomplish this, it was necessary for the experimental procedures to permit the collection of data with the least possible disturbance to the natural group processes being observed. The importance of collecting data in social innovative experiments without disturbing the naturalistic setting of those processes has been discussed elsewhere (Fairweather, 1967, p. 127). One of the best methods for minimizing interference with the ongoing group processes is to collect the data as an integral part of the daily routine of the small-group ward program at the hospital (pp. 37–39). Even when the administration of questionnaires was necessary, they were given to the members of a patient group every three months during regularly scheduled meetings. These meetings and the collection of information during them had also been made an integral part of the ward program from the outset of the experiment (pp. 45–47).

For the analysis, variables were chosen that covered as many aspects of group functioning as it was practical to measure under the circumstances of the field experiment. The variables included the members' own histories of institutionalization, group size, turnover of group membership, information and problem input to the group, leadership, cohesiveness, role clarity, morale (including attitudes, satisfactions, and expectations), group performance, rewards and punishments, and intragroup choices of companions. Group size was held nearly constant during the measurement period, with the number of members ranging from 13 to 20; usually the groups contained from 15 to 17 men. The variance in group size was so small that it could be considered a constant in the present study; therefore, no analysis of the effect of the group size variable was made. The measure of group cohesiveness was based on the theoretical notions of Jackson (1959), who defined cohesiveness to be a combination of a member's attraction to the group and his acceptance by that group. Jackson proposed that these two factors were independent. This proposition was tested in the present experiment by the inclusion of two separate variables: "attraction to the group" and "acceptance by the group," as well as by a separate score combining these two scores into a measure of "cohesiveness."

The investigation began when four new patient task groups were formed from the patients living on the experimental ward (pp. 45–47). These patients were matched in groups of four on social activity and each of the four patients was then randomly assigned to one of the four experimental task groups. Thus, the four groups were similar in social activity—a variable previously found to affect group performance (Maynard, 1964; Sanders, MacDonald, and Maynard, 1964). The formation of new groups permitted the measures to be taken during the developmental stages of group processes. Immediately upon formation, the new groups completed the research forms which were given them. This procedure yielded initial measures on the variables that were given to all groups at intervals of about three months. These repeated measurements every 90 days occurred at what will be called "time periods," with the initial testing being called period I, while the others were given consecutive Roman numerals, that is, period II, period III, and so on. Nine time periods encompassing 24 months' time were included for the analysis of hospital group processes.

A total sample of 315 persons participated in the task groups while the study was in progress. All participants resided on the ward for at least five working days before their first test responses were obtained. This requirement was adopted because Sanders and MacDonald (1963) found that the roles and attitudes of new group members are relatively stable by the end of only one week on the small-group ward. Most of the participants bore the diagnosis of "schizophrenic reaction." Because the experimental units were naturalistic, open social groups in the hospital setting, their membership changed progressively over time to the point where it had changed completely by time period IX.

The data were analyzed by the method of cumulative communality cluster analysis developed by Tryon and his associates at the University of California, Berkeley (Tryon, 1964; Tryon and Bailey, 1965). A cluster analysis was completed for each period to obtain a "snapshot" of the group processes at that time. After all nine periods had been clustered, an analysis comparing all nine time periods revealed the main generalized dimensions of group functioning for the entire 24 months of the experiment.

The Dimensions of Patient Group Processes

The comparative analysis produced seven clusters. The first three clusters account for 92 per cent of all the variance contained in the matrix of correlations at the beginning of the comparative analysis. These three define the main dimensions of group processes emerging from all nine periods of the study.

Table 15.1 summarizes variables constituting the content of the three main dimensions, in addition to showing their presence or absence at each time period. The content of these three dimensions concerns (1) group

Table 15.1 Variables Comprising the Dimensions at Each Time Period

	Time Period								
Dimension	*I (0 days)*	*II (90 days)*	*III (180 days)*	*IV (270 days)*	*V (360 days)*	*VI (450 days)*	*VII (540 days)*	*VIII (630 days)*	*IX (720 days)*
1. *Group Cohesiveness*									
Cohesiveness	X	X	X	X	X	X	X	X	
Morale	X	X	X	X	X	X	X	X	X
Attraction to group	X	X	X	X	X	X	X	X	X
Satisfaction with leader	(X)	(X)	X	X	X	(X)	X	(X)	X
Expectancies	X	(X)	X	(X)	(X)	X	X	X	X
Choice of others		X	(X)	X	(X)	X		(X)	X
2. *Group Performance*									
Performance			X	X	X	X	X	X	X
Reward	X		X	X	X	(X)	X	X	X
Problem input				—X		—X	—X	—X	X
Information input				X			X	X	X
Information input÷ Total input				X	X	X	X	X	X
Percent turnover of membership						X	X	(X)	X
Variance of performance			—X	(X)	—X	X	X	X	—X
Variance of reward			—X			—X	X	X	X
3. *Leadership and Role Delineation*									
Leadership		X	X	X	X	X	X		
Role clarity		X	X	X	X	X			X
Acceptance by group		X		X	(X)	(X)	X		X
Diagnosis and chronicity			X			(X)	X		
Time in group				(X)		(X)			

cohesiveness, (2) group performance, and (3) leadership and role delineation. The marks in the body of the table show the presence of each variable at each period, either as a variable strongly associated with a cluster at that period as X, or as a variable which is more weakly associated with the cluster at that period (X in parentheses). A variable which is negatively related to a cluster is denoted as $-X$.

Table 15.1 shows that highly cohesive groups are composed of members who are attracted to the group; who choose many of their fellows to share in their time, abode, and work; who are satisfied with their group's leaders and have positive attitudes toward its customs (high morale); and who have high positive expectations about their future life outside the hospital. These variables constitute dimension 1. Dimension 2 shows that groups having the most adequate performance receive greater rewards (or less punishment); receive fewer notices of rule infractions by their members (problem input); receive more purely informative input and a high proportion of information in their total input; and have a higher turnover of membership. In the context of the experimental ward, this last characteristic reflects a higher rate of group members leaving the hospital. Such groups, however, are *not* consistently less variable in performance, as might be expected from a previous study (Maynard, 1964). Dimension 3 reveals that a group in which members have well-defined roles also has a high average level of leadership in its total membership and tends to be composed of less disturbed psychiatric patients. Such groups also show a higher degree of acceptance by their members.

The Independence of the Dimensions

The relations among the three dimensions found in the analysis are as interesting as their content. The correlations in Table 15.2 show the degree to which the dimensions approach complete independence or orthogonality. Inspection of Table 15.2 shows that the three dimensions are relatively independent of each other. The low correlations shown in Table 15.2 indicate that highly performing groups need not be highly cohesive or have high morale; nor do such groups require members to have clear social roles or high leadership potential. Good performance, however, *is* associated with reward and punishment and with the sheer amount of information a group receives. This finding is supported by recent studies with similar groups (Maynard, 1964; Sanders, MacDonald, and Maynard, 1964) and with groups of servicemen in a different setting (Sampson, 1963). It should be noted that this link between group performance and reward does not imply causality, and is not directly relevant to theoretical questions about the role of reward in learning and behavior change. In this case, the relationship simply reflects the consistency of the ward social system: good performance by a group was usually followed by the reward of more money and passes to

Table 15.2 Correlations among the Three Main Clusters

	1	2	3
Cluster	*Group Cohesiveness*	*Group Performance*	*Leadership and Role Delineation*
1. Group cohesiveness		.13	.19
2. Group performance	.13		.00
3. Leadership and role delineation	.19	.00	

leave the hospital groups, while poor performance usually resulted in less money and passes.

Previous studies have failed to find a direct relationship between group cohesiveness and group performance (Darley, Gross, and Martin, 1952; French, 1951) or have shown that the former may raise or lower the latter, depending on other circumstances (Schacter, Ellertson, McBride, and Gregory, 1951). The present study does *not* support the idea that cohesiveness, satisfaction, and morale are completely independent of performance in a group. But the relative independence of these two dimensions (cohesiveness and performance) is important because both of them might be used as common outcome criteria in experimental social innovation studies (Fairweather, 1967, pp. 81–85). The results here do imply that such criteria must be *equally* stressed and *independently* measured, since group conditions which will generate the desired levels on one dimension will not necessarily do so on the other. Natural examples of the relative independence of group performance from the satisfactions and attitudes of group members have always been evident wherever men live as slaves. The results only verify this, therefore, and stress the importance of having at least these dual criteria in mind for establishing and evaluating such new social systems.

The orthogonal (independent) relationship between group performance and group leadership is not clear by itself, but prior work and additional data from the present study make it more understandable. Groups varying in composition with respect to the social activity of their members do not show performance which is directly related to the average social activity score of the group. Rather, certain optimal ratios of highly active to minimally active members mark the most productive groups, and performance decreases as the ratio departs from the optimum in either direction (Maynard, 1964; Sanders, MacDonald, and Maynard, 1964). The measure of group leadership used in this study is strongly related to the social activity measure used in prior studies. Therefore, the relation of average group leadership to group performance must tend toward the shape of an inverted U-curve, producing the very low correlations found in the present study (the average correlation was .03 over all nine time periods).

It is possible, therefore, that the measure used to represent "leadership" in dimension 3, that is, the "amount" of leadership possessed by each member of the group, might not depict the possible effect on a group of having a single, strong leader. Many students of group processes hold that it is the presence of a single leader which is the critical factor in the performance of a group. To test for this "great man" effect, the single, highest leadership score for each group at a particular time period was determined and a rank correlation coefficient (*rho*) was computed between it and the group's performance score for that same period. This was done for each time period independently, since the conditions at different periods may not have been identical. Only at the first two time periods did there seem to be a significant relationship—the value of *rho* at period I was .95, and at period II it was 1.00. The second of these values is statistically significant at the .05 level of confidence and the first approaches this situation, but at no other period is there a significant relationship between performance and the single highest leadership score in a group. Thus, in the results from this study, there appears to be no consistent relationship between a group's performance and the fact that it may have one outstanding leader.

Another aspect of the relative independence of the three dimensions involves the measures of group cohesiveness used in this study. As explained earlier, the measure derives from a theoretical proposition by Jackson (1959) that group cohesiveness is a function of the two orthogonal (independent) dimensions—"attraction to the group" and "acceptance by the group." Both of these variables, as defined by published instruments (Jackson and Saltzstein, 1956; Jackson and Snoek, 1959) appear in the present study, as well as the measure of "cohesiveness" based on an additive combination of them. In the cluster analysis, the measure of "attraction to the group" was assigned to dimension 1, but the measure of "acceptance by the group" was placed in dimension 3. Since the correlation between these two dimensions is .19 (Table 15.2), it would seem that Jackson's assumption of orthogonality is essentially correct. However, because the "cohesiveness" variable which was based on the two relatively independent Jackson measures falls in dimension 1, it appears that "attraction to the group" is far more important than "acceptance by the group" in determining group cohesiveness and high morale—at least as these three variables were defined in the present study.

The Development of the Dimensions

The three main dimensions presented in Table 15.2 seem to be basic throughout the measurement span of nine time periods, with variations occurring at each period according to the conditions prevalent at that time. These variations have to do with the presence or absence of variables in a particular dimension from one period to another. Since the three main dimensions appear to represent stable group processes, the dimensions can be used as "templates" to compare the clusters actually obtained at each period. In this way an estimate of the variability of the clusters from these "standards" at each time period can be made.

To make these estimates of cluster variability, all variables which appear in Table 15.1 as members of a cluster at least four times during the measurement span will be taken as dimension *definers*. A count will be made to find the *proportion* of total definers missing from each dimension at each period. This proportion serves as a score—the highest value indicating the least variability or the greatest stability, that is, the closest fit to the total number of dimension definers. Figure 15.1 presents a comparison of the stability of the three main dimensions for the nine time periods that are involved.

Figure 15.1 shows that the groups experienced a period of development which was completed by period III. Their group processes then remained relatively stable for the remaining six times periods. An exception occurred, however, at time period VIII. At that time such stability dropped to the level of the developmental phase at time period II. The state of the group processes at these two time periods seems to be outside the ordinary variance of those processes, since at both points there is the total loss of a dimension ("group performance" at time period II; "leadership and role delineation" at time period VIII). This loss is accompanied by one of the rare occasions of instability in dimension 1 (time period VIII) after stabilized group processes had been achieved. The fluctuation at time period VIII appears to be the result of unrepresentative measurement procedures, a matter discussed elsewhere (pp. 287–291).

The most stable dimension over the entire period of measurement was "group cohesiveness." It emerges strongly even during the developmental phase and is comprised of three exceptionally strong variables (morale, cohesiveness, and attraction to the group; two of these three appear at each time period as shown in Table 15.1. The second dimension, "group performance," was slow to develop but, once established in time period III, gained stability during the rest of the measurement time. Dimension 3, "leadership and role delineation," was fully developed by period II but never attained the stability of the first two, primarily because it consisted of only three defining variables.

Earlier, the correlations of group performance with the highest individual leadership score in each group were discussed (pp. 283–284). By themselves they were not significant findings, but with this new information about the developmental phase during time periods I and II, they suggest that a strong single leader (or a small group of leaders) has more effect on group performance when group processes are less well developed than when such processes are fully formed and stable. A narrative description of the impact of such a leader (the peer coordinator of the lodge) on the

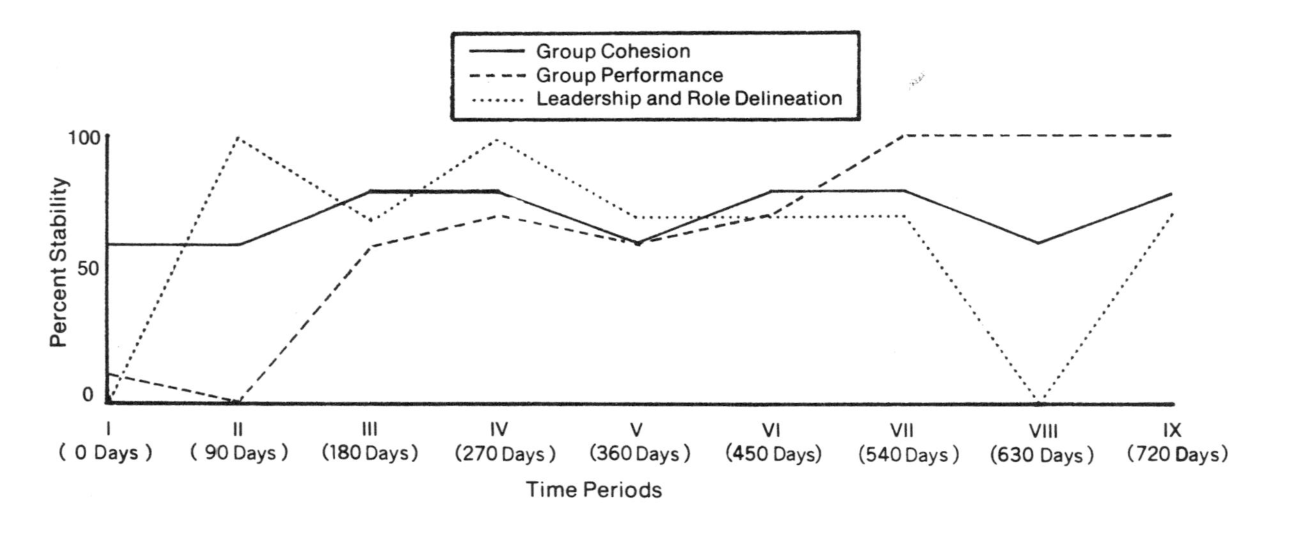

FIG. 15.1.—*Relative stability of the dimensions at each time period.*

performance of a new group appears elsewhere (pp. 64–69), where it is noted that the demise of this leader after the group had become better organized did not result in a drastic loss of group organization. Further support for this notion is to be found in an earlier study by Fairweather and his associates (1964, p. 182) where it is shown that a poorly performing (and perhaps disorganized) patient group is markedly improved by a good leader and that even when the leader leaves the group, performance does not drop to previously attained levels.

Effect of Change in Group Membership

The changes in group processes during the early part of the measurement period are understandable because in the new groups they were becoming stabilized. Thus, a relatively stable period following such development might also be expected. There still remains, however, the question of whether the instability after the developmental phase is due entirely to normal variability or whether any deviations can be associated with particular events. This is especially the case for the great drop in stability at period VIII, shown in Figure 15.1 by the discrepant levels of the three dimensions at that time.

The instability at period VIII seems partly artifactual, being most likely the result of atypical testing procedures and hence not entirely due to the actual relationships among the variables which might have prevailed at that time. Because of administrative changes, both the persons administering the tests and the procedure of collecting the completed forms were modified for this test session. This modification apparently had the effect of generating enough atypical responses from men on the ward to give this somewhat distorted picture of the group processes. Two sources of evidence support this explanation of the increased variability at period VIII. One factor is the continued stability of dimension 2, which is mainly defined by variables measured directly from the day-to-day operating of the groups. Such measurements do not depend on the responses at particular testing sessions. The second piece of evidence for this interpretation is the unusually high amount of variance remaining after the computer-programmed cluster analysis for period VIII was completed. The amount of variance unaccounted for at period VIII is much greater than at any other time (even greater than the amount during the development phase). It seems likely, therefore, that the testing procedures at time period VIII produced so many random or atypical responses that the automatic cluster analysis presented a distorted picture of the group processes for that point in time.

The major factor affecting the dimensions of group processes observed during the study was the source of variation already described in this chapter: changes in the particular variables constituting a dimension. This effect is linked with a concurrent change in membership over time.

Table 15.3. Number and Per Cent of Sample from Time Period I Remaining at Each Subsequent Time Period

Number and Per Cent	*Time Period*								
	I (0 days)	*II (90 days)*	*III (180 days)*	*IV (270 days)*	*V (360 days)*	*VI (450 days)*	*VII (540 days)*	*VIII (630 days)*	*IX (720 days)*
Remaining N	63	39	27	27	20	3	7	2	0
Remaining %	100	62	43	43	32	5	11	3	0

Table 15.4. Number and Per Cent of Sample That Are New Members at Each Time Period

Number and Per Cent	*Time Period*								
	I (0 days)	*II (90 days)*	*III (180 days)*	*IV (270 days)*	*V (360 days)*	*VI (450 days)*	*VII (540 days)*	*VIII (630 days)*	*IX (720 days)*
Total Number	63	60	60	55	58	60	70	75	75
Number of New Members	63	20	27	17	26	40	31	38	52
Per Cent of New Members	100	33	45	31	45	67	43	51	68

The details of membership change appear in Table 15.3 and 15.4. Table 15.3 presents the overall turnover of the sample during the whole experiment. It shows the number and percentage of persons beginning the study who remained at each period. By time period IX, none of the initial 63 men remain. Thus, by the end of the experiment the original sample of members had been completely replaced by new members. The turnover rate for successive periods can also be shown as a percentage of the sample at each time period that consisted of new members entering the groups. Table 15.4 presents this information. Thus the group processes that were analyzed at each period were based on groups whose membership constantly changed rather drastically. Any consistency or continuity in group processes from one time period to another occurred in measurement samples of group processes under conditions where membership turnover between measurement points was never less than 30 per cent and sometimes reached as high as two-thirds of the members (periods VI and IX in Table 15.4). Taken together, Table 15.3 and 15.4 stress the degree of openness of the social system on the experimental ward and the changing group membership conditions under which the data of this study were collected. Relative stability of group-process dimensions was observed despite severe fluctuation in group membership. Actually, the two sources of dimension variation are directly linked.

Figure 15.2 displays the overall stability of the dimensions over time, as shown in Figure 15.1, along with the concurrent state of group membership. Once stable processes have been achieved at time period III, the relative stability of the dimensions usually fluctuates directly with the change in membership. Generally, the dimensions become less stable, in terms of a loss in defining variables, when there is a significant loss of original members together with a large influx of new members. Conversely, the dimensions become more stable if the percentage of original members remains steady or increases, accompanied by a decrease in the percentage of new members. The only apparent exception to this rule occurs at time period VI, where a great change in membership followed by a move to a new ward location is linked with an increase in the stability of the dimensions.

But a closer inspection of the data shows that the exception at time period VI is only apparent; a different kind of instability in the dimensions appears at this time. This type of instability is not detected by the measure used for Figure 15.1, that is, the number of missing definers, but it is more important than a simple loss of defining variables from a particular group-process dimension. A glance at Table 15.1 reveals that the group-performance dimension has lost one of its major definers (reward) at time period VI. This is the only time period when such a loss occurs after the developmental phase of time periods I and II had been completed. Even more important, the cluster analysis at time period VI shows that this "missing definer" has

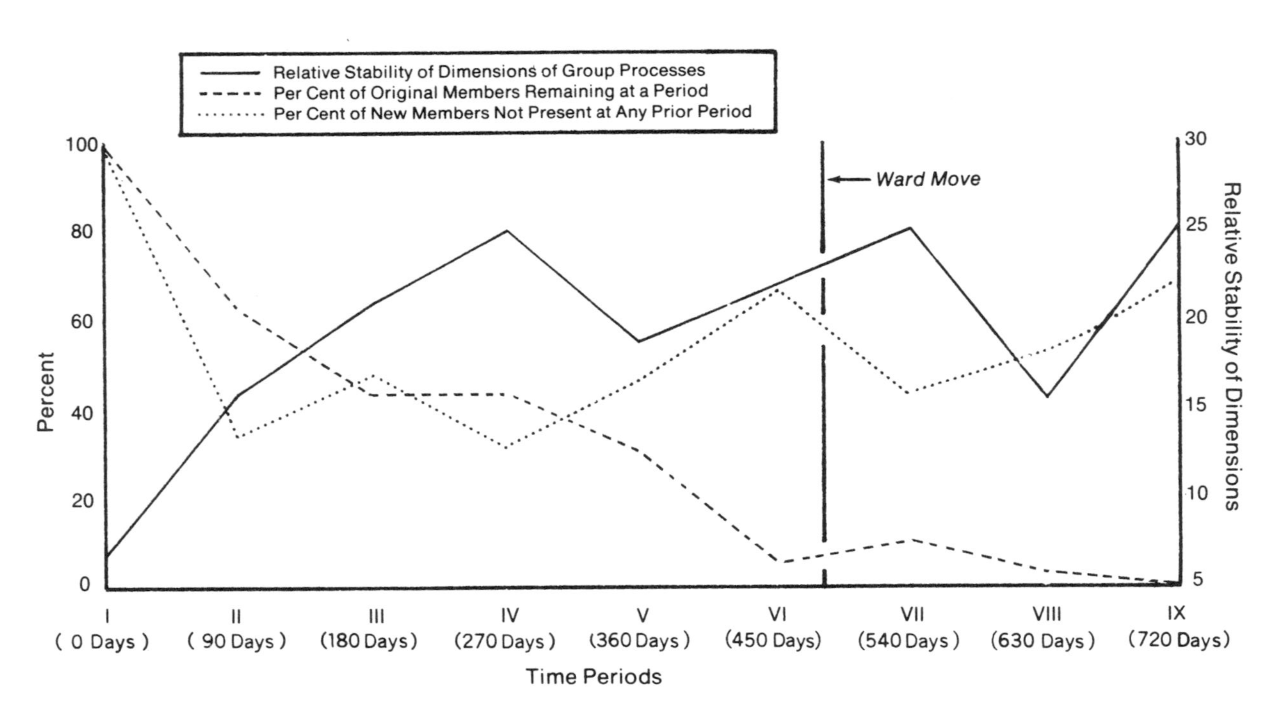

FIG. 15.2.—*Relative stability of the dimensions of group processes and the concurrent change in group membership at each time period.*

moved toward a configuration of variables found only during the developmental phase. These two facts indicate a tendency for the group performance dimension at period VI to regress toward the configuration characteristic of the developmental phase. This regression coincides with the largest absolute drop in original group members (Table 15.3) during the study and with a large influx of new members (Table 15.4).

However, the characteristic pattern of the developmental phase did *not* reappear subsequently, in spite of the tendencies in that direction at time period VI. Thus, it appears that the stable processes of an established group might be shaken by a turnover of membership, and even severely shaken by a large change over a short time, but the tendency of the group processes to remain stable allows for a considerable change in membership to occur without breakdown into a new developmental phase. The results also imply that group performance is the group-process dimension most sensitive to a change in membership. It proved to be the most variable dimension during the first six time periods, when the greatest change in membership occurred, and it was the one at time period VI which showed the most definite regression toward the initial phase of group development.

This exploration of patient small-group processes in the hospital ward situation can be summarized as follows:

1. Patient group processes in the ward situation develop over a period of three to six months from the time the group is assembled and are relatively stable thereafter.

2. Such group processes can be defined by three dimensions which are relatively independent. They are: (1) group cohesiveness, (2) group performance, and (3) leadership and role delineation. These three dimensions constitute the minimum measurement requirements for observing and conceptualizing group processes in a reliable fashion.

3. Change in patient group membership affects all three types of processes but does not destroy them; the dimension of group performance is the most affected by such changes and the dimension of group cohesiveness is the least.

4. The two dimensions of group cohesiveness proposed by Jackson (1959) are relatively orthogonal (independent), as he assumes in theory, but a measure of group cohesiveness additively derived from them is more associated with "attraction to the group" than "acceptance" by it.

5. Patient group performance during a period of development or instability of group processes may be more affected by the ability of a single strong leader than when the processes are fully formed and stable. This statement should probably be qualified by the conditions of heterogeneity of group member characteristics extant in the group being observed, as established in prior studies (Maynard, 1964; Sanders, et al., 1964).

Group Processes in the Lodge Society

In the community lodge society, an observer might reasonably expect that small group processes would vary from those observed in the very different social situation of the mental hospital ward. In order to explore systematically group processes as they developed in the lodge society, the research staff employed the same methods of data collection and analysis as were used in studying such group processes on the hospital ward. Hence, measures were taken every 90 days and their relationships were again determined through the use of cluster analysis methods (Tryon, 1964; Tryon and Bailey, 1965). However, the group process variables measured at the lodge were not measured in the same way they were on the hospital ward, because of important differences in the two social situations. The measuring instruments for some of the variables in the hospital simply could not be used to measure the same variables in the experimental lodge society. When this happened, new and appropriately pretested assessment devices for the same variables were created. Thus, each new instrument was created, at least rationally, to measure the same variable and dimension as its hospital counterpart. This change in the operations of measurement for some of the variables is the most important difference in the procedures for observing group processes in the two different social situations.

In relation to such differences, the two variables of performance and reward, which were the main definers of the group performance dimension in the hospital ward (p. 281), could not be measured in the same way at the lodge. In the hospital setting, performance was measured by having the ward staff rate the general performance of the group for the week preceding such a staff evaluation. At the lodge, there were no such evaluations, both because there were no staff there and because the autonomy of the group precluded such an arrangement. Instead, the measure of group performance which was adopted consisted of a staff person's assessment of the quality of work done by the janitorial and gardening service. Thus, the staff coordinator inspected the jobs done by the work groups in the community and rated them on a work performance checklist. A score, derived from this instrument, assessed the performance of the janitorial crews on each job and a mean score combining a number of these ratings provided a measure of overall performance by the lodge group for any particular period of time. This comprises the measure of group performance used for the analysis of group processes in the lodge society.

Defining performance in this manner was appropriate to the social setting at the lodge. The definition of reward followed the same logical development. The measure of the variable adopted for the community situation was the actual amount of money paid to each of the lodge members for a week's work. In contrast, on the hospital ward this variable was measured by the particular combination of money (in the form of weekly cash withdrawal from the patient's funds), and freedom (in the form of the length of pass time allowed away from the hospital), corresponding to the patient's level of achievement within the ward program. At the lodge, freedom was equivalent for all, since there was no restriction on the movement of the members after the usual eight-hour work day. Hence, pass time could not serve as a reward to lodge residents; only money remained as a viable reward.

These two measurement redefinitions of variables serve as concrete illustrations of the difference between the social situation of the hospital and the lodge. One may gain a full appreciation of this difference by comparing the description of the experimental ward (Fairweather, 1964) with the account of the lodge given earlier in this book (pp. 45–126). The following sections will permit the achievement of the main object of analyzing group processes in these two social situations: to discover what similarities and differences occurred as a result of this change in social situation. It is important to recall in this connection that all of the men who lived in the lodge had come initially from the experimental ward at the hospital. Thus, all of the group members at the lodge who provided the data used in the analysis presented in this section were some of the men who had also formed the groups that were studied in the first section of this chapter. (A full account of the lodge population characteristics was given in chapter 3).

Experimental Procedure and Data Analysis

In most respects, the experimental procedures for collecting and analyzing the data were identical with those for the hospital ward (pp. 37–39). Aside from the change in measurement of the two variables already described, only one important change was made to adapt methods to the difference between the hospital and lodge settings. This change concerns the number of measurements during which data were collected, and the way in which those data were grouped for analysis.

At the lodge, group process data were collected every 90 days on nine different occasions. Thus, data were available for only eight measurement time periods instead of the nine used in the hospital. The reason for this was that the initial testing of the group of men going to the community was done on the hospital ward and, as such, it did not measure the social processes of the lodge. A new grouping of the data was necessary because of the smaller number of participants living in the lodge. Since only 75 persons were participants in the lodge society over 42 months, compared with 315 men in the hospital ward analysis, a problem for data analysis was created by the consistently small number of persons that were involved at any one time period. With numbers at particular time periods of less than 20 persons, it was impossible to make reliable analyses of the group processes by the exact methods used for the hospital data (pp. 279–280). To solve this dilemma, the time periods were pooled into three time blocks. The first block consisted of measures from the 90- and 180-day time periods, the second block of those from the next three 90-day periods, and the last block from the last three 90-day time periods in the study. By this method, the number of persons in the three blocks increased to 21, 29, and 35 persons, respectively.

But combining time periods into blocks entailed the risk that a developmental period in the earlier stages of the group processes might be missed because of the inability to trace such developing processes through separate analyses of each of the earlier time periods. From the results of the ward analysis, it seemed a good possibility that such developmental stages would appear, and they will be discussed subsequently (pp. 298–300). Following the procedure already described (pp. 279–280), a separate cluster analysis for each block of three time periods established the dimensions of group processes in the community lodge situation. Finally, an overall comparison of these three cluster analyses was made.

The Dimensions of Group Processes at the Lodge

The cluster analysis produced three clusters of group process variables. The first two represent clear, solid dimensions of group processes in the lodge setting, while the third is essentially a residual cluster with very little coherence and stability. There is quantitative evidence that this last cluster has relatively little meaning. Together, the first two dimensions account for about 95 per cent of all the variance contained in the matrix of correlations at the beginning of the analysis. The two dimensions divide this variance about equally. The third dimension accounts for only 1 per cent of that same pool of variance.

Table 15.5 summarizes the content of the three dimensions produced by the cluster analysis and shows which variables belong to different blocks of time. The *X* markers in the body of the table show the presence of a variable that is positively related and the $-X$ markers show the presence of a variable which is negatively related to the other variables in the same cluster. In the third block of time, the analysis combined two related clusters into a more general dimension. The variables which were members of one cluster at the third block of time are presented simply as *X*'s while those from the second cluster are shown with an asterisk as X^*.

Even a casual study of Table 15.5 reveals two important differences between the group processes on the hospital ward and in the lodge society. The ward analysis showed that groups in the hospital required three distinct dimensions to account adequately for their processes (Table 15.1); Table 15.5 shows that an essentially complete description of group processes at the lodge are encompassed by only two. This is the first major difference between the two social situations.

The second difference is equally important. Similar to the hospital group

Table 15.5. Variables Comprising the Dimensions at Each Block of Time in the Community Lodge Situation

	Time Block		
Dimension	*I* (*180 days*)	*II* (*450 days*)	*III* (*720 days*)
1. *Group cohesiveness*			
Cohesiveness	X	X	X
Morale	X	X	X
Attraction to group	X	X	X
Satisfaction with leader	X	X	X*
Time in the group	—X		
2. *Group performance and leadership*			
Leadership	X	X	X
Performance	X	X	X
Sociometric choice by peers	X	X	X*
Acceptance by the group	X	X	X
3. *Residual dimension*			
Reward	—X	X	
Diagnostic category		X	

analysis, the first dimension of group processes at the lodge is one of morale, group cohesiveness, satisfaction with the group leader, and attraction to the group as defined by Jackson (pp. 279–284). But unlike the hospital groups, the second dimension at the lodge links leadership of the group with its performance. One of the important findings about hospital groups is that group performance in the hospital is not related to group morale and cohesiveness or to group leadership. At the lodge, the former appears to be true but not the latter. At the lodge, groups showing high performance also enjoyed a high level of leadership and contained members who were often chosen by their fellows as preferred companions in a variety of situations and who also had wide acceptance in the group. Such groups tended to have members who had spent a relatively short time in the group.

Dimension 3 appears in Table 15.5 only for the sake of completeness. The table shows fully its residual nature. It does contain the reward variable, which was an important dimension-defining variable in the hospital analysis (pp. 280–282). The reward variable as it appears in Table 15.5 should not be confused with the term as it is used in various theories of learning in the field of psychology. As in the hospital, its relationship to group performance simply reflects the consistency with which it was linked with that variable. Any effect which associated rewards might have had on the group's performance cannot be determined from this analysis. What this information does stress is that the system of rewards at the lodge through weekly wages did not correspond well to the performance of the group from week to week in its janitorial business. This fact was apparent to anyone familiar with the operation of the janitorial service: the weekly payroll was dependent on receipts from customers for the week and payment was often delayed for various reasons. Thus, money earned in one week might or might not be paid to the workers during that week, depending on the efficiency of the business manager and the outstanding bills.

The Independence of the Dimensions in the Lodge Situation

In the hospital ward analyses, the three group-process dimensions were almost completely independent of each other. The same degree of independence reappears in the analysis for the lodge data. Table 15.6 shows that the two dimensions of group process at the lodge were almost completely orthogonal (independent), and that even the residual dimension had very little relationship to the other two. It is interesting to note that the residual dimension, which contains the reward variable, is most closely associated with the group-performance dimension. The degree of association is greater than that of any two dimensions in the hospital analysis (p. 283). This fact provides a certain perspective on the combined results of both analyses, since dimension 2 from this analysis contains the variables of performance and leadership, while the residual dimension contains "reward." It seems that the main definers of dimensions 2 and 3 in the hospital analysis (p. 281) have separated and regrouped themselves into different dimensions under the social conditions of the community subsystem, but that enough communality between them remains to be reflected in the −.23 correlation between the residual dimension (containing "reward") and the group-performance dimension.

Data gathered in the hospital setting showed that there was no relationship between the morale and group cohesiveness variables and the group's performance on the ward. The same finding for the community situation reappears in Table 15.6, as shown by the low correlation of −.08 between dimensions 1 and 2. However, the independence of leadership from group performance observed in the hospital did not carry over into the lodge setting. The independence of leadership and performance for the ward situation was explained by similar findings in prior studies which showed that the relationship of mean group leadership and group performance tended to resemble an inverted U-curve (p. 283). The results from the lodge data

Table 15.6. Correlations Among the Three Dimensions for the Lodge Situation

	1	*2*	*3*
Dimension	*Group Cohesiveness*	*Group Performance*	*Residual Dimension*
1. Group cohesiveness		−.08	.05
2. Group performance	−.08		−.23
3. Residual dimension	.05	−.23	

show that in the community situation the relationship tends to be positive and linear in form. The difference seems to be a function of the differences in the two social situations. The studies mentioned earlier all took place in a hospital setting, either similar or identical to the ward situation analyzed here. The congruence of the results from the several studies completed in the hospital setting most logically must derive from similarities in the hospital social situation, contrasted with that of the lodge society in the community.

It is relatively simple to outline the major differences in the hospital and community social situations. In the hospital, the groups performed on the ward. No matter how great their efforts to become autonomous, they could only exercise limited discretion in managing their affairs. Inevitably this must have tended to discourage effective leadership and to decrease its observable effect on performance. In the hospital, the effects of poor leadership were offset to a great degree by the presence of the ward staff itself, especially when the performance of the group deteriorated badly. Thus, through bolstering patient group performance, the hospital staff would not and realistically could not permit totally autonomous leadership to emerge in patient groups, no matter how well intentioned it might have been. Furthermore, even if the staff did relinquish control, the larger social organization of the hospital was likely to fill in the breech and act in its place.

At the lodge, there was admittedly some degree of control over the men's fate exercised by the staff coordinator, particularly at the outset of the experiment (pp. 45–69). Even then, however, the coordinator did not have the pervasive dominance accorded to professional persons by hospital routine. Furthermore, his activities were directed consciously at greater and greater autonomy for the group members. For this reason, there were far greater opportunities for peer leadership to emerge within the group and, in turn, for such leadership to have an effect on group performance, particularly since the groups worked on their janitorial jobs in physical isolation from the lodge and the staff coordinator. Under these conditions of performance, the completion of the task in a satisfactory way was immediately dependent on peer leadership in the work group as the job was being completed. Any exertion of leadership by the coordinator could occur only after the job was finished by the work crew but found to be undone or done poorly. Effective peer leadership may thus have arisen to avoid re-doing jobs or to avoid other consequences which arose in such cases (pp. 64–69).

The independence of the group process dimensions in the community is similar to the finding made in the analysis of the ward data. Similarly, the orthogonal (independent) relationship between the two Jackson measures of "attraction to the group" and "acceptance by the group" (pp. 279–284), as in the hospital analysis resulted in these two variables belonging to two different dimensions, supporting Jackson's theoretical assumptions (Jackson, 1959). Replicated in the lodge analysis also was the association of the variable "cohesiveness," derived additively from the two Jackson measures, with the variable "attraction to the group"; both variables belong to the dimension of cohesiveness.

The Development of the Dimensions in the Lodge Situation

Earlier, a dilemma was mentioned concerning the arrangement of the lodge data analysis so that the dimensions would be based on large enough numbers of persons so as to be reliable (p. 293). The problem involved the combination of time periods into three blocks of time, which might not allow the detection of a developmental phase in the group processes similar to that observed in the hospital analysis (pp. 284–287). Some information about the development of group structure can be found in Table 15.7. It summarizes the "completeness" of the dimensions at each block of time, based on the proportion of the defining variables for each dimension which are present at each time block. For the purpose of this analysis, a defining variable is classified as one that appears as a cluster definer in two or more blocks of time. The table shows that the dimensions are fully formed and stable by the second block of time (450 days) and continue to be in the remaining block.

The 90 per cent "completeness" of the dimensions at the first block of time suggests that a developmental phase might be taking place during these first three time periods (180 days) in the lodge setting, but it is only suggestive. By itself, this evidence would not be a sufficient basis for claiming that such a development was actually occurring. But in view of the results from the hospital analysis which showed just such a developmental phase during the early life of the patient group, it is worth further exploration.

To find an answer, separate analyses were performed for the first three time periods at the lodge, using the small number of participants available, in order to discover if some evidence for a developmental process could be found. The number of participants for the three analyses were 12, 15, and 17 persons, respectively. As stated before (p. 293), the reader should bear in mind that the first measurement time period at the lodge covered the three months *after* the group in the community lodge subsystem had left the

Table 15.7. Relative Completeness of Dimensions at Each Block as a Per Cent of Defining Variables Present (Lodge Situation)

	Time Block		
Dimension	*I (180 days)*	*II (450 days)*	*III (720 days)*
Dimension 1	100	100	100
Dimension 2	80	100	100
Overall completeness	90	100	100

hospital. The first testing of this group had been done in the hospital and clearly could not be taken as data in the community setting to be used in an analysis of social processes at the lodge. Thus, the analysis of the first time period at the lodge encounters the members three months into living in the community as a group. This fact will be important in any comparison with the results found in the hospital analysis.

The results of the three exploratory cluster analyses are presented in Table 15.8. As in Table 15.1, the presence of highly related variables at the three different time periods are shown as X's, and those in weaker association with the cluster definers appear as X's in parenthesis.

The information in Table 15.8 indicates that there *was* a developmental phase in the group processes at the lodge similar to the stage found in the hospital analysis (pp. 284–287). The evidence for this is more easily grasped by seeing the data presented in another way. Table 15.9 shows the percentage of all the variables in each of the block dimensions in Table 15.5 that are represented in each of the clusters found in the three time period analyses. For example, cluster 1 at time period I of data collection contains three of the four variables which define the block dimension of "group cohesiveness" (p. 295): thus it is 75 per cent complete; cluster 2 at time period I shows three of five definers of the block dimension "performance and leadership," (p. 295), so that it is considered 60 percent complete, and so on. The mean percent of completeness for all clusters at each time period is presented in the third row of Table 15.9. Below these figures, for comparison, are placed the corresponding figures for completeness for 90, 180, and 270 days in the hospital analysis. In both cases, one can observe progression toward more and more complete-

Table 15.8. Variables Comprising the Clusters Found for the First Three Time Periods at the Lodge

		Time Period		
		I	*II*	*III*
Cluster	*Variable*	*(90 days)*	*(180 days)*	*(270 days)*
Cluster 1:	*Cohesiveness	X	X	X
	*Morale	X	X	X
	*Attraction to group	X	X	X
	*Satisfaction with leader		(X)	X
	Time in the group		X	(X)
Cluster 2:	*Leadership	X	X	X
	*Performance	X	X	X
	*Acceptance by the group	X	X	X
	*Sociometric choice by peers	(X)	X	X
	*Time in the Group			
	Reward		(X)	X

* Designates a defining variable from the Time Block Dimensions (Table 15.5).

Table 15.9. Relative Completeness of Clusters at Each of First Three Time Periods as Per Cent of Defining Variables Present (Lodge Situation)

	Time Period		
Cluster	*I* *(90 days)*	*II* *(180 days)*	*III* *(270 days)*
Cluster 1	75	75	100
Cluster 2	60	80	80
Mean per cent completeness at each time period in lodge situation	68	78	90
Mean per cent completeness at same time periods in hospital groups	53	67	83

ness in the dimensions of group process for the three corresponding time periods, that is, after the same length of time for group development.

This percentage comparison in Table 15.9 between the development of group processes in the hospital and community social settings suggests that the developmental phase proceeded at a more rapid pace in the lodge. It also seems true, by considering both Tables 15.7 *and* 15.9, that the dimensions at the lodge were more complete and stable after the first 90 days than were those in the hospital situation. However, these inferences are only tentative, since the small numbers on which the group process dimensions were compared in the lodge time-period analyses do not allow as much confidence that the results are as reliable as those obtained with the hospital data. Similarly, the analysis of the lodge data by blocks does not give as much detailed information about group processes at the lodge as was obtained from the time period analyses of the hospital information. Nonetheless, the possibility that group development proceeded from a socially amorphous to a more structured situation in the lodge as well as in the hospital is very plausible. Indeed, it appears to support the detailed narrative observations presented about lodge societal development in chapters 4 through 7.

The Effect of Changing Membership and Staff Coordinator Leadership

When Table 15.5 was introduced earlier in this chapter, it was indicated that the cluster analysis for the third block of time (720 days) created two separate clusters that were assigned to a more general dimension. This happened with both dimensions of group process at the lodge at this point in time and asterisked *X*'s were adopted in Table 15.5 to distinguish the variables from the two clusters. Plainly, this situation must be explained. It is true that the variables included in the two clusters did not separate enough to escape being included in the general dimensions produced by the cluster analysis, since a correlation of −.70 represents the strength of their relationship to each other. Nonetheless, it is still significant that there was enough shift in the variables comprising these two dimensions so that two clusters were created at the last block of time where there had been only one in previous blocks. Also, in the case of both dimensions, definers of the dimension are affected: in the case of the "leadership—performance" dimension, two definers are involved.[1]

A similar kind of variation in the dimensions of the hospital groups was accounted for by a concomitant change of membership as the measurement periods progressed (p. 287). A similar explanation seems reasonable for the lodge situation. Figure 15.3 shows two measures of group membership for the three blocks of time: the percentage of the block sample who are original lodge members, and the percentage of new members who arrived at the lodge during the interval between each of the time blocks. In the first two blocks of time, the percentage of original members exceeds the percentage of new ones; but by the final block, the trend lines have crossed and original members are in the minority. This phenomenon is one possible explanation for the change in the two dimensions observed in the last time block. Further, another influence which might have played a part here concerns the nature of the leadership at the lodge. All the observations providing the data for the analysis at the last time block were made during the tenure of the lay leaders at the lodge (pp. 88–100). The account in chapter 6 of the shift from professional staff to lay leaders and observations of the effects of the change described there suggest that the arrival of the lay leaders affected the group processes in a number of significant ways (pp. 88–90). Hence, this change in leadership may also have been reflected in the lodge-group members' responses on the assessment devices administered during the last time block.

The results of the analysis from the lodge-group process data can be summarized as follows:

1. Group processes at the lodge develop over a period of three to nine months from the time the group is first formed and these social processes are relatively stable thereafter. This finding is similar to that encountered with the hospital groups (p. 291).

2. The processes are defined by two major dimensions rather than by the three found in the hospital analysis. They are: (1) the group cohesiveness dimension found in the hospital groups, and (2) group leadership and group performance combined as a single dimension.

3. As with hospital groups, a change in membership appears to affect both dimensions of group processes, but it does not destroy them. Such processes might also have been affected by the change from professional to lay leaders at the lodge during the last block of time analyzed.

4. The same orthogonality (independence) of Jackson's postulated

1. In cluster analysis, a definer is either the "pivotal variable with the highest variance of squared correlation coefficients" or a variable most highly related to the pivotal variable (Tryon and Bailey, 1965, p. 58).

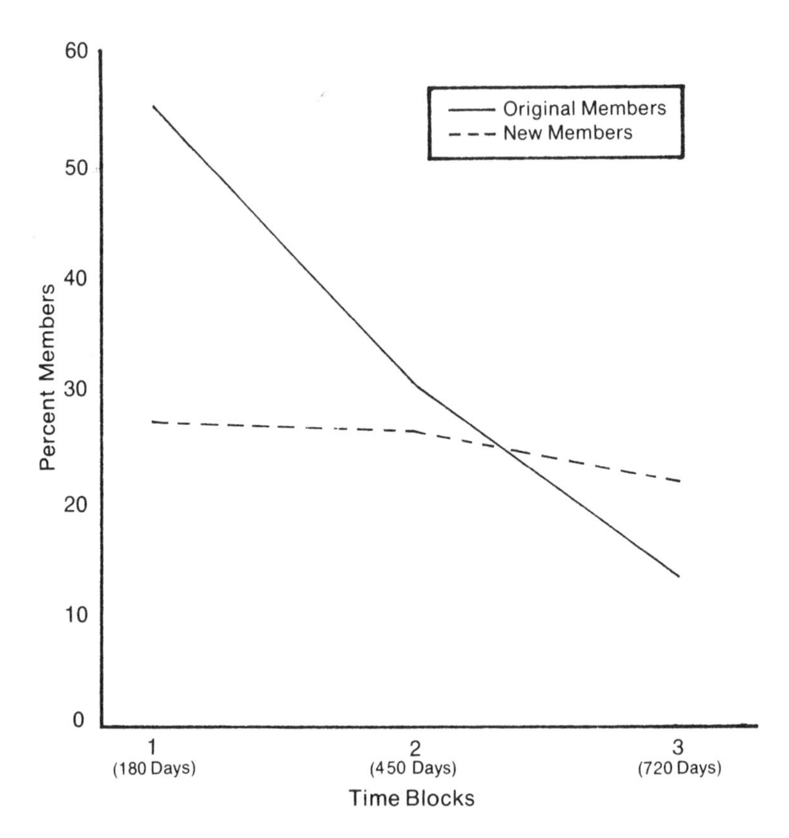

FIG. 15.3.—*Per cent of original and new lodge members at three time blocks.*

two dimensions of group cohesiveness (1959) found in the hospital groups reappears in the lodge data; again, attraction to the group was more strongly associated with a measure of group cohesiveness additively derived from both his proposed dimensions.

5. It is possible that group processes pass more rapidly through the developmental phase in the lodge setting and that the processes are more stable after formation than in the hospital environment. On these points, data of the present analysis are not conclusive and inferences drawn from them must remain as suggestive hypotheses for future experiments to explore more fully.

PART V. IMPLICATIONS FOR INNOVATIVE RESEARCH WITH THE MENTALLY ILL AND OTHER MARGINAL GROUPS

16 STAFF AND PATIENT VIEWS OF INNOVATIVE HOSPITAL AND COMMUNITY TREATMENT PROGRAMS

The federal hospital where the present study was conducted includes two divisions of about one thousand beds each, assembled under a single administrative unit. A recently built hospital division dealt mainly with admission and short-term treatment of mental patients. It also included a large general medical and surgical service. The older division, commonly referred to as the "continued treatment service," housed a population of mental patients almost entirely chronic, as that term was defined in earlier work (Maynard, 1964)—that is, hospitalized for two years or more. The experimental ward which served as the "feeder" to the experimental community lodge was located in the older division.

To measure knowledge of the experimental program by the staff and patients in the hospital, and to gauge their attitudes about the project, a series of questionnaires, and structured taped interviews were administered at the hospital throughout the study. Two questionnaires, one dealing with attitudes toward the ward program and the other with attitudes toward the community lodge, were completed by the management personnel of the hospital and the professional staffs of psychiatry, psychology, social work, and nursing at three different times: at the beginning of the lodge program; when the lodge had been operating for a year; and just before the end of the research. The same questionnaires were completed by a random sample of hospital patients at the same three times that they were administered to the hospital's staff members. Two tape-recorded interviews were completed by all staff and patients in the questionnaire sample concurrent with each of the last two questionnaires.

Taped, structured interviews were the other source of information about staff and patient attitudes. Such interviews were completed with the chief administrative personnel in the hospital, the staffs of neuropsychiatric (NP) wards, and selected patients from those same wards in both divisions of the hospital (p. 37). Some of these persons had also responded to the questionnaires. The staff members interviewed were the psychiatrist, psychologist, social worker, head nurse, secretary, and a nursing assistant on each ward. Patients interviewed on each neuropsychiatric ward were randomly selected, with the constraint that they could not be members of the experimental sample. Because of the smaller patient populations on the wards at the new division of the hospital, two patients from each of its wards were interviewed, compared to four from each ward in the older division. The interviews were presented to the interviewees as an attempt to find out how much was known to the hospital about the experimental programs on the research ward and in the community. The interview was held at a time most convenient to the interviewee. There was very little resistance to this research procedure by any of the groups interviewed, with the exception of two persons, one at each of the two divisions.

At the new division, a psychiatric resident working on one of the teaching wards used by the university medical school objected to his patients being interviewed, on the basis that his patients had been research subjects too often. He also believed that his ward staff should be informed of the details of the research before any interviewing was done on the ward. He was soon joined in these views by other residents with patients on the same ward. Although his demands were reasonable, meeting them would have made the ward atypical in comparison to others on which interviewing had been completed. Consequently, no further interviewing was conducted on that ward.

At the older division, a group of ward psychiatrists refused to be interviewed because they did not wish their comments to be tape-recorded. It was their view that they had insufficient information about the programs and consequently were concerned that they might be misquoted. This reaction originated with a protest by one of the psychiatrists at a regular staff meeting. He became quite upset when it became known to him that psychiatrists were being asked to submit themselves to tape-recorded interviews. Anxiety increased among the group, with the resulting refusals, although none refused to allow patients or other staff members on their wards to be interviewed if those persons were willing. Interestingly, the doctor who first became quite vehement about the interview procedure allowed himself to be interviewed in the first series but refused an interview in the second one.

Staff and Patient Attitudes Toward the Two Hospital Divisions

Since the research activity of this study was centered at the older division of the hospital, the attitudes toward the two divisions held by personnel throughout the hospital were of considerable interest. At the start of the project there was a functional difference between the two divisions. The newer one was the admitting division and had an affiliation with a university medical school. In fact, one of the buildings where university personnel and residents administered wards affiliated with the medical school was known throughout the hospital as "the university building." The new division also was the location of all the women's neuropsychiatric wards in the hospital, all the general medical and surgical wards, and all of the top-level administrative offices. The older division, described earlier in this chapter (pp. 305–306), was the continued treatment center for chronic psychiatric patients. This was true for most of the study, but by the last year of the project this function was somewhat modified by the direct admission of a few patients from state hospitals to the older division.

Aspects of this functional difference between the two parts of the hospital usually appeared in answers by the administrative and professional staff when requested to compare the two. Their comparative statements often contained either the implication or the outright statement that the division in which the respondent worked was the better of the two. But the general opinion was held by both groups of respondents that the old division was a "disadvantaged" part of the hospital. Not unexpectedly, this attitude was especially prevalent at the new division. For example, one of the administrative staff saw "striking contrasts . . . visible contrast in the patient group in terms of chronicity and age . . . above all there is a feeling . . . in [the old division] that they are poor relations or stepchildren . . . harder to maintain sort of an electrical excitement in a situation where you are dealing with more chronic patients and the risk is of chronicity in staff. . . . An administrator has to work very hard to make sure that the staff does not develop a chronic orientation. . . ."

There was also concern on the part of some ward staff members at the new division that "many patients perceive [the old division] as being negative, as having connotations of being bad. . . ." As one social worker at the new division said:

> A lot of our patients, when they are told they are going to be transferred feel that they're being rejected, are being sent to a bad place where maybe they are going to get beaten up or ignored, and [where] there are a lot of old, not-very-well-cared-for men. . . . Part of this is a feeling of rejection, as very often [we] do send people to [the old division] when we get disgusted with them, and many of the staff look on [it] as a place to send patients to get rid of them—or to punish them, . . . and this feeling is conveyed to the patients.

Personnel at the old division usually shared this view. While they generally saw their work environment as preferable to the other part of the hospital because of its friendlier, more relaxed, and pleasant atmosphere, many of them resented what they felt was its "stepchild position." They disliked the old division's image as a place to which patients came as punishment, or as a depository for all of the "patients they don't want" in the rest of the hospital, meaning by this the newer division.

Despite the generally negative attitudes toward the old division, the experimental programs located there were usually held in high regard; indeed, they served to improve the image of the division by their presence. An example of this appears in the views of the administrator already quoted (p. 307). He commented: "If it had not been for [the research] program, which has been the only breath of professional adventure and innovation over there . . . it would be even more of a sleepy hollow . . . if it hadn't been for this program which generates excitement and results." Much of the professional staff felt the same way. One psychologist working in the new division summed it up as follows:

> I feel that the [experimental] program is very exciting and [I] send a lot of patients over there. . . . [I] regret there is a considerable prejudice against [the old division] in this hospital among patients and staff members alike. Very often patients are threatened with [going there], and in many cases it does seem to be . . . the end of the line. . . . Certain parts of [the old division] are acting as a domiciliary at the present time and we send patients from this ward when we feel that there is not much [more] that we can do for them. . . . The [experimental ward] program is an exception and we see this as a forward step for the men we send over. . . . [I] feel this offers them something that we can't offer them over here. Staff-wise and in many ways, I feel that [the old division] has been getting the short end of the stick for a long, long time. . . . Many of the psychiatric staff are not on the same level of competence as over here. . . . I feel that morale among staff is lower than it is here . . . with [the] exception of [the experimental ward].

In contrast, some professionals preferred the old division. One psychologist working at the old division who had spent an equal amount of time in both locations said:

> I find things quite different over here . . . in spite . . . of a smaller staff, things are more relaxed and the staff is in general much more enthusiastic over here. . . . More freedom to develop conceptually unified and consistent programs over here. . . . Over there we spent an infinite amount of time in meetings because of having to communicate with so many people and so many different points of view. At [the old division things are] more oriented toward improving the patient's behavior and toward getting them out of the hospital equipped to get along in some fashion with some support outside the hospital . . . rather than trying to make him well in some idealistic sense of the word that bears little relationship to what a usual,

chronic schizophrenic, nonmiddle-class person needs to get along in his limited borderline world outside.

One could summarize the attitudes of the administrative and professional staff in the following way. They perceived the two divisions as functionally different: Those at the new division saw it as the active, progressive teaching unit which sent recalcitrant or hopeless patients to the old division's chronic wards; they usually exempted the experimental programs from such an assessment of the old division, holding them in high esteem. Those at the old division shared these views with minor reservations, but believed that they worked in a friendlier, more cooperative and more relaxed atmosphere. The general attitudes of these personnel toward the two parts of the hospital remained fairly constant during the entire study. But there was a slight shift in the last few months in the new division staff's image of the old one, particularly by members of the ward staffs. Several of them mentioned that they were impressed by what they had heard of the active experimental treatment programs at the older division. Some thought the morale was better there, since the staffs were more interested and involved in their programs. One physician even mentioned the development of a "step-child feeling" within the new division, based on the feeling he perceived on the regular psychiatric wards that the university wards there were getting the "best" patients.

The views of the two divisions prevalent among the nonprofessional staff of the hospital were generally the same as those described for the administrative and professional personnel. However, some details of the nonprofessional staff's attitudes were different and interesting enough to deserve comment. At the time of the first series of interviews, the ward secretaries' attitudes toward the two divisions were more or less predictable. At each division, they either could make no comparison, believed there was no real difference between the two, or preferred the division at which they were working. New division secretaries preferred their work setting because of its faster pace, and commented they had heard that the old division was "depressing" and "patients were hesitant about going [there] because [it was the] end of the road." Secretaries at the old division preferred its warmer, friendlier, more relaxed atmosphere.

But by the time of the second series of interviews, the new division's secretaries responded quite differently. Fifty per cent of those interviewed said that they did not like working there or would prefer the older division. One summed up her feelings by saying that "the new division's atmosphere is terrible . . . no politeness or kindness." Others said that at the new division there was a "lack of communication;" that the old division was "closer knit," "warmer, less impersonal." Specific reasons for the prevalence of this bitter attitude at this particular time remain unknown. The secretaries denied any recent occurrence which might account for this attitude. At this time there was no such dramatic change in the attitudes of the old division's secretaries, although one did complain that the new division was, in her opinion, better staffed.

Nursing aides (nursing assistants) at the new division frequently saw no great difference between working in the two sections of the hospital. Some had heard that it was better to work at the old division, but that patients did not like to be transferred there. In the first interview series, one aide said that he hears that "[the old division] is the fear park . . . punishment to go there . . . but I also hear good things about the programs." Those who definitely preferred the new division felt that it was more of a hospital and had heard that the other division was old, dirty, and "a back ward." A few would have preferred being at the old division, as they thought it was less "chaotic" and there was not as much supervision over their work.

The majority of the old division aides definitely preferred their work setting because of the more relaxed, friendlier atmosphere, and because they felt the aides were treated better by other staff members and had more responsibility. A small percentage would have preferred to be at the new division because it was "more of a hospital." One such aide remarked that "[the old division] is just a retirement place."

Patients' responses to a request for comparison on the two divisions divided into three general categories. They either saw one division or the other as better or they thought there was no essential difference between the two. At both divisons, there were patients who said they neither knew nor had heard about the other division and hence did not volunteer comparison. At the time of the first interview series, none of the new-division patients expressed a preference for the other division. Eighteen per cent of those interviewed not only preferred their location but felt that the older division was "bad," "a snake pit," "the end of the line," and were frightened at the possibility of a transfer to it. In the second interview series, some of the new-division patients expressed negative attitudes toward the older division, claiming that it was "more restrictive" or "depressing" and that "the worst patients are sent there." At this point, such a feeling did not appear to be as extreme as previously; one patient at the new division actually expressed a preference for the older one. Negative attitudes toward the older division also stemmed from some patients who had been transferred there from the newer part of the hospital. While some in this group preferred the new division because it was "newer," "more modern," and "more active," one stated that he preferred it because they have "more success with patients . . . but I failed there." Another said that he had been "transferred here for disciplinary reasons" and that in his former ward he had been "recognized as a person . . . everything [is] better there." This belief about having been transferred for reasons of failure or discipline seemed less prevalent in later interviews; if expressed, it seemed to have less importance to the patient making the response.

Staff and Patient Knowledge about the Experimental Programs

During the collection of the attitude questionnaires, there were occasional complaints from some of the hospital staff who resisted completing forms concerning "programs we know nothing about." Despite this, Table 16.1 shows that fully 84 per cent of the management and ward staffs who were interviewed at the time of the first interview series admitted to some knowledge of the ward program, while 89 per cent had knowledge of the lodge. This was at a time about midway in the lodge study. By the time of the second interview series, 81 per cent of this group had some knowledge of the ward program and 98 per cent knew of the lodge. Overall, there was a decrease in the knowledge of the ward program in the hospital among administrative and professional staff. However, Table 16.1 shows that this decrease in knowledge was due entirely to the staff at the newer division of the hospital; at the older division the knowledge of both programs, already very high at the first interview, increased even more by the second, with a knowledge of the lodge reaching 100 per cent. The explanation for this phenomenon resided in the fact that the actual location of the experimental unit was at the old division, but this result also highlights another factor affecting the results, namely, the relatively separate working lives which the staffs led at the two divisions. At a time when fully 93 per cent of the professional and administrative people at the old division knew of the experimental ward, the knowledge of the same program at the new division had dropped to 72 per cent.

Among the nonprofessional staff, only 21 per cent of the ward secretaries interviewed had any knowledge of the ward program at the first interview, while 43 per cent knew of the lodge; in the second series of interviews, the comparable figures were 27 per cent for the ward and 55 per cent for the lodge. Table 16.2 shows that here, too, this type of staff person at the old division was more aware of the experimental programs than the same kind of staff at the new division. It also shows that the lodge program was better known. Midway in the study at the time of the first interview series, only one secretary had made an actual contact with the janitorial service. She had called them about a job but had not gone any further, since they would

Table 16.1. Percentage of Administrative and Professional Staff Having Knowledge of the Experimental Programs at First and Second Interviews

	Knowledge of Ward Program		*Knowledge of Lodge Program*	
Hospital Division	*1st interview*	*2nd interview*	*1st interview*	*2nd interview*
New division	82	72	86	97
Old division	89	93	93.5	100
Both divisions	84	81	89	98

Table 16.2. Percentage of Ward Secretaries Having Knowledge of the Experimental Programs at the First and Second Interviews

Hospital Division	*Knowledge of Ward Program*		*Knowledge of Lodge Program*	
	1st interview	*2nd interview*	*1st interview*	*2nd interview*
New division	14	10	29	40
Old division	33	50	66	75
Both divisions	21	27	43	55

not give her an hourly rate and she could not be home during the day for an estimate. At the time of the second interview series, one of the secretaries knew two people who had used the service and had been very satisfied with it; another had actually used and been satisfied with it herself. During the second series of interviews, some uncertainty showed itself among the secretaries with respect to their knowledge of the ward program, since they confused it with another program, recently put into operation, which included small patient groups and a token reward system. In spite of this, there was a gain in knowledge of the research programs overall. The increase in information was greatest at the old division; only one secretary there had no knowledge of either program at the second interview. In part, of course, this was an effect of the first series of interviews, but there also seemed to be somewhat more contact established with the project in other ways.

One secretary learned of the lodge project in an interesting way. Her husband had met a lodge member at a bar and had agreed to drive him to his home which was about 40 miles away. Before doing so, he accompanied the lodge member to the motel, expecting that it would be like any other motel. He realized that it was "peculiar" because of the way the other lodge residents were acting. Although he was becoming frightened, not understanding the living situation, he still drove the lodge member home, as he felt he could not do otherwise. Upon his return home, he told his wife of his terrifying experience, and this impelled her to ask some of the hospital staff if they knew anything about this group. In this way she learned about the program.

As expected, more of the nursing aides interviewed at the old division knew about the experimental programs than those at the newer division, but the degree of knowledge was surprising. At the first interview series, 100 per cent of the aides at the old division knew of both programs and at the second interview series, the figure lowered to 93 per cent. At both times there was not one aide at the old division who had not heard of at least one of the programs. Table 16.3 gives information on the overall degree of knowledge of the programs among the aides at the hospital at both interviewing times.

Table 16.3. Percentage of Nursing Aides Having Knowledge of the Experimental Programs at the First and Second Interviews

	Knowledge of Ward Program		*Knowledge of Lodge Program*	
Hospital Division	*1st interview*	*2nd interview*	*1st interview*	*2nd interview*
New division	29	27	36	64
Old division	100	93	100	93
Both divisions	62	64	66	80

Table 16.4 describes the knowledge about the experimental programs held by patients in the hospital. The familiar pattern of a higher level of awareness of the experimental programs in the old hospital division, and an increase in knowledge of both programs over time emerges in the group as a whole. At the new division, patients gave as their sources of information either staff or other patients and, in the second series of interviews, several mentioned former lodge members as their informants. Some patients mentioned that there had been discussions in their ward community meetings about these two programs. One of the women patients mentioned that, although her ward was aware that the lodge program was not available to female patients, in one of their community meetings they had discussed the desirability of such a program for women.

There are several possible reasons for the increase in patient information at the old division. During the two-year period between interviews, there were quite a few patients who had gone through the ward program, increasing such sources of information for this division. A number of wards had incorporated certain aspects of the experimental *ward* program into their own routines, so that this had led to more widespread knowledge of the older experimental program in the old division. By far the largest number of older division patients had heard of the ward program from other patients, frequently in negative terms. The typical comment was: "Fellows don't like it." If patients elaborated this comment, they stressed that the ward program was "too strict" and that the "whole group suffers for what one [per-

Table 16.4. Percentage of Patients Having Knowledge of the Experimental Programs at the First and Second Interviews

	Knowledge of Ward Program		*Knowledge of Lodge Program*	
Hospital Division	*1st interview*	*2nd interview*	*1st interview*	*2nd interview*
New division	14	29	7	19
Old division	37.5	66	12.5	11
Both divisions	29	55	11	13

son] did." Positive statements by patients were phrased generally in terms of the ward and lodge being "rehabilitative" and that the ward was "good for motivating the patients . . . [it] keeps them on their toes."

Staff and Patient Attitudes Toward the Experimental Programs

Results from the questionnaires showed that there was a significant difference between staff and patient attitudes toward the ward program ($\chi^2 = 6.40$, 1 df, $p < .01$). Patients held more positive attitudes toward the program than did the staff. There was no similarly significant difference between patients and staff with respect to the lodge program. A glance at the mean values presented in the last column of the bottom two sections of Table 16.5 shows this effect very clearly. Furthermore, no significant differences in attitudes toward the ward obtained among the five staff groups—psychiatrist, psychologist, social worker, nurse, and administrator. But significant differences did occur with respect to the lodge program ($\chi^2_r = 9.87$, 4 df, $p < .05$). Psychologists and social workers held more positive attitudes toward the lodge, followed by those of psychiatrists, administrators, and finally, nurses.

Examining Table 16.5 in detail, it is evident that the most positive attitudes toward the ward program were held by two of the three patient groups in the research sample at the time they were leaving the ward and the hospital ("terminal" column). Since the attitude scales were given when the patients were leaving the ward, it seems apparent that these groups felt the ward program had been beneficial to them. As one might expect, the lodge group was most positive toward the lodge program on the eve of their departure for the community, while the attitudes of the volunteer nonlodge group toward the community project were somewhat more negative, possibly because they could not go to the lodge. The most negative patient group was the nonvolunteeer patient group which had refused to go to the lodge. They apparently did not see the community subsystem as desirable or helpful for them (pp. 245–248). The nursing, psychiatric, and administrative staffs were somewhat neutral toward both programs. Generally speaking, these groups are primarily concerned with in-hospital treatment and the maintenance of institutional processes. It is perhaps no wonder that they were more positive toward the community program which was not likely to be too threatening to their hospital roles.

The most startling reversal of attitude toward the two programs occurred among psychologists and social workers. Table 16.5 shows that their attitudes were the most negative toward the ward program but were among the most positive toward the experimental community lodge. From informal contacts during the experiment, it seemed clear that these two groups had more knowledge of the research project than other professional groups and also showed the most sustained interest in both programs. The most likely

Table 16.5. Mean Scores on Attitude Questionnaires at Three Testings for all Patient and Staff Groups

Program and Personnel	Testing Time			
	Initial	*Intermediate*	*Terminal*	*Mean*
WARD PROGRAM				
Staff Attitudes				
Administrator	28.76	25.64	27.62	27.34
Psychiatrist	26.66	27.70	28.91	27.76
Psychologist	25.29	25.08	24.55	24.97
Social Worker	25.00	26.40	25.31	25.57
Nurse	26.35	27.18	26.67	26.73
Staff Mean				26.45
Patient Attitudes				
Nonvolunteer	26.96	29.62	30.51	29.03
Volunteer/Nonlodge	28.50	34.14	31.57	31.40
Volunteer/Lodge	30.09	32.70	32.76	31.85
Patient Mean				30.76
LODGE PROGRAM				
Staff Attitudes				
Administrator	31.79	30.76	32.94	31.83
Psychiatrist	32.50	32.56	32.83	32.63
Psychologist	34.39	33.71	35.19	34.43
Social Worker	33.75	34.38	33.00	33.71
Nurse	32.12	30.88	32.11	31.70
Staff Mean				32.86
Patient Attitudes				
Nonvolunteer	31.38	31.28	30.59	31.08
Volunteer/Nonlodge	31.27	35.40	33.25	33.31
Volunteer/Lodge	33.24	34.40	35.44	34.36
Patient Mean				32.92

explanation for this reversal of attitudes is that it may have resulted from the artifact of distributing the ward and lodge questionnaires at the same time. This procedure may have elicited a comparison of the two programs instead of an independent evaluation of each. If this were true, then such a reversal of rankings might become understandable. For the psychologists, the effectiveness of the ward had already been demonstrated by prior research (Fairweather, 1964) and the emphasis of the present experiment was upon the lodge. For the social workers, since one of their primary functions at the hospital was discharge planning, they were especially aware of the problems of chronic mental patients in returning to community living, and may have recognized the need for supportive living and working situations in the community. Hence, both groups might have concluded that the lodge provided a highly desirable, much-needed, community resource. If either of these groups were forced to choose one program over the other in a direct comparison such as may have been provoked by the questionnaire distribution, the lodge program would be the victor.

Since attitudes toward the lodge were elicited in terms of respondent expectancies about the lodge's success, it is important to note that the patient groups clearly had more positive attitudes than the staff. These results have an interesting parallel in prior work done by MacDonald, Sanders, and Fairweather (1962). In that study, predictions of the posthospital adjustment of mental hospital patients by staff and patient groups were analyzed and compared with follow-up measures of the actual adjustment of each patient for whom a prediction was made. Although no group emerged as a successful predictor of such posthospital adjustment, it was clear that staff members were the most pessimistic in their expectancies for discharged patients, while peer members of patient task groups to whom each of the patients belonged were the most optimistic. Optimism of other patients who were not members of the task group but were measured fell between these two extreme positions. The present results seem, therefore, to reflect the same staff "pessimism" and peer-group "optimism" observed in this prior investigation.

Most of the administrative and professional staff felt that the experimental programs had had no effect on their work at the hospital. At both the first and second interviews, 65 per cent of this group took this view of the ward program. At the first interview, 79 per cent of the same group had a similar opinion of the lodge experiment, but by the second interview the percentage had dropped to 71 per cent. Apparently, in spite of the more generalized positive change in attitude over time toward the lodge program by many staff members, most of these in-hospital professionals felt that the lodge program had less effect on their work than did a hospital ward program.

It is interesting to note that those who felt that neither of the programs had affected their work *adversely* were either administrators who were in a position to receive patient or community complaints, or those who were concerned about getting patient help assigned to their hospital departments. One such person revealed that he generally heard about the ward "from those who do not like it; relatives and patients . . . who don't like it come to see me." The hospital librarian complained that she had "had a patient assigned to work here whose psychologist insisted that he be transferred to the experimental ward and, we know, he was miserably unhappy there and was soon transferred off the ward . . . now we have no patient help." The dietician complained that "when we try to get patient assignments . . . they say they don't have patients to assign to the dietetic service." She felt this was because the best patient workers were in the experimental ward program, and therefore had been given group-work assignments.

Those who felt their work had been changed in some positive way by these two programs fell into two general groups: Those who saw the ward and lodge as useful potential referral resources; and those who felt that they were exciting, stimulating programs which had affected their thinking and their approach to their own treatment programs. One ward psychologist saw the effect of the lodge "in terms of us being more aware of certain criteria . . . that chronic patients are rehabilitatable under certain circumstances . . . gave us a good grounding as a means of approaching our own project . . . in general just sobered us."

There were rather neutral attitudes expressed toward the lodge by some hospital physicians, and some negative reactions from a group of physicians at the old division. But there were also exceptions. One of the physicians at the new division remarked that the lodge was, "one of the really significant programs in rehabilitation that's going on. I feel that the social system developed there is going to be able to maintain these men . . . I feel that most of the men we have . . . at [the old division], in the right sort of situation, . . . can become productive, and this has a great degree of rehabilitative effect." The psychiatrist in charge of the university research and teaching unit at the hospital saw the main effect of the lodge to be on his thinking: "In regard to programs we might be trying out here . . . [the experimental lodge] work had been very inspiring and stimulating in thinking about programs . . . to establish an industry program . . . to continue the same group outside . . . [and] very influential in some of our research thinking."

Social workers at the hospital seemed especially to consider the lodge study of value to the hospital. At the time of the second interview series, the end of the research phase at the lodge was approaching and there were already rumors about the lodge's closing among all the professional staff. One psychiatrist expressed wonder at "discontinuing such a successful enterprise"; but the social workers seemed especially distressed. One remarked that he had "recently heard that the life of the lodge was in jeopardy. This came with a feeling of much disappointment and despair, since I see the lodge as a step forward." Another said, "I heard that the whole thing is in doubt now that the grant has run out and there is some question about whether it will just die off. . . . [I] would hate very much to see that happen."

Table 16.6 presents a summary of the attitudes toward both the ward and community experimental programs that was expressed in the interviews by all the hospital staff. It provides this information for both the old and

Table 16.6. Percentage of Administrative and Professional Staff at the Hospital Positively Evaluating the Two Experimental Programs at the First and Second Interviews

	Positive Evaluation Ward Program		*Positive Evaluation Lodge Program*	
Hospital Division	*1st interview*	*2nd interview*	*1st interview*	*2nd interview*
New division	23	20	20	21
Old division	31	30	18	28
Both divisions	26	24	19	24

new divisions separately and for them combined. The most revealing aspect of the table is the small percentage of positive responses elicited from administrative and professional hospital personnel. Whereas 81 per cent of the administrative and professional staff had knowledge of the small-group ward program at the end of the second interview (Table 16.1), only 24 per cent positively evaluated it (Table 16.6).[1] Similarly, 98 per cent of this staff had a knowledge of the community lodge program by the time of the second interview (Table 16.1) and, again, only 24 per cent evaluated the program positively (Table 16.6). Thus, with both the hospital small-group and community-lodge innovative programs about which most of the professional staff had some knowledge, only about 18–31 per cent viewed these new programs positively. This information suggests that awareness of innovative research activity within an institution by no means generates positive support among its administrative and professional personnel.

Hospital Staff Contacts with the Lodge

Only four of the staff people interviewed in the first interview series had used the lodge's janitorial service.[2] Of these, three were very satisfied; one had found the job adequate and was willing to try them again. One social worker who had been very satisfied described her reactions as follows: "Only one I saw was the guy who came to do the estimate. . . . He sure looked like a mental patient. . . . He did a good job . . . price quite reasonable. . . . I really was amused because they rearranged the furniture and we always used to joke about how the patients would fix up the day room like a bus station so none of them would have to look at each other—they fixed my living room like that." Several others in the first interview series mentioned that they had heard from people who had used the service and been satisfied. One psychologist said that he had heard mixed reports on the janitorial service, that while some people were very satisfied, others said that they would not use the service again. These were all employees of the hospital who had been hesitant about voicing their complaints directly to the lodge supervisor at the time their grievances occurred.

Five of the people interviewed at the second series had used the janitorial service. Three were very satisfied, although one of them said he was now displeased because his home could no longer be serviced, since it was considered outside the area where the members would undertake work. One said that he had used the service twice, that neither time had it worked out too well but that he would be willing to have them again. Another, a social worker, described her contacts with them as follows:

1. The average per cent of agreement reached by two raters was 92 per cent by classifying interview responses as positive, negative, or neutral.

2. For lodge members' attitudes about hospital personnel as mental health workers, see pages 150–152.

> I started using them on a weekly basis and at that point they apparently had a psychologist . . . he would come in and check their work and if I ever did have a complaint, which was rare, I would talk with him. Their work was satisfactory—it wasn't the greatest, but was satisfactory. . . . [Then] they brought in an outside nonprofessional man to oversee the work and the work deteriorated greatly . . . and finally about three months ago, I fired them. . . . I think the project is a great thing, but from a personal viewpoint, I didn't think the janitorial service was too good. . . . The gentleman . . . who was managing them kept boasting to me that he was treating them more like human beings and they were making more money, but, it seems to me they were doing poorer work. He wouldn't check their work, because he felt it might offend them and wouldn't ask them to do corners because they might have to get down on their knees . . . so I was very disappointed in them. But, professionally, I think that the whole idea is very good that a group of fairly chronic patients can maintain themselves independently.

Several mentioned during their second interviews that they had heard reports on the janitorial service from various sources. One said that he had "heard mixed reports from the nonprofessional community about the janitorial service . . . [from] two neighbors who use them, one of whom said it was kind of adequate. . . . Someone came back in response to a complaint and made good on the contract. [I] heard of another neighbor who was disappointed and said she wouldn't have them back." One nurse knew two people who had used the service. "They thought it was amazing how so many people could stand around. . . . They seem to get things done, but it took them so long to do it. . . . [They] advised that if anyone had them to be sure to get out of the house, because if you didn't, it would drive you crazy." Both of these people had been quite satisfied with the end product.

The following report by one of the hospital social workers demonstrates both her own mixed feelings about the lodge as a resource and the reactions of some mental health people "who did not get out of the house":

> [I] heard some very good things and some things that weren't very complimentary. . . . I heard from people who had used the service in the past and were very satisfied and then one person who used it again and was not. . . . I had a friend who used it and was very dissatisfied in the last four or five months. . . . Her general complaint was that the group took on something it couldn't do and that the person who seemed to be supervising them was scattered and had little understanding of what he was doing. . . . I don't know whether he was an ex-patient or a full-time employee. I got the impression he was a full-time employee. . . . This was a person who, I felt, would have a great deal of understanding and be reasonably tolerant in that she had supervised a mental health clinic herself. . . . She called them in to do some house cleaning and garden work and I think they finally ended up just leaving the job. She had to get someone else to do it. . . . I hear a good deal about it from patients who come back

> from the lodge. . . . We frequently got patients who were rejects from the lodge. . . . Of course, you get a little of it colored through a person's illness, too, but some had a little sense of exploitation and some a sense of disappointment.

Staff contacts with the lodge's janitorial service were thus few and far between. Opinions of hospital staff members seemed to be focused mainly on the business aspect of the program, and were liberally mixed with rumored satisfaction and dissatisfaction with the service. In general, it may be said that lodge members functioned in the community substantially outside the purview of staff members at the hospital from which they departed for the lodge. Such a situation, reflecting general lack of involvement by members of a social institution in the activities which may lead to its improvement and change, suggests the need for more active participation in innovative programs by those persons within the institution, some of whom have the authority to change its practices and most of whom have the responsibility to implement them.

17 OPERATING PRINCIPLES FOR COMMUNITY TREATMENT SUBSYSTEMS

This study was carried out as a direct result of preceding studies which showed a high recidivism rate among hospital patients who had been institutionalized for considerable periods of time (Fairweather, 1964). It was designed to test several hypotheses mainly concerned with the effects that a living and working situation established in the community might have upon reducing this high recidivism rate and enhancing the chronic mental patients' social status. A working-living social subsystem was established which linked the hospital to a dormitory located in the community. Here the individuals lived and operated a business.

By establishing such a dual-purpose residence in the community, return to or remaining in the hospital were both drastically reduced and employment greatly improved. But a reduction in recidivism and increased employment were not the only benefits. Such constructive living was accompanied by strong feelings of pride that the members had about the organization, themselves, and their accomplishments. And these accomplishments were attained with little professional support and at a minimum cost to the public when contrasted with the cost of mental hospital care. More important, perhaps, the new working-living subsystem was integrated into society without encountering difficulties with other members of society. Most members of society accepted the ex-patients and respected them as responsible citizens. But perhaps the most important result of this study was that the newly created participating social statuses for the ex-patients generated an identification with the usual goals of the society by a group of its members who previously had been generally isolated from it and who in the past had little regard for it. This study created a living system which largely negated the social marginality which was such a characteristic feature of the background of most of the lodge members. In addition to recognizing these concrete benefits, it is also important to place these results in a broader prospective, especially since this experiment has shown that new social statuses *can* be created for the mentally ill and that such persons *can* live durably in the community. The question naturally arises: What principles of organization can be abstracted from the experience of operating this new social subsystem that may help future workers with this or other marginal social groups? Certain features undoubtedly created this successful outcome. These features may be viewed as operating principles for social subsystems that can be established to provide a more responsible and rewarding social position for chronic mental patients.

The *first principle* that is of primary importance in creating such a new status concerns the degree of ego-involvement that the participants must develop in order to make the subsystem work. The experimental evidence clearly suggests that ego-involvement is directly related to *the "stake" that the participants have in the social subsystem.* The tasks performed by the members must be meaningful to them. Throughout the course of the experiment presented here the lodge members typically thought their work was important and they became increasingly proud of their organization. They wanted the organization to succeed. The members often remarked that the janitorial and gardening service was *their* business. The feeling of identification with the success of the organization was enhanced by their ownership of the business. Such ownership is important when placed in the perspective of contemporary American culture. In America, great value is placed upon the ownership of property. Individuals who have *not* achieved a rewarding social status in this culture—such as the chronic mental patients described here—tend to attach great importance to the ownership of property. Thus, an organization which they manage and control leads to perceptions of personal success in terms of social values that are an accepted part of the culture. When such perceptions occur, the feelings of personal accomplishment are often positive and intense.

Within the context of the social organization, each individual should develop a personal sense of his own worth. This enhances identification with the organization and its goals. Such a sense of personal worth was exemplified in the perception of those marginal workers who believed they were indispensible to the lodge organization, even though they did not contribute nearly as much to the total work effort as the workers or crew chiefs. Nonetheless, their positive perception of their own contribution and their belief that the organization needed their services resulted in identification with the organization and its goals. They often openly declared their pride in the lodge, and some even bragged about its accomplishments. They told others of their very important role in the organization. Even though the work of these marginal members often was inferior to that of others, the fact that they were permitted to remain in the organization in full participating statuses brought about a personal commitment to it. These marginal members often chose not to participate totally in work or decision-making, but the fact that they could, if they chose to do so, contributed to their feelings of acceptance.

A *second principle* derived from the research results is that *any subsystem must give as much autonomy to its members as is possible, consistent with their behavioral performance.* While autonomy of action contributes to each member's "stake" in the organization, it is such an important aspect of the conduct of social subsystems that it is treated here as a separate and independent principle. When the participants in any developing social organization are not initially capable of assuming full autonomy, organizational procedures must be structured by someone else who does not "belong." The leadership roles of such "outsiders," however, should be relinquished as quickly as possible. The degree of autonomy that members of a social organization can assume must be based upon empirical testing of their capacities for responsibility, rather than arbitrary guesswork. This is especially important with members of the mental health professions who often perceive the chronic mental patient as being far less capable than he actually is (p. 151). Only when real-life trials indicate that the members of such a subsystem are incapable of performing responsibly should the professional staff assume responsibility for them. When they do, repeated trials aimed at more complete autonomy for the members should be immediately instituted and continuously maintained.

Thus, in accordance with this principle, control over lodge affairs was gradually given to the members. By the end of the study the group had become completely autonomous. Such a procedure stands in direct contrast with the social status usually ascribed to participants in "total institutions" such as hospitals, prisons, rehabilitative camps, and the like (Goffman, 1962). The members living in these societies typically are not allowed to assume a completely responsible role because the statuses of the professional staff are usually defined as the superordinate ones and those of the inmates as the subordinate ones. In such lowly social positions members cannot assume responsibilities that are delegated to others in superior statuses through institutional practice. Despite this, once such a person is discharged from a total institution, irrespective of the time he has spent in such an assigned subordinate status, he is typically expected by society to assume full citizenship responsibilities immediately upon his return to the community. Redelegation of citizenship responsibilities gradually and by continuous trial is one way to find the maximum possible level of responsibility for each such person participating in a social subsystem. Such trials can ascertain the level of autonomy that is possible for each individual, without inviting the personal failure which has always been observed to have such a disastrous psychological and social impact upon former inmates of such total institutions.

There are several practical ways in which staff authority can gradually be transferred to subordinate members. Jurisdiction over disciplinary problems among peers can be turned over to a committee of the membership. Such matters as who should hold particular statuses within the organization, such as crew chief and worker statuses in the lodge, can be determined by the membership. They can also be charged with the responsibility for handling the financial affairs of the organization and altering organizational procedures when necessary to meet the changing needs of its members. The administration of rewards and punishments should be put in the hands of the members as quickly as possible. Autonomy can also be achieved by placing operations that are essential to the daily functioning of the subsystem, such as bookkeeping, the dispensing of medication, and the purchase of food in the case of the lodge, under the direct control of the membership.

Not all these responsibilities can or need to be delegated at once. They can and probably should be delegated gradually, so that the assumption of a second set of responsibilities is contingent upon adequate performance in carrying out the first, the third upon adequate performance of the second, and so on. Such a step-wise system of progressive and graded responsibility was a feature of the hospital ward from which the lodge members came (Fairweather, 1964). However, it should not be overlooked that the delegation of *all* responsibilities should be the ultimate goal of the staff. This should be completed as quickly as possible because autonomy increases the "stake" that each member has in the social organization of which he is a member. The foresighted professional staff will not hesitate to turn over to the members of any such social organization those activities which its members are capable of assuming when determined by actual trial. Such a method of determination gives confidence in the members' capabilities to the staff as well as to the members. At the same time, the responsible staff must itself be willing to assume responsibility in those areas where the members demonstrate an incapacity to do so, and without using failures at such independent attempts as an excuse to perpetuate the members' subordinate status.

The subsystem should have a vertical organization so that both a division of labor is possible and a meaningful role can be found for all members. This *third principle* was exemplified in the vertical social organization of the lodge, which permitted upward mobility *within* the lodge society. Those members who were motivated and capable of assuming higher social statuses did so and, at the same time, a meaningful social position was established for those members who were not capable or did not aspire to higher social positions within the organization. Thus, it was possible for each member to find a social position commensurate with his abilities and interests. Any particular social status, however, was not permanent and changes continuously occurred in the social position of lodge members—workers became crew chiefs and crew chiefs became workers.

Different types of work for the participants should be provided within the subsystem. The greater the diversity of tasks involved, the more likely it is that work which has meaning for every member can be found. In the lodge, the diversity of tasks was pronounced. Jobs for the kitchen crew included cooks, helpers, and the administrator of the kitchen; janitorial crews had crew chiefs, workers, and marginal workers; gardening crews had the same three work statuses; other jobs such as bookkeeper and truck driver provided so much diversity of employment that every member of the lodge society found a job that was acceptable to him.

A social subsystem with vertical mobility also provides a social organization whose different statuses can be ranked in order of their degree of responsibility. The highest statuses can be given the highest rewards, so that motivation toward more responsible social positions can be maintained. Each member can thus aspire to the highest status of which he is capable and can be rewarded accordingly. It is also important to note here that when higher rewards are linked with higher statuses, it is much easier for the participants within the subsystem to deal with the jealousies and rivalries that inevitably occur. Because the rewards are attached to the status, the individual occupying a given status receives the rewards commensurate with it, irrespective of who he might be.

Any created social subsystem must be compatible with the environment in which it is implanted. Its internal social organization and its physical location must be compatible with the broader society, according to this *fourth principle.* The entire social organization of any potentially successful new social subsystem must be as close a facsimile of the broader society as it is possible to make it, consistent with the capabilities of its participants. This is necessary because some individuals who participate in such organizations will leave and reenter the larger society. For this reason, life in the subsystem must stress those behaviors that will permit any resident of the subsystem to make this transition without undue stress. The more identical the subsystem is to the society, the easier such transitions become.

For example, vertical organization and division of labor just mentioned are modeled upon the larger society. A meaningful system of rewards and real-life tasks were also attributes of the lodge society that were compatible with the larger society. The type of work done by members of such a subsociety should be work for which society has a need. In such cases, those behaviors learned while the person is a participant in the subsystem can be directly transferred to other community situations. It is, therefore, important that the social organization of the created subsystem represent statuses and role behaviors that exist and are accepted in the society at large.

Social subsystems established to give new social statuses and roles to the mentally ill will typically not be completely identical with those in the society. Certain behaviors that are acceptable within such model societies may not be compatible with the behavioral norms of the larger society. As an example, the establishment of the lodge executive committee which dealt with violations of norms internal to the subsystem was the means by which the behavior of its members was regulated so that the larger society would not reject it. Few homes or organizations in the larger community have such specifically organized regulatory social processes. From this example, however, it may be inferred that social processes solely internal to a social subsystem do not have to be compatible with the greater social environment, but social processes that cross the boundaries into the community must be compatible with the larger society. As another example, despite differences between the lodge and the surrounding community in the methods for distribution of income, a bookkeeping procedure was established in the lodge which was the same as bookkeeping procedures everywhere. This was necessary because auditors from the community supervised the lodge's business books. It is at such points of contact with the community that practices which are compatible with the larger society must be maintained.

Subsystem compatibility with the geographical location in which it is implanted is also necessary. It is highly questionable whether the lodge could have survived if it had been implanted at the outset in an upper middle-class neighborhood. Although it was unusual, some members did venture into the surrounding community evidencing odd behaviors which were either ignored by the neighbors or were considered not much different than that which might be expected from any resident there. Trucks and other heavy equipment were commonplace in the neighborhood. Thus the appearance of trucks filled with workers was not perceived as different from what might occur at any place of business in the locale. The group was also racially integrated, and racially mixed groups were common in the area where the lodge was located.

It seems logical that while every social subsystem for chronic mental patients that is implanted in the larger community will necessarily differ from the community itself in certain respects, there is only a certain degree of deviation that can occur at any one time without so disrupting the typical social processes of its locale that antagonism against the subsystem will occur. In instances where these tolerances are exceeded, the implanted subsystem may be rejected or destroyed.

Since chronic mental patients often exhibit behavior that is not acceptable in society at large, the *fifth principle* requires that *subsystems de-*

signed for mental patients must establish internal norms that are tolerant of the deviant behavior that is normative for that particular population. Many mentally ill persons do not behave in ways that are acceptable to the society at large, but such behavior is normative for them. It is difficult, if not impossible, for individuals who have been continuously hospitalized to discard aberrant behaviors immediately upon entry into a community if, indeed, such behavior can be totally extinguished at all. The members of the subsystem must be tolerant of these behaviors. In the lodge, for example, members often hallucinated while talking with other members within the confines of the lodge itself. To take an extreme example of such toleration, one member who openly hallucinated within the lodge and enroute to work was informed by his crew chief upon arrival at the work site that no talking was permitted on the job. Usually he was silent during work hours but upon entry into the truck for the trip back to the lodge, he began hallucinating again—an acceptable behavior for his peers.

Leaders of such subsystems should be able to differentiate clearly the behavior norms of the greater society from those of the subsystem. Eventually the behavior within the subsystem tends to become somewhat similar to that required for community living. There was a trend in this direction from the opening of the lodge to the eventual assimilation of its members into the community. But it does appear from this experience that some persons may never be able to assume completely the responsibilities of full citizenship. Each person within the subsystem should be expected to contribute whatever he is capable of giving but, at the same time, other members of the subsystem must be aware and understanding of the fact that some persons have certain rather permanent incapacities which prevent them from active and full participation in the usual citizen's role.

A specific communication system needs to be devised for each subsystem, according to a *sixth principle*. The importance of continuous information feedback to members of such social subsystems about their performance cannot be overstressed. An almost continuous input of information to lodge members was necessary in order for them to achieve acceptable job performance and to maintain such performance. The curve of performance for all members was variable. According to the lodge experience, therefore, it is at the point of a generalized downturn in performance that information about such a decrement in performance is urgently needed. The input of information should be maximized at the point where deterioration in performance begins, because such information often prevents further deterioration of performance and aids in reestablishing more adequate levels of performance that have often been achieved in the past.

In the lodge subsystem, the dining area of the lodge served as the place for continuous exchanges of informal information about one's self and others. This continuous informal communication served to clarify interpersonal conflicts that might otherwise have become serious threats to the continuation of the organization. Information about problems among members was presented to the executive committee by lodge members and by the professional staff. Once the executive committee assumed its proper role, it almost always arrived at adequate solutions when the board of peers had accurate factual information about such real-life problems. As time passed, these solutions became more and more appropriate in terms of society's mores. In the initial stages of the lodge's operation, the staff supervisor retained a veto power over the executive committee's decisions and, in the infrequent case where their decision was unacceptable, his veto created an atmosphere for further deliberation which eventually resulted in an acceptable solution. Thus, through continuous information feedback, (including the fact a veto had been used), the executive committee eventually reached a level of judgment so reasonable that supervisory vetoes became unnecessary (pp. 86–87).

Other forms of communication can also be used to provide such needed information. For example, the consultants to the lodge were a constant and valuable source. The janitorial consultant gave the lodge members continuously updated information about the use of new janitorial techniques that could be of use to the organization. The crew chiefs inspected the work of each crew and rated their performance. Their ratings were in turn evaluated by a staff member, particularly during the developmental stages of the organization. For the first six months of the lodge's operation, weekly meetings were held in which any personal problems that the members had were discussed and reviewed. This meeting served initially as a source of information to the participants in the lodge which eventually was no longer needed (p. 49). Another form of information feedback was the annual customer questionnaire, which requested information from them about the adequacy of the work performed by the janitorial and gardening service. Of course, the immediate feedback by customers while the work crews were on the job was perhaps the most valuable source of information. And information feedback from crew chiefs to new members during work training sessions was helpful in creating good work habits.

Some persons will want to enter and some will want to leave such a subsystem. *Mobile entry and exit from the subsystem should be possible without penalty to the individual* is the *seventh principle* of subsystem operation. If the community subsystem is voluntary, there will be continuous entry into and exit from it. Free access to the larger community should be provided for residents in such social subsystems. For this reason, training for living in the larger community should be one of the primary aims of the subsystem. A social atmosphere conducive to venturing forth into the community without attaching penalties to such movements should be provided. This is important because the member leaders of such autonomous social subsystems will often feel an obligation to their group. This sense of obligation may cause them to hesitate in leaving the group, even though they are capable of such a move into the larger society. The social norms of the subsystem should encourage such departures when they are clearly warranted and it can do this by attaching no sanctions to exit from it.

But it is equally important that no penalty be attached to remaining in the subsystem if a person is incapable of completely independent living. The research results of this study showed that certain members were able to perform quite adequately in the lodge setting but rapidly became disorganized or otherwise incapacitated when they attempted to live independently in the community. It seems plausible, therefore, that for some individuals a dormitory type of life constitutes maximally independent living for them. It is therefore critical that the norms governing movement into the broader community also do not punish those who have achieved their highest level of adjustment within the created social subsystem, in acknowledgement of the fact that their probability of movement into the broader community is slight.

The *eighth principle* for such subsystems requires that *persons should perform as groups wherever possible.* From earlier studies and the one presented here, it appears that membership in a reference group is very important in maintaining the chronically disturbed person in the community as well as in the mental hospital (Fairweather, 1964). Furthermore, the norms of such groups reflect realistic performance standards for the members. This is essential with chronic mental patients, who often are unable to behave within socially acceptable limits without the support of a group. Many examples can be cited from life at the lodge. The work crews comprised of three or more men were able adequately to perform on the janitorial or yard job. Each member of the crew had a particular task which he typically completed. The usual composition of such a crew was a leader (crew chief), worker, and a marginal worker. It was the marginal worker whose work was constantly brought up to acceptable standards by the working example of the supervisor and worker. Without the framework of the group and the supervision and help of the crew chief, the marginal worker often failed.

But it was not in work alone that the group served to structure the social situation, for the group improved decision-making processes as well. The executive committee, which made the major decisions concerning the lives of the members, was an excellent decision-making group. The consensus arrived at through their discussions of the problems facing the members was often more realistic than one individual's opinion. And, in addition, such discussions focused on decisions about real-life problems also brought about group cohesiveness. Group decision-making and mutual work led to shared pride in the organization, which emphasized the worth of every individual and resulted in high group morale.

Only a limited number of people should participate in any subsystem constitutes the *ninth principle.* It is important that close interpersonal contact be established for the members of such a subsystem because it promotes identification with the subsystem and its goals. Interpersonal experience with others also yields a personal knowledge of them which can serve as the basis for decision-making by peers. Large organizations tend to become impersonal. For example, the greatest number of individuals at the lodge at any one time was 33. When the number of 33 was reached, the lodge members own executive committee asked that it not be exceeded, because the organization was becoming "large like the hospital." Even though a different physical plant might have permitted more participants while still maintaining its home-like social atmosphere, it seems clear that too many people would have tended to make the organization too impersonal for the members both to perceive their peers as a reference group and to identify with the organization and its goals.

New social subsystems need to be implanted in the community so that they are not dependent for their existence upon the good will of the community in which they are implanted. The *tenth principle* stresses that while it is important that the social subsystem be compatible with the environment in which it is placed, it is also important that it should be financed and supported by agencies or groups who are *not* directly dependent upon the immediate neighborhood for their financial support. Chronic mental patients who return to the community need time to become self-sufficient and they also need protection against community pressures that might destroy the embryonic social organization to which they belong. The lodge did not become self-sufficient until its fourth year of operation. The members were sustained through the formative stages, when great insecurity prevailed, by the strong support of two interested and devoted staff coordinators. The financial support, work organization, and relations in the community were established through a federal agency, a local university, and a rehabilitative nonprofit corporation. It was the combined efforts of these three organizations that offered support for the fledgling organization when it could have been most easily destroyed.

The social organization of the social subsystem must be so arranged that individuals may substitute for other individuals when required. It was a recurrent experience in the community-lodge work situation that a particular person might not be available for work on a particular day. That experience is the source of this *eleventh principle.* It was most important that another person be able to take his place when this occurred, in order that lodge operations not suffer. In order to appreciate the significance of this, one needs to imagine the entire group as a work force where several individuals are trained for the same role and each one is capable of assuming it on short notice. For example, it was not uncommon that an alcoholically inclined person would not be available for work on a particular day because of excessive indulgence, although he might have been perfectly capable of working the following day and for several days thereafter. Psychotic persons with psychosomatic complaints often were unable to work on a particular day or during a particular time period. On the other hand, such persons frequently recovered quickly and asked to be returned to their work. It is, therefore, essential that every function in the social subsystem be so organized that any person can be replaced by another on very short notice. In other terms, this might be called the *principle of substitution* (p. 78).

A social subsystem for the chronically disturbed person should emphasize equally both rehabilitative and work norms. This represents the *twelfth principle* of subsystem operation. The history of the lodge revealed that in the initial stages of development the emphasis of the members was upon a deep concern for the adjustment of their fellows. Thus, in the early days of the lodge, it was a common practice for the members to try to persuade any member who wanted to return to the hospital that he should make a more diligent attempt to remain in the community. Helpfulness among the members was common and a bond of being adventurers together in a new situation was the *Zeitgeist.* As the lodge became more and more similar to the community, work norms became the dominant behavioral guide lines. There was less and less concern for one's fellows. Eventually, it was necessary for the lodge supervisors to reestablish the work-rehabilitation balance in values. If social subsystems are to be established that adequately meet the needs of the total chronic ex-patient population—a goal that seems both realistic and desirable—a continuing balance between rehabilitative and work norms seems essential.

The *thirteenth principle* is: *Any social subsystem for chronically disturbed persons must establish an appropriate mechanism for handling medication.* Shortly after the lodge was activated, one member failed to take his medication and was returned to the hospital. From that point on, the members themselves assumed the responsibility for seeing that the offending members took their prescribed medication. When any member was not taking his medication, it soon became obvious to the residents of the lodge, because his behavior became more disorganized. The members then quickly informed the offender that his medication would be given to him. After this plan was developed, little further difficulty was experienced with members failing to take their medication.

The thirteen principles set forth here are a synthesis of the information gained from study of the lodge society. These principles may have general applicability to the entire national population of hospitalized mental patients. Two examples provide the evidence suggesting this possibility. During the latter stages of the lodge society's existence, one of the investigators was requested by a large hospital in a predominantly rural southern state to work with their staff toward establishing a community work-living situation. Through the use of funds from different sources than the lodge's research staff had used, a program in the community was established for persons who averaged 13.8 years of previous psychiatric hospitalization. Both men and *women* patients are included in the nine groups which have been formed up to the present time. Through close consultation with the person who helped establish the prototype lodge society itself, the hospital personnel were able to adapt most of the lodge procedures to the new setting. Men and women lived in dormitories in the community. Men worked at golf courses and other such places in teams doing gardening, landscaping, and groundskeeping work. The women worked in groups at several nursing homes, as well as in motels and restaurants in the local area. They have all provided much needed services for the local society. So much so, that requests from other potential employers, such as large hotels, federal natural resource agencies, and farm operators, could not be filled in favor of requests by the original employers for additional groups of workers. Some of the outcomes of this program, which at this writing has been in existence more than 24 months, have been: 72 such chronic patients have left the hospital; of the 8 who have returned to the hospital since the beginning of the program, 6 have remained there but 2 have again reentered the community; 6 have gone on to other community-living situations from their community dormitories.

Another program was established in an urban setting in a different part of this country. In this case, the hospital staff and patients established a work and living situation modeled directly upon the prototype lodge program reported in this book. This new lodge program was established in a growing urban center precisely because its own program had failed to meet the needs of discharged chronically hospitalized patients (Kraft, Binner, and Dickey, 1967). Hospital experience with these patients strongly suggested that its usual methods of treatment would merely result in an accumulation of such ex-patients as a growing casework load for its social workers, without adequately meeting the basic needs of such persons for survival in the community. Accordingly, a community lodge similar to the one reported in this study was established. The major features differentiating the new lodge program from its prototype were that lodge members from the outset had to contribute one-half of their board and room expenses, and the hospital provided no small-group ward experience for its patients admitted to the new lodge in the community. After the institution of the lodge, 20 members were admitted, most of whom had been previously failures in the usual psychiatric aftercare programs such as day care, outpatient care, halfway house residences, and family care. According to recent information, of the 20 patients who were initially admitted to the lodge, 14 are still there, one has died, three have returned to the hospital. The remaining two are currently living in the community while working—one on a full-time basis and one in part-time employment.

These two examples strongly indicate the generalized utility of the prototype lodge society for meeting the needs of chronically hospitalized mental patients. They show that such useful situations can be established in both rural and urban areas for both men and women discharged from state as well as federal hospitals, following the 13 principles set forth in this chapter. Furthermore, these two examples demonstrate clearly that traditionally trained mental health workers can change their own roles to meet the needs for establishing and maintaining such social subsystems both useful and beneficial to the majority segment of the mental patient population.

But the fact that the lodge prototype seems adaptable to widely differing circumstances of treatment, particularly when one considers the degree of incapacity of those ex-patient participants who were able to live within the broader society without the need for the large mental hospital, questions the very utility of the large mental hospital itself. Since continuous hospitalization may be the end result of the interaction of a total institution with emotionally unstable and dependent persons, a new program can be envisioned which might prevent such lengthy hospitalization. This might be done by replacing the mental hospital with a new community social subsystem for behavioral deviants. Such a new subsystem might include a psychiatric treatment ward in a general medical-surgical hospital where persons would arrive who are in an acutely agitated psychotic state. As soon as mitigation of their acute symptoms has occurred, a behavioral change that often develops rapidly with tranquilizing medication now available, the hospitalized person could be sent to a "diagnostic center" located in a member-governed community dormitory. Other persons who needed help but who were not acutely disturbed could come directly to the self-governing dormitories for admission without having to enter the treatment ward in the general hospital. Residents of the "diagnostic" dormitory could participate in making plans that would provide each person with a social situation which would allow him the maximum possible arena for personal and social adjustment on a flexible basis.

No emphasis would be placed upon formal diagnostic labels and other traditional admission procedures in this kind of "diagnostic center." Rather, "diagnostic" procedures would involve a shared, group decision-making activity aimed at creating for each person the most challenging social environment possible. After such a decision was made, the "diagnosed" person would be sent to the social situation deemed most appropriate for him. For example, a married individual who had a supportive living situation at home and a job might be returned to his home almost immediately, with plans made for outpatient treatment of a kind meeting his particular needs. Other persons with less supportive family situations, particularly those young people whose histories include chronic behavioral and emotional maladjustment, could be sent to other self-governing dormitories in the community where programs specially designed for their well-being would be available.

Institutions already established in the community could also provide needed services. For example, an individual could live in the member-governed dormitory and attend school, take on-the-job training, or be employed full time. Training for skilled and unskilled work as well as academic course work could be offered these persons. Whenever an outside community organization, such as a school, offered a needed educational or training opportunity, the person could participate in such an already established community institution. His medical needs could be met by local physicians working in clinics. When the situation warranted, such a person could leave the dormitory for a more independent existence of his choosing. If he was unable to survive in the more independent situation, he could return to the dormitory. Whether or not he returned to the neuropsychiatric admissions ward in the general hospital before returning to the dormitory would depend on the degree of behavioral disorganization at the time he wished reentry into the dormitory. If his behavior was severely disorganized, he could return to the hospital ward and leave again as soon as his behavior improved. If his behavior was not disorganized, he could return directly to the dormitory. Thus, rehabilitative efforts would center around each person's needs at the time, with the aim of full citizenship for all. In this manner, a social subsystem which maximized the potential of each person while at the same time providing a supportive situation without which some could not maintain themselves would be developed. Such self-governing dormitories could be established for both men and women residents, along the lines of dormitory residences at many major universities today. For instance, they could have common dining and recreational areas, much like such college residences have.

This spectrum of new social situations covering the needs of important segments of that part of our population defined as mentally ill would, of course, require very different professional staffing patterns. Professional staff could serve in their usual role as therapists for those living in family situations and at the same time as consultants to the lodge societies. On the other hand, the role of some might be entirely to create a social climate for group decision-making. It would be clearly incumbent upon those acting as consultants to establish programs which would allow the maximum possible autonomy for the participant group members in whatever social situation they find themselves. The relative autonomy of the small group in the hospital (Fairweather, 1964), and of the members of the lodge society described here, may serve as prototype examples of what can be accomplished when the philosophy of the rehabilitative organization is to maximize the independence and creativity of each participant.

The community program of self-governing dormitories for emotionally disturbed persons just described ought to be most effective if it is instigated before people become chronically hospitalized mental patients. If successful, such a community-based program could replace the large mental hospital. Since the essential emphasis would be upon creating the opportunity for the maximum adjustment possible for any person at any one time, a subsystem guided by this goal is not likely to become severely regulatory or overly controlling, because such authoritarian social processes would not permit the development of responsible individual behavior. Of course, such a treatment subsystem would have to be empirically developed by establishing it as a small model program and comparing it with current psychiatric practices in order to determine whether or not it would result in the elimination of chronic hospitalization. Such an outcome ought to lead to the dissolution of the large mental hospital, since the large mental hospital's primary goal as a social institution would have been displaced into the community by newer, more useful institutions. However, comparative evidence demonstrating the effectiveness of any treatment program such as these community dormitories is essential before such programs can be placed in existence at the service of the community and its emotionally disturbed members.

It has become clear from the research results of this study that new and meaningful participating social statuses can be created for mental patients in American communities. Historically, such persons have been labeled as "mentally ill," and removed from the community, usually by legal devices. It is this label of "mental illness" which has come to be associated with a lowly social status in our society. For example, this study has shown that many mental health hospital personnel, as a consequence of unintentionally adopting this concept, perceive the hospital patient as ill and hence unable to achieve adequately in his environment (p. 151). Such a perception more often than not restricts treatment programs by placing the patient in a relatively subordinate social position, one which contradicts even the patients' own expectancies (p. 316). Patients frequently perceive themselves as being able to succeed. This study has shown that when the appropriate social situation exists, they often do. Such successes in turn reinforce these positive perceptions and expectations and often lead to additional personal gains. It therefore seems important for each person to have the opportunity to perceive himself as capable of achievement. This study suggests that a participating social situation can lead to such a perception regardless of a person's emotional handicaps. Owning and operating a business, as the ex-mental patients did at the lodge, gave great prestige to those who participated in it. Many consequently perceived themselves as successes, mainly because being a member of the lodge society was a signal that they had been integrated into their society as participating persons.

The results of this study indicate that the traditional concept of mental illness needs to be replaced. A more meaningful, action-directed concept that could lead to more general social acceptance of those who are emotionally different would simply define each person's adjustment as the degree to which he was a responsible, participating member of his society. In such a case, the emotionally disturbed person could be viewed as having certain social deficits that a particular social situation could be created to alleviate. This conception would not fail to recognize the utility of medication or other new biochemical agents for permitting greater accessibility to that specially devised social situation.

With these assumptions about emotional disturbance, the goal of rehabilitation would become the maximization of such a person's participation in the larger society to the extent possible at a particular time, without punishing those not currently capable of it. Such a change in conceptual direction is urgently needed in order for such programs to be successful, for the results of this study show that chronic schizophrenic ex-patients only slightly modify their actual behavior. This slight modification, however, is sufficient for living in the society if the person's perception of himself is positive and the social situation in which he finds himself is adequately planned to take account of his personal deficiencies. Whatever new treatment programs *are* developed for the emotionally disturbed, especially those more severely afflicted, it seems clear that they should provide each person with maximum participation in the decision-making processes of the program. Such processes as assuming responsibility for fellow members, developing work techniques, and having control of money allow such persons to participate more realistically in their ongoing life situation. Participation in such processes is the very essence of citizenship which has so often eluded the returning mental patient. It is to be hoped that the operating principles outlined in this chapter will encourage many responsible persons in our society to work toward providing such responsibilities to these persons who can now be looked upon as capable of holding them alongside any other citizen they may encounter in the community.

18 A RECURRENT SOCIAL PROBLEM: CHANGING THE SOCIAL STATUS OF MARGINAL MAN

This study of the lodge society has brought into sharper focus a number of current social issues. The subordinate social position of the mental patient, from the time he comes to the attention of the community because of his aberrant behavior until he leaves the treatment subsystem itself, is not his exclusive possession in this society. With the disappearance of the frontier, technological advances, urbanization, and persistent prejudices, relatively nonparticipant social positions, or at least substantially marginal social statuses, have developed for many other citizens. Persons who occupy this type of lowly position are often involved in the social problems of our time. These members of our society may be ascribed such a marginal social status because they are elderly, alcoholics, drug addicts, criminals, delinquents, the physically incapacitated, those with "different" skin colors, or—in latest vogue—the socially and culturally disadvantaged. In a recent publication, Fairweather (1967) describes such marginal members of society as follows:

> . . . marginal man is the product of his society. He exists as such because his social status and role are clearly defined at the fringes of social organization. This status effectively isolates him from meaningful social participation. He therefore has little commitment to or identity with the generic goals of his society. The permanent social problem of marginal groups therefore is their need for new social statuses and roles which will bring

about their integration into the social life of the community accompanied by some personal feelings of achievement.

Much of the information from this study of a lodge subsociety indicates that a marginal person must have a sense of his own worth in order to identify effectively with his society. For this reason, many current social and economic programs for marginal persons which maintain them in subordinate social statuses by regulations relating to their eligibility or qualification for various forms of public assistance fail to enhance the substantive accomplishments of this segment of our society. Furthermore, programs which typically establish the subordinate and superordinate statuses and roles of the medical community, as well as many of the aid programs designed for marginal groups by sociologists, psychologists, social workers, and other interested professional persons must inevitably fail because the programs themselves are not the outgrowth of a marginal population's needs and active participation. For example, after the Watts riots in Los Angeles, an involved black person told about encountering social workers, sociologists, and other professional people who had been sent to the area to remedy the situation by "telling us what to do." Under these conditions, a sense of accomplishment or involvement can hardly exist. Participation in planning their future by representatives of marginal groups can be a critical and essential form of social action directed toward eliminating the subordinate social statuses of such persons.

This study has also shown that, for certain persons, employment is possible only under specially designed supportive conditions in the community. Such persons are, at least initially, unable to assume the full employment responsibilities required by the ordinary work role in our society. This problem is critical not only for discharged chronic mental patients, but also for other marginal groups, such as ex-prisoners and uneducated persons. If industry selects its employees solely on the basis of their ability to produce, what role is the larger society then willing to provide for those persons not only incapable of meeting such industrial role requirements but also not sufficiently disabled to require continuous care? The problem of meeting the needs of such persons has been made all the more pressing because of current advances in the automation of work. It would appear that increasingly greater numbers of people may become unemployed for this and other reasons in future years unless society plans meaningful programs for them as an integral part of their living situations. The experimental work completed in this book clearly shows that the role that society prescribes for these people is not but should be as meaningful and productive as possible. It has become obvious that it is only by a feeling of contribution to the society at large and to those of its members one contacts that persons identify intensely with their society and become its supporters rather than its willing or unwilling destroyers.

In this increasingly urban society which emphasizes productivity and work and in which wealth is an important measure of personal achievement, it is very difficult for any person to achieve this sense of personal accomplishment unless business and industry are willing to hire him so that he is afforded an opportunity to accumulate wealth. Traditional industrial practices in this country, however, have tended often in precisely the opposite direction. More and more emphasis has been placed upon the prior qualifications of the worker. By this emphasis upon efficiency and production, substantial groups of persons who are unable to meet such qualifications are effectively eliminated from the labor market. In fact, in many large industries uneducated persons or those who are easily emotionally upset often fail to attain successful scores on screening devices such as psychological tests that are often used nowadays as one criterion for employment itself. It is of paramount importance, therefore, that the hiring practices in this culture be altered to include individuals who can make a personal contribution to the business or industry even though they might not be able to meet the rigorous standards often required to attain employment in it. However, it is questionable whether such practices can and will be adopted primarily because of the need to maximize financial profit. If they cannot, it certainly becomes appropriate to recommend that industries owned and operated by such persons as the lodge members discussed in this book be created for them. For example, it might be possible to organize cooperative industries or businesses which could eventually become independent organizations administered and operated by persons who were previously marginal members of their society.

But new and more participating social statuses for marginal persons need not be restricted to citizens with physical or emotional problems. They could be extended to all types of marginal people living in our society. Black people living in the ghettos and socially deprived persons living in Appalachia could both become more participating citizens who might then have a stronger interest in their society. The blind, the criminal, the drug addict, and the delinquent could become more constructive, participating members of their society if appropriate social positions were established by those more powerful and wealthy members of our society who could provide the resources to create new social situations where such participating statuses could exist. Alternatives to this type of development are already being created, most notably in the black communities, where a strong emphasis upon solution of their problems through social and political organization and control of ghetto enclaves by black people themselves is being increasingly advocated and, in some cases, implemented. It apppears that if the dominant segment of our society will not engage in helping to establish more participating social positions for such marginal persons, they will set about to accomplish these goals by themselves, no matter how forlorn their accomplishment may appear to be. Such attempts, often in the face of seemingly impossible odds against unyielding efforts at retention of local political and social control by members of dominant groups in our society, could only arise from a courage born of despair with the life which such marginal social positions breed.

On the other hand, should the dominant members of our society decide to set about including marginal persons in more participative roles, however limited their contributions initially might be in view of their previously disadvantaged status, the new social statuses that could be created might revitalize our society in an extremely rewarding fashion. Such unity would be especially important at the present time in the face of the increasing polarity of thought and action which the persistent social problems of marginal persons induces. Nevertheless, implementation is not as simple as the decision to adopt such a new course of social action. This can most logically proceed by building and comparing different small-scale social models that might incorporate such marginal persons into more contributing roles in their society. Such new social statuses cannot in the long run be realistically and meaningfully established without the type of evaluation presented in this book. Experiments which establish new innovative models for the solution of a particular social problem and then compare them for their effectiveness in solving such problems are mandatory first steps in creating such new social positions. It is only through successive approximations at problem solution from such comparative experiments that meaningful new community subsystems that genuinely solve the problems of marginal persons can be found. One methodology to do this has already been proposed in a recent book entitled *Methods for Experimental Social Innovation* (Fairweather, 1967).

Another broad social issue raised by this study concerns the degree of voluntary participation which should be considered in such newly created programs. For example, volunteering is an exceedingly important issue in community mental health programs as they are conducted today. In this study, 50 per cent of all the patients that might have benefited from the living and working situation of the lodge in the community did not volunteer for such an opportunity. Yet the follow-up information gathered throughout the study showed that nonvolunteers, despite the claims of many that they had jobs assured them in the community, were in fact rarely employed and were, at the very most, no more satisfied with their life's situation than the lodge members who did volunteer. This information raises the issue of the responsibility a society has to those who are relatively incapacitated but who do not volunteer to participate in community subsystems that are designed to benefit them. It can, of course, be argued that any such involuntary membership is a violation of the democratic ideals of this society. Thus, it would be argued that it is more important for the society to support in other ways those members who do not participate in such programs, even when the programs might benefit them, than to jeopardize the important principle of voluntary membership. On the other hand, it can also be argued that such citizens may be incapable of making a rational decision at the moment it is offered and that they therefore should participate in programs found to be beneficial to others like themselves. Such an issue cannot be debated within the scope of this book. But it is clear that in the near future our society will have to make this kind of moral determination as treatment programs are moved further and further into the community and away from the large mental hospital, and as new and innovative programs are created for the disadvantaged. It is for this reason that this important moral issue is broached here.

The discussion contained in these pages has included some suggested changes in the ways in which marginal persons could be treated in this society. Further, some ideas have been offered about the ways in which contributing social roles for marginal persons could be created and tested for their effectiveness in achieving the goal of their increasing participation. But the process of innovating such changes in our society is fraught with many problems, not the least of which is resistance to changing the practices of the concerned social institutions. The problem of how institutions can be persuaded to alter those of their methods for solving problems which have become inadequate may be the foremost social problem of our time. Certainly, one of the most important findings of this study was the failure of an existing institution to change its methods of operation, even though direct empirical evidence showed rather conclusively that a new treatment program was more beneficial to its members than the ones it currently was using to meet the same needs of the persons it was designed to serve. Despite the empirically demonstrated fact that the lodge members assumed far more responsibility, gained greater self-enhancement from their work, and did so at a greatly reduced cost than their counterparts receiving regular aftercare services, the hospital from which all the patients for this study came was unwilling or unable to change its procedures and incorporate this new beneficial community innovation into its treatment programming. In fact, the hospital that administratively supported the research project from its inception did not incorporate the innovation into its service program, even though its administrators had evidence of its beneficial effects at least one year before the program was discontinued. Nevertheless, members of the research staff did consult with other hospitals and subsequently helped two interested hospitals in other parts of the country to establish community programs similar to the one reported here.

Innovative treatment program research is therefore not enough. Even though such experiments can demonstrate more advantageous programs, experiments cannot establish them as service programs. This must always be done by those members of our society charged with responsibility for the operation, maintenance, and improvement of its social institutions.

But how are new approaches to the problems of social marginality that are discovered by research activity then to be incorporated into the appropriate institutions of our society? Surely future research will have to be aimed at discovering how to effect social change in such large social institutions as the mental hospital. Members of American society have already become accustomed to making a heavy investment in research for space and military hardware. Substantial investments are also becoming customary in studying our society's social problems. However, the need to utilize scientific knowledge in bringing about effective social change must be recognized. Until methods are developed to aid our society in adapting its institutions to ever-present changing conditions of its life, all such social research investment will have gone for naught. Recognition of this need and the determination to create effective methods for such social changes may be financially expensive in the short run, but they will probably be socially inexpensive in the long run.

It is most likely that social organizations with this sole mission need to be created. Institutes for experimental social innovation may have to be formed. An example of such an institute has been proposed in a recent book (Fairweather, 1967). Since marginal persons would need to be involved in all phases of such innovative research because of their first-hand knowledge of a particular social problem, such institutes for experimental social innovation would bring together researchers, marginal members of society, and its decision-makers. Using them as a common meeting ground for planning research and discussing results could make such institutes powerful instruments for creating needed social change. If those responsible for changing public policy, the persons who would be affected by such a change (often members of a marginal population), and social innovative researchers themselves were involved in planning such experiments to investigate alternative solutions to pressing social problems, each group would be in some measure already committed to implementing a course of social action where the results were definitive. Perceiving such research as *their* research and its experimentally validated results as *their* results would markedly enhance a commitment to social change, if indeed the research results showed that a new solution would demonstrably better the lives of the participants. Of course, such institutes could also serve as communication centers for disseminating information to the very legislators, administrators, and other persons and agencies already charged with the responsibility for the orderly social change of our society's institutions in response to changing needs.

Adopting such a route to the solution of our social problems today requires an act of faith, on the part of every concerned citizen, namely, that it is valuable for deviant members of our society to have as broad an opportunity for participative interaction in it as is consistent with their capacities. It would be necessary that our society be willing to devote substantial amounts of its resources toward providing the facilitative social conditions which will capitalize on the behavioral potential of such marginal persons while giving them something of value in return for their participative effort. This includes extending to them trust rather than suspicion in relation to their potential capabilities, since this is clearly essential for the psychological survival of such deprived persons, if not for every human being. It is possible that this kind of focus on social-problem solution will turn attention once again to the creation of social systems which are fitted to human needs, rather than the fitting of human beings with their diverse needs into already-established social statuses in ongoing and unchanging social institutions. Historically, such institutions are beginning to show themselves inadequately prepared, because of their size, complexity, and rigidity, to take account of those needs in a flexible and responsive fashion. Only cooperative effort can create a social atmosphere in these institutions that will benefit all concerned. It may be, however, that this society cannot mount a cooperative effort to change its social institutions. Issues of power and control may so preoccupy its decision-making members that improving the social position of its marginal members will continue to be given a low priority. If such is the case, no research, however valid, can change those aspects of the society that are inhumane and unjust.

REFERENCES

ANGRIST, S. S. See Lefton, Dinitz, Angrist, and Pasamanick, 1967.

BAILEY, D. E. See Tryon and Bailey, 1965.

BALLACHEY, E. L. See Krech, Crutchfield, and Ballachey, 1962.

BEAN, L. L. See Myers, Bean, and Pepper, 1965.

BEARD, J. J., PITT, R. B., FISHER, S. H., and GOERTZEL, V. Evaluating the effectiveness of a psychiatric rehabilitation program. *Amer. J. Orthopsychiat.*, 1963, 33 (4), 701–12.

BELLAK, L. and BLACK, B. J. The rehabilitation of psychotics in the community. *Amer. J. Orthopsychiat.*, 1960, 30 (2), 346–55.

BINNER, P. R. See Kraft, Binner, and Dickey, 1967.

BLACK, B. J. See Bellak and Black, 1960.

BLACK, B. J. See Kase, Gadlin, and Black, 1966.

BLEULER, E. *Dementia praecox, or the group of schizophrenias.* (1911) trans. by Zinken, J. New York: International Universities Press, 1950, 474–75.

BLUMENTHAL, R. L. See Meltzoff and Blumenthal, 1966.

BOOTHE, H. See Schooler, Goldberg, Boothe, and Cole, 1967.

BROWN, G. W. *Experiences of discharged chronic schizophrenic patients in various types of living groups.* Milbank Memorial Fund Quarterly, 1959, 37, 105–31.

BUREAU OF THE BUDGET. *Standard industrial classification manual.* Washington, D.C.: U.S. Government Printing Office, 1957.

BUREAU OF THE BUDGET. *Standard industrial classification manual, supplement.* Washington, D.C.: U.S. Government Printing Office, 1963.

CARR, L. J. *Situational analysis: an observational approach to introductory sociology.* New York: Harper & Brothers, 1948.

CAUDILL, W. *The psychiatric hospital as a small society.* Cambridge, Mass.: Harvard University Press, 1958.

COLE, J. O. See Schooler, Goldberg, Boothe, and Cole, 1967.

CRUTCHER, H. B. Family care. In Arieti, S. (Ed.), *American handbook of psychiatry.* New York: Basic Books, Inc., 1959, 1877–84.

CRUTCHFIELD, R. S. See Krech, Crutchfield, and Ballachey, 1962.

CUMMING, E. See McCaffrey, Cumming, and Rudolph, 1963.

CUMMING, E. Allocation of care to the mentally ill. In Zald, M.D. (Ed.), *Organizing for community welfare.* Chicago: Quadrangle Books, 1967, 109–59.

DARLEY, J., GROSS, N., and MARTIN, W. Studies of group behavior: factors associated with the productivity of groups. *Journal of Applied Psychology,* 1952, 36, 396–403.

DAVIS, A. Caste, economy, and violence. *Amer. J. Sociol.,* 1945, 51, 7–16.

DEMARCHE, D. F. See Robinson, DeMarche, and Wagle, 1960.

DICKEY, B. A. See Kraft, Binner, and Dickey, 1967.

DINITZ, S. See Lefton, Dinitz, Angrist, and Pasamanick, 1967.

ECONOMIC REPORT OF THE PRESIDENT, 1967. *House Document No. 28, 90th Congress, 1st Session.* Washington, D. C.: U. S. Government Printing Office, 1967.

ELLERTSON, N. See Schacter, Ellertson, McBride, and Gregory, 1951.

ERIKSON, K. T. Patient role and social uncertainty: a dilemma of the mentally ill. *Psychiatry,* 1957, 20, 263–74.

FAIRWEATHER, G. W., SIMON, R., GEBHARD, M. E., WEINGARTEN, E., HOLLAND, J. L., SANDERS, R., STONE, G. B., and REAHL, G. E. Relative effectiveness of psychotherapeutic programs: a multicriteria comparison of four programs for three different groups. *Psychol. Monogr.,* 1960, 74, No. 5 (whole no. 492).

FAIRWEATHER, G. W. See Forsyth and Fairweather, 1961.

FAIRWEATHER, G. W. See MacDonald, Sanders, and Fairweather, 1962.

FAIRWEATHER, G. W. See Lerner and Fairweather, 1963.

FAIRWEATHER, G. W. and SIMON, R. A further follow-up comparison of psychotherapeutic programs. *J. Consult. Psychol.,* 1963, 27, 186.

FAIRWEATHER, G. W. (Ed.), *Social psychology in treating mental illness: an experimental approach.* New York: John Wiley & Sons, Inc., 1964.

FAIRWEATHER, G. W. *Methods for experimental social innovation.* New York: John Wiley & Sons, Inc., 1967.

FERGUSON, C. A. *The legacy of neglect.* Fort Worth, Texas: Industrial Mental Health Associates, 1965.

FISHER, S. H. See Beard, Pitt, Fisher, and Goertzel, 1963.

FORSYTH, R. P. and FAIRWEATHER, G. W. Psychotherapeutic and other hospital treatment criteria: the dilemma. *J. Abnorm. Soc. Psychol.,* 1961, 62, 598–604.

FREEMAN, H. E. and SIMMONS, O. G. *The mental patient comes home.* New York: John Wiley & Sons, Inc., 1963, 2–3.

FREEMAN, H. E. Social change and the organization of mental health care. *Amer. J. Orthopsychiat.,* 1965, 35 (4), 717–22.

FRENCH, R. L. Sociometric status and individual adjustment among naval recruits. *J. Abnorm. Soc. Psychol.,* 1951, 46, 64–71.

GADLIN, W. See Kase, Gadlin, and Black, 1966.

GEBHARD, M. E. See Fairweather, Simon, Gebhard, Weingarten, Holland, Sanders, Stone, and Reahl, 1960.

GOERTZEL, V. See Beard, Pitt, Fisher, and Goertzel, 1963.

GOFFMAN, E. The characteristics of total institutions. In *Symposium on preventive and social psychiatry.* Washington, D. C.: Walter Reed Army Institute of Research, 1957, 43–84.

GOFFMAN, E. *Asylums* (essays on the social situation of mental patients and other inmates). Chicago: Aldine Publishing Company, 1962.

GOLDBERG, S. C. See Schooler, Goldberg, Boothe, and Cole, 1967.

GREENBLATT, M. See Landy and Greenblatt, 1965.

GREGORY, DORIS. See Schacter, Ellertson, McBride, and Gregory, 1951.

GROSS, N. See Darley, Gross, and Martin, 1952.

GUREL, L. and JACOBS, D. A critical survey of vocational rehabilitation of the psychiatric patient. *Psychiatric Evaluation Project: Background Paper No. 61–4,* Washington, D. C.: Veterans Administration, 1961.

HALL, J. C., SMITH, K., and SHIMKUNAS, A. Employment problems of schizophrenic patients. *Amer. J. Psychiat.,* 1966, 123, 536–40.

HILLER, E. T. *Social relations and structures.* New York: Harper and Row, 1947.

HOLLAND, J. L. See Fairweather, Simon, Gebhard, Weingarten, Holland, Sanders, Stone, and Reahl, 1960.

JACKSON, J. M. and SALTZSTEIN, H. D. *Group membership and conformity processes.* Ann Arbor, Mich.: University of Michigan, Research Center for Group Dynamics, Institute for Social Research, August, 1956.

JACKSON, J. M. and SNOEK, J. D. Effect of invidious exclusion from a group on feelings toward self, others, and on tendencies to conform. *American Psychologist,* 1959, 14, 335 (abstract).

JACKSON, J. M. A space for conceptualizing person-group relationships. *Human Relations,* 1959, 12, 3–16.

JACOBS, D. See Gurel and Jacobs, 1961.

KASE, H. M., GADLIN, W., and BLACK, B. J. *Directory of sheltered workshops serving the emotionally disturbed, 1965.* New York: Altro Service Bureau, 1966.

KRAFT, A. M., BINNER, P. R., and DICKEY, B. A. The community mental health program and the longer-stay patient. *Arch. Gen. Psychiat.,* 1967, 16, 64–70.

KRECH, D., CRUTCHFIELD, R. S., and BALLACHEY, E. L. *Individual in society.* New York: McGraw-Hill, 1962.

LAMB, H. R. Release of chronic psychiatric patients into the community. *Arch. of Psychiat.,* 1968, 9, 38–44.

LANDY, D. See Wechsler and Landy, (Eds.), 1960.

LANDY, D. and GREENBLATT, M. *Halfway House.* Washington, D. C.: Vocational Rehabilitation Administration, 1965.

LANDY, D. H. Rehabilitation as a sociocultural process. *J. Soc. Issues,* 1960, 16 (2), 3–7.

LEFTON, M., DINITZ, S., ANGRIST, S. S., and PASAMANICK, B. Former mental patients and their neighbors: a comparison of performance levels. In Weinberg, S. K., *The sociology of mental disorders.* Chicago: Aldine Publishing Company, 1967, 255–62.

LERNER, M. J. and FAIRWEATHER, G. W. The social behavior of chronic schizophrenics in supervised and unsupervised work groups. *J. Abnorm. Soc. Psychol.,* 1963, 67, 219–25.

LEVINSON, D. See Pine and Levinson, 1961.

MCBRIDE, DOROTHY. See Schacter, Ellertson, McBride, and Gregory, 1951.

MCCAFFREY, I., CUMMING, E., and RUDOLPH, C. Mental disorders in socially defined populations. *Amer. J. Pub. Health,* 1963, 53 (7), 1025.

MACDONALD, W. S., SANDERS, D. H., and FAIRWEATHER, G. W. *The validity of staff, peer, and nonpeer predictions for the posthospital adjustment of mental patients.* Unpublished manuscript, 1962.

MACDONALD, W. S. See Sanders and MacDonald, 1963.

MACDONALD, W. S. See Sanders, MacDonald, and Maynard, 1964.

MARTIN, W. See Darley, Gross, and Martin, 1952.

MAYNARD, H. *The effect of group composition on task performance.* Unpublished Master's Thesis. University of Oregon, Eugene: 1964.

MAYNARD, H. See Sanders, MacDonald, and Maynard, 1964.

MECHANIC, D. Some factors in identifying and defining mental illness. *Ment. Hyg.,* 1962, 46, 66–74.

MELTZOFF, J. and BLUMENTHAL, R. L. *The day treatment center.* Springfield, Ill.: Charles C Thomas Press, 1966.

MUTH, L. T. *Aftercare for the mentally ill—a world picture.* Philadelphia, Pa.: Mental Health Education Unit. Smith, Kline, and French Laboratories, 1957.

MYERS, J. K., BEAN, L. L., and PEPPER, M. P. Social class and psychiatric disorders: a ten year follow-up. *J. Health and Hum. Beh.,* 1965, 74–79.

NUNNALLY, J. C. *Popular conceptions of mental health.* New York: Holt, Rinehart, and Winston, Inc., 1961.

OLSHANSKY, S. The transitional sheltered workshop: a survey. *J. Soc. Issues,* 1960, 16 (2), 33–39.

PASAMANICK, B. See Lefton, Dinitz, Angrist, and Pasamanick, 1967.

PATTON, G. O. Foster homes and rehabilitation of long-term mental patients. *Canad. Psychiat. Assoc. J.,* 1961, 6, 20–25.

PEPPER, M. P. See Myers, Bean, and Pepper, 1965.

PINE, F. and LEVINSON, D. A sociopsychological conception of patienthood. *Int. J. Soc. Psychiat.,* 1961, 7 (2), 106–22.

PITT, R. B. See Beard, Pitt, Fisher, and Goertzel, 1963.

REAHL, G. E. See Fairweather, Simon, Gebhard, Weingarten, Holland, Sanders, Stone, and Reahl, 1960.

ROBINSON, R., DEMARCHE, D. F., and WAGLE, M. K. *Community resources in mental health.* New York: Basic Books, Inc., 1960.

ROSS, H. A. Commitment of the mentally ill: problems of law and policy. *Mich. Law Rev.,* 1959, 57, 945–1018.

RUDOLPH, C. See McCaffrey, Cumming, and Rudolph, 1963.

SALTZSTEIN, H. D. See Jackson and Saltzstein, 1956.

SAMPSON, E. D. Individual and group performance under reward and fine, *J. Soc. Psychol.,* 1963, 61, 111–25.

SANDERS, D. H. See MacDonald, Sanders, and Fairweather, 1962.

SANDERS, D. H. and MACDONALD, W. S. *Exploratory analysis of role differentiation and group processes in heterogeneous groups.* Unpublished manuscript, 1963.

SANDERS, D. H., MACDONALD, W. S., and MAYNARD, H. The effect of group composition on task performance and role differentiation. In G. W. Fairweather (Ed.), *Social psychology in treating mental illness: an experimental approach.* New York: John Wiley & Sons, Inc., 1964, 196–209.

SANDERS, R. See Fairweather, Simon, Gebhard, Weingarten, Holland, Sanders, Stone, and Reahl, 1960.

SCHACTER, S., ELLERTSON, N., MCBRIDE, DOROTHY, and GREGORY, DORIS. An experimental study of cohesiveness and productivity. *Human Relations,* 1951, 4, 229–38. Also Chap. 27 in D. Cartwright and A. Zander (Eds.), *Group Dynamics.* Evanston, Ill.: Row, Peterson, 1953.

SCHEFF, T. J. The role of the mentally ill and the dynamics of mental disorder: a research framework. *Sociometry,* 1963, 26, 436–53.

SCHEFF, T. J. *Being mentally ill: a sociological theory.* Chicago: Aldine Publishing Company, 1966.

SCHEFF, T. J. The societal reaction to deviance: ascriptive elements in the psychiatric screening of mental patients in a midwestern state. *Soc. Problems,* 1964, 2 (4), 401–13. In Weinberg, S. K., *The sociology of mental disorders,* Chicago: Aldine Publishing Company, 1967, 184–92.

SCHOOLER, N. R., GOLDBERG, S. C., BOOTHE, H., and COLE, J. O. One year after discharge: community adjustment of schizophrenic patients. *Amer. J. Psychiat.,* 1967, 123, 986–95.

SCHWARTZ, C. G. See Schwartz and Schwartz, 1964.

SCHWARTZ, M. S. and SCHWARTZ, C. G. *Social approaches to mental patient care.* New York: Columbia University Press, 1964.

SHIMKUNAS, A. See Hall, Smith, and Shimkunas, 1966.

SIMMONS, O. G. See Freeman and Simmons, 1963.

SIMON, R. See Fairweather, Simon, Gebhard, Weingarten, Holland, Sanders, Stone, and Reahl, 1960.

SIMON, R. See Fairweather and Simon, 1963.

SIMON, W. B. On reluctance to leave the public mental hospital. *Psychiatry,* 1965, 28 (2), 145–56.

SMITH, K. See Hall, Smith, and Shimkunas, 1966.

SNOEK, J. D. See Jackson and Snoek, 1959.

STEINBACH, M. See Vitale and Steinbach, 1965.

STONE, G. B. See Fairweather, Simon, Gebhard, Weingarten, Holland, Sanders, Stone, and Reahl, 1960.

TRYON, R. C. Domain sampling formulation of cluster and factor analysis. *Psychometrika,* 1959, 24, 113–35.

TRYON, R. C. *The component programs of the BC TRY system.* Dittoed manuscript, Project CAP, Department of Psychology, University of California, Berkeley, 1964.

TRYON, R. C. and BAILEY, D. E. *User's manual of the BC TRY system of cluster and factor analysis (tape version for IBM 709, 7090, 7094 programs in Fortran II)*. Berkeley, Calif.: University of Calif. Press, 1965.

U. S. BUREAU OF THE CENSUS. *U. S. Censuses of Population and Housing: 1960. Census Tracts. Final Report PHC (1)–137*. Washington, D. C.: U. S. Government Printing Office 1962a.

U. S. BUREAU OF THE CENSUS. *U. S. Censuses of Population and Housing: 1960. Census Tracts. Final Report PHC (1)–138*. Washington, D. C.: U. S. Government Printing Office, 1962b.

U. S. BUREAU OF THE CENSUS. *County Business Patterns, 1964. Part 1—U. S. Summary*. Table 1 A. Washington, D. C.: U. S. Government Printing Office, 1965a.

U. S. BUREAU OF THE CENSUS. *County Business Patterns, 1965. California CBP–65–6*. Table 1 B. Washington, D. C.: U. S. Government Printing Office, 1965b.

U. S. BUREAU OF THE CENSUS. *County Business Patterns, 1965. California CBP–65–6*. Table 1 B. Washington, D. C.: U. S. Government Printing Office, 1966.

VITALE, J. H. Mental hospital therapy: a review and integration. In Masserman, J. H. (Ed.), *Current Psychiatric Therapies*. Vol. II. New York: Grune and Stratton, 1962, 247–65.

VITALE, J. H. and STEINBACH, M. The prevention of relapse of chronic mental patients. *Int. J. Soc. Psychiat.*, 1965, 11, 85–95.

WAGLE, M. K. See Robinson, DeMarche, and Wagle, 1960.

WALDRON, J. Clinical signs in chronic schizophrenia: their importance in resettlement. *Amer. J. Psychiat.*, 1965, 121 (9), 907–9.

WECHSLER, H. The ex-patient organization: a survey. *J. Soc. Issues,* 1960, 16 (2), 47–53.

WECHSLER, H. and LANDY, D. (Eds.) New pathways from the mental hospital. *J. Soc. Issues,* 1960, (2), whole issue.

WEINGARTEN, E. See Fairweather, Simon, Gebhard, Weingarten, Holland, Sanders, Stone, and Reahl, 1960.

INDEX

Made in the USA
Columbia, SC
24 April 2020